Permar's

Oral Embryology and Microscopic Anatomy

Frontispiece. A photomicrograph of a ground section cut faciolingually through a human maxillary first premolar. The enamel has a deep fissure in the central developmental groove. At the entrance to the fissure, on the triangular ridge of the buccal cusp, there is a barely visible dark area which is probably the beginning of a caries lesion. There is no evidence of caries at the bottom of the fissure.

In the enamel on the buccal and on the lingual surfaces of the crown there may be faintly seen near the dentinoenamel junction the narrow light and dark areas which are the bands of Hunter-Schreger.

Notice the curvature of the dentinal tubules in the crown of the tooth. Notice the configuration of the pulp chamber: the pulp horn in the buccal cusp extends much farther occlusally than the pulp horn in the lingual cusp. The pulp cavity here is empty because the pulp tissue was destroyed in the preparation of the section. Notice the relatively narrow root canals. It is difficult to determine the thickness of the cementum on this section at this magnification. (As seen under very low power of the microscope.)

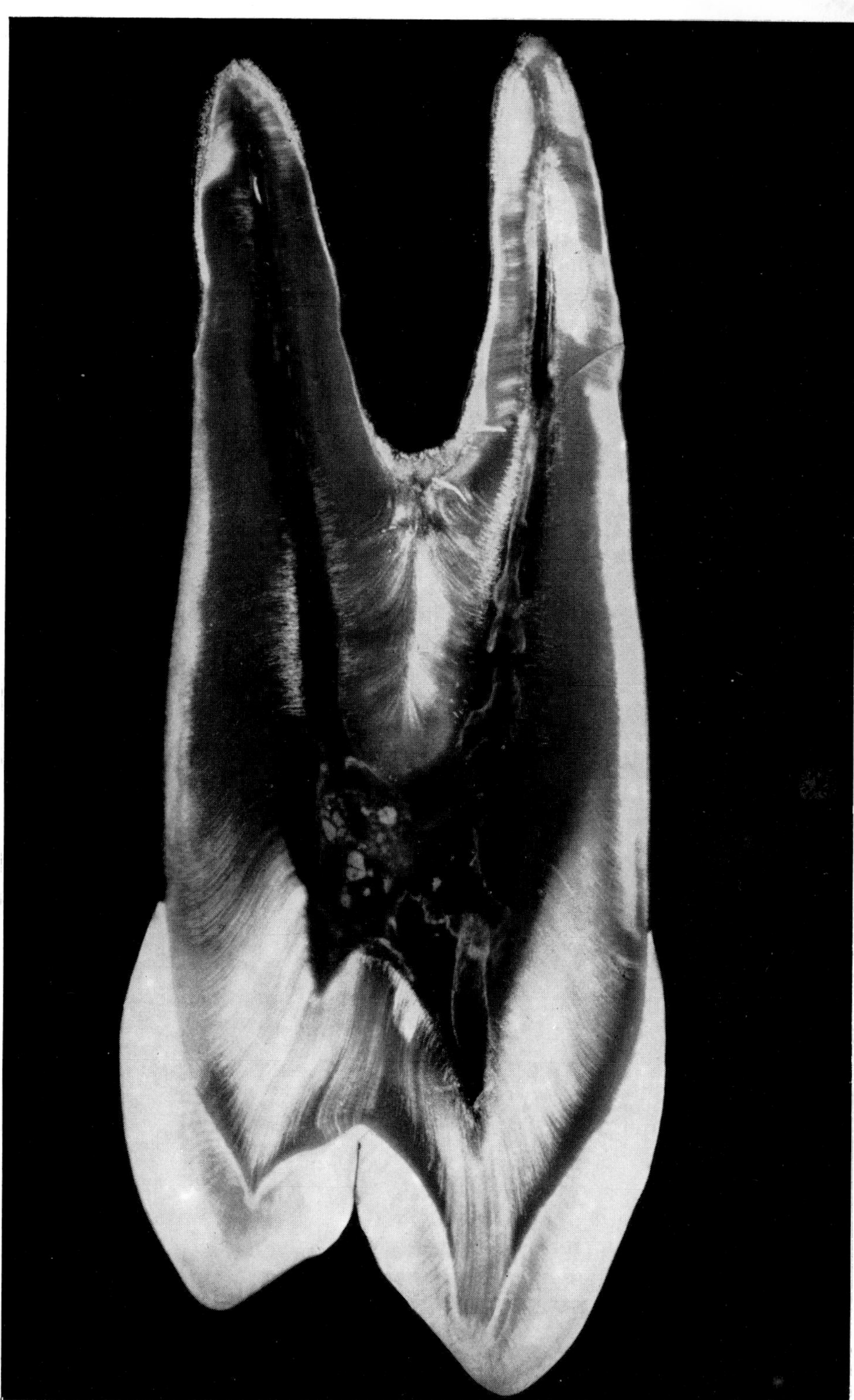

Frontispiece

Permar's

Oral Embryology and Microscopic Anatomy

A Textbook for Students in Dental Hygiene

RUDY C. MELFI, D.D.S., Ph.D.

Professor of Dentistry (Oral Biology), College of Dentistry, The Ohio State University, Columbus, Ohio

EIGHTH EDITION

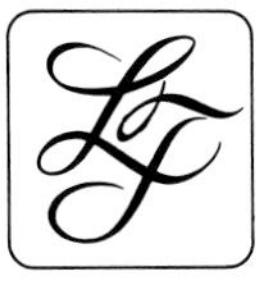

LEA & FEBIGER • Philadelphia •

Lea & Febiger
600 Washington Square
Philadelphia, PA. 19106-4198
U.S.A.
(215) 922-1330

Library of Congress Cataloging-in-Publication Data

Permar, Dorothy.
[Oral embryology and microscopic anatomy]
Permar's oral embryology and microscopic anatomy: a textbook for students in dental hygiene.
p. cm.
Includes bibliographies and index.
ISBN 0-8121-1063-3
1. Teeth. 2. Mouth 3. Mouth—Diseases. I. Melfi, Rudy C. II. Title. III. Title: Oral embryology and microscopic anatomy.
[DNLM: 1. Mouth—embryology. 2. Tooth—anatomy & histology. WU 101 P451m]
RK280.P4 1988
611'.31—dc19

First Edition, 1955
Second Edition, 1959
Third Edition, 1963—Reprinted, 1965
Fourth Edition, 1967—Reprinted, 1969
Fifth Edition, 1972—Reprinted, 1973, 1975
Sixth Edition, 1977—Reprinted 1979, 1980
Seventh Edition, 1982—Reprinted, 1985
Eighth Edition, 1988

Printed in The United States of America

Print number: 4 3 2

For

DOROTHY PERMAR

Late Professor of Dentistry

The Ohio State University

Preface

This book was written for students who have selected Dental Hygiene and Dental Assisting as career goals. It is understood that these students have so much to learn, in so many subjects, that to confront them with detailed accounts of complicated physiologic processes would not serve to broaden their education. Instead, it would place them in a maze. With this in mind, the text has been kept simple enough to be understandable and comprehensive enough to be useful.

It is assumed that the student who uses this book has had a course in biology and has some knowledge of both mammalian anatomy and human tooth morphology. Although it would be helpful, comprehensive instruction in histology or embryology is not necessary.

The subject matter includes an introduction to general histology; the embryologic development of the face and oral cavity; development of teeth and their eruption, and in the case of primary teeth, their shedding; tooth enamel, dentin, cementum, and pulp; periodontal ligament; oral mucosa and salivary glands; developmental tooth anomalies; dental caries; and a chapter on the temporomandibular joint.

This edition has been revised and updated to reflect new concepts and developments that have occurred in the subject. The incorporation of additional photomicrographs and diagrams is intended to aid the student in the interpretation of the text and to emphasize the relevant information.

For those students interested in exploring the literature for information in greater depth, the references in the footnotes and at the end of chapters will be helpful. Selection of the references has been made from publications usually available to students in dental fields. The references are by no means exhaustive. The ones cited are considered guideposts for the beginning student who wants more information on a particular subject.

I am grateful for the courtesies of my associates. Their names appear in association with figures throughout the book. A special appreciation is extended to Donna Smith for secretarial assistance.

Columbus, Ohio Rudy C. Melfi

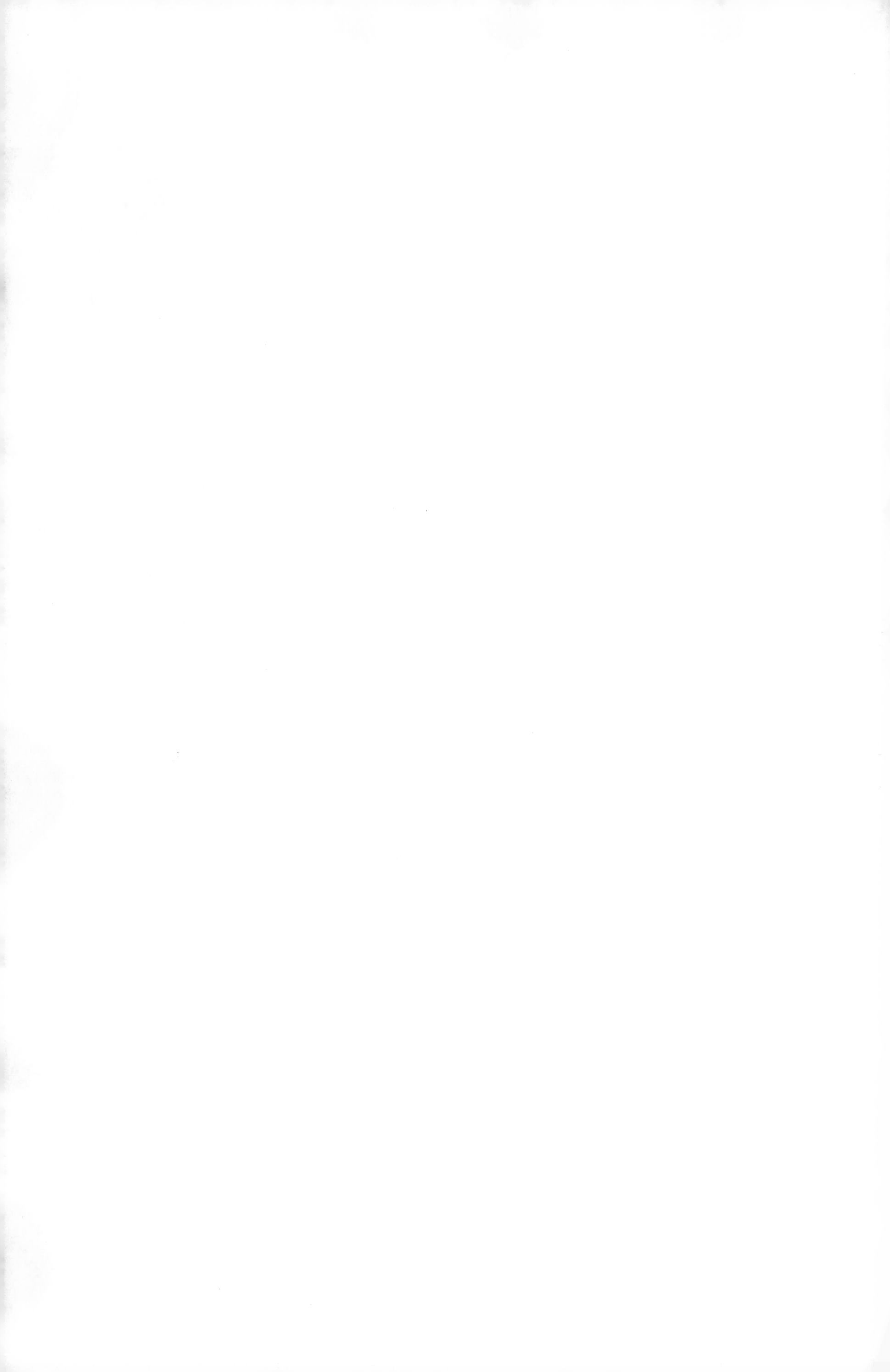

Contents

Chapter 1

INTRODUCTION TO HISTOLOGY

GENERAL HISTOLOGY

The Nature of Histology

Histology is the science of tissues (histo = tissue; logy = the science of). Of particular interest in Dentistry are the tissues of the oral cavity.

A *tissue* is sometimes defined as a group of more or less similar cells with intercellular substance and tissue fluid, combined in a characteristic manner and performing a particular function. Some examples of human tissues are muscle, bone, blood, epithelium of the skin and mucous membrane, connective tissue of the skin and of the mucous membrane, and the pulp of a tooth. The hard components of a tooth—enamel, dentin, and cementum—are also tissues, although enamel and dentin, and some cementum, have exceptional characteristics.

Tissues vary greatly in appearance and in structure. Some are hard (bone); some are soft (muscle). Some are sturdy and withstand wear and injury (surface layer of the skin); and some are delicate and serve as linings (lining of the respiratory tract). Some are secretory in function (salivary gland tissue); and some are nutritive in function (blood).

How Tissues Are Studied

Microscopic examination of tissues started in the early nineteenth century, and study has been extended and developed as improvements have been made in the construction of microscopes and in the techniques of tissue preparation. Usually tissues must be stained in some manner in order that their different components may be seen clearly with a microscope. Sometimes dyes are injected into the blood stream of a living animal, and the tissues which have taken up the stain from the blood are subsequently removed from the animal and cut into thin sections. Or tissues may be grown in artificial nutrient media in a glass tube, and their growth and development observed from hour to hour or from day to day. The most usual method of tissue preparation is probably that of removing a small piece of tissue from the body, embedding it in paraffin, sectioning it, and staining it.

Let us suppose, for example, that a dentist wants to examine the microscopic structure of the soft tissue surrounding the teeth. A small piece of this gingival tissue is carefully removed from the mouth with a sharp instrument and is immediately placed in a bottle containing a fixative. In this solution it is sent to a microtechnique laboratory. When the specimen is received in the laboratory, it is dehydrated in absolute alcohol, allowed to stand in xylene, and then placed in a dish of melted paraffin which is kept in a warming oven. In a few hours the paraffin will have completely permeated the tissue. The paraffin and tissue are then poured into a small container. Hardened in cool water, the paraffin becomes a firm block which contains the specimen in its center. The paraffin block is then cut into sections (slices) with an instrument called a microtome. Each paraffin section is about 8 micrometers (μm) thick and has in its center, of course, a section of the embedded specimen which is the same in thickness. The paraffin sections are arranged on glass microscope slides, with egg albumin used as an adhesive. The slides are then passed through xylene which dissolves away the embedding paraffin, leaving the thin section of tissue attached to the slide. In order that the structure of the tissue may be studied, it is necessary now to pass the slides through appropriate tissue stains.

There are innumerable kinds of tissue stains. One of the common combinations of stains is hematoxylin and eosin. When the slides bearing the sections of tissue are immersed in the hematoxylin the nuclei of the cells will take up the stain and become deep blue. Subsequent immersion in the eosin stain will cause the cytoplasm of the epithelial cells to become a pinkish color and the intercellular substance of the connective tissue to become pink. Stains other than hematoxylin and eosin are used to bring out different tissue structures. After they are stained the tissue sections are covered with a small, very thin cover glass. In this way the slides are permanently preserved.

Specimens which contain mineralized tissue such as bone and teeth must be demineralized in a weak acid before they can be cut with the sharp knife of the microtome. The demineralization process is the removal (dissolving) of the mineral material from the organic material of a tissue. As a result of this demineralization process, changes are inevitable in certain tissues. Tooth enamel, for instance, is usually entirely lost when a tooth is allowed to stand in acid. Tooth enamel is about 96% mineral material and only 4% organic material and water. When the mineral is removed by the acid, the delicate organic portion of the enamel is mechanically washed away unless special techniques for its preservation are employed. Other kinds of mineralized tissues retain their form when they are demineralized. Dentin, cementum, and bone, because they contain a much greater proportion of organic material, are not thus destroyed when the mineral material is removed in the process of demineralization. Completely demineralized dentin, cementum, or bone will retain its original shape, although it can be easily pierced with a needle.

The enamel of a tooth may be preserved for study if instead of using the demineralizing, embedding, and sectioning procedures the tooth is merely ground down to one thin section. This is done on a lathe with a revolving stone. With this technique it is not difficult to obtain a tooth section less than 20 μm thick. Specimens of teeth prepared in this way are referred to as *ground sections* (see Frontispiece). Ground sections are mounted on glass slides and covered with a cover glass in the same way that other types of sections are preserved.

Components of a Tissue

Tissues are made up of *cells, intercellular substance,* and *tissue fluid.*

A *cell* is a unit of living substance (protoplasm), usually having cytoplasm and a nucleus. It may exist as an individual, as in unicellular animals, or it may be part of a tissue of a large animal or plant and be dependent upon other cells for existence.

Cells show an almost infinite variation in size, shape and structure. In animals the largest of cells is an ovum: a chicken egg, or even a human ovum (120 μm in diameter). In contrast to these cells, a human red blood cell is about 8 μm in diameter.

Circulating human red blood cells have lost their nuclei; white blood cells contain one or several nuclei. Muscle cells are distinctive because their cytoplasm has the power of strong contraction. Fat cells contain large amounts of fat, which push the nuclei away from the center of the cells and against the cell walls. There are many kinds of cells which, along with varying kinds and amounts of intercellular substance and different amounts of tissue fluid, determine the nature of the various kinds of tissues.

Intercellular substance is a product of living cells and is distributed among the cells in all of the tissues of the body. It holds the cells together and provides a medium for the passing of nutrients and of waste materials from capillaries to cells and from cells to capillaries. The amount and kind of intercellular substance differ in different tissues. In some human tissues, such as bone, intercellular substance is the predominant element. In other human tissues, such as the epithelium which makes up the surface of the skin, intercellular substance is small in amount and the cellular elements predominate. Intercellular substance occurs in two forms: one form is *fibrous* in nature and the other is *amorphous* in nature (a = without; morphous = form) (Fig. 1–1).

The fibrous part of the intercellular substance, formed by cells of the tissue, is also referred to as *formed elements.* Four types of these fibrous or formed elements are found in the human body—*collagen, reticulum, elastic,* and *oxytalan.* Reticulum fibers are considered to be younger forms of collagen fibers, and oxytalan fibers younger forms of elastic fibers.

The amorphous part of the intercellular substance is commonly referred to as *ground substance.*It functions as a molecular sieve, allowing the passage of metabolities between the blood and tissues; it also serves as a physical barrier to prevent the spread of foreign elements such as microorganisms. The ground substance is a complex of chemical substances known as mucopolysaccharides (also called *glycosaminoglycans* and *proteoglycans).* Students who are interested in the structural, physical, and chemical features of the fibrous and ground substance types of intercellular substance should consult standard general histology textbooks.

Tissue fluid is that part of the blood plasma which can diffuse through the walls of capillaries. In the tissue fluid nutrients are carried out through capillary walls to the surrounding intercellular substance and then to the cells; and waste products of the cells are returned in the same manner from the intercellular substance to the capillaries. Tissue fluid may be present in a tissue in relatively small proportions, as in the epithelium of the surface of the skin; or it may form a large proportion of the tissue, as in blood. The tissue fluid of epithelium, of bone, and other tissue is, of course, derived from blood.

Classification of Tissues

In their gross and microscopic appearance, and in their function, tissues vary so widely that the beginning student may well feel that there is little or no

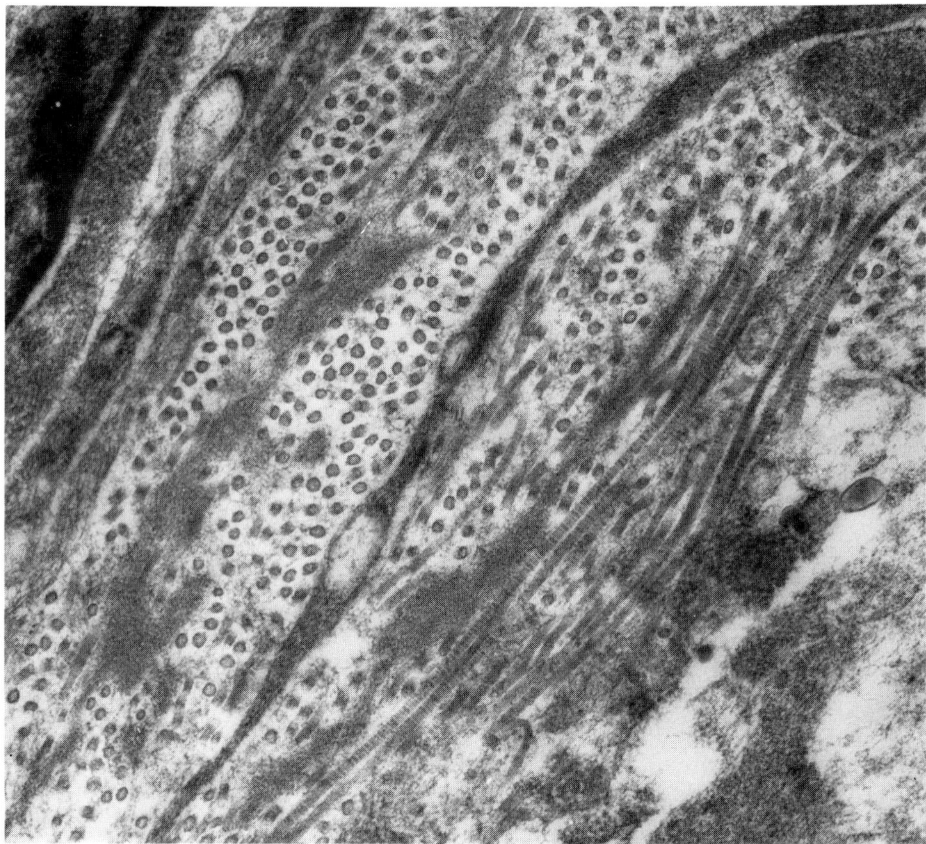

Fig. 1–1. Electron micrograph of connective tissue showing the two forms of intercellular substance. The fibrous form here is *collagen* fribils cut in cross and longitudinal sections. A close look at the longitudinally cut fibrils, running diagonally from top to bottom on the right side, will reveal crossbanding; this is a characteristic of collagen fibrils. The amorphous or ground substance is seen as clear areas around the collagen fibrils. (Courtesy Dr. Dennis Foreman, Collage of Dentistry, The Ohio State University.)

relationship among them. This seeming confusion grows less, however, when it is discovered that for purposes of easier study and better understanding histologists have developed a classification for tissues. Tissues are alike in that they are made up of cells, intercellular substance, and tissue fluid. Tissues differ in the form and number of cells, in the type and amount of intercellular substance, and in the amount of tissue fluid. It is on the similarities and differences of tissues that the histologist has based his classification.

Human tissues have been assorted into *four primary groups: epithelial tissue, connective tissue, muscle tissue* and *nerve tissue*. The tissues of each of these primary groups have certain major, fundamental characteristics in common. But there are also differences within the groups; and so each of the four primary groups has been subdivided. The subdivisions are based on structural differences which clearly distinguish one tissue from another.

A brief classification of human tissues is presented in Table 1-1.

Tissues are combined in characteristic ways to form *organs*, such as heart,

Table 1–1. Classification of Tissues

Epithelial Tissue	1. Surface cells of covering and of lining membranes (as of skin of mucous membranes) 2. Glandular tissue
Connective Tissue	1. Fibrous (as in skin beneath the epithelium) 2. Loose areolar (as in thin membranes between various layers of tissue) 3. Adipose (fat) 4. Hemopoietic (= blood-forming: bone marrow, lymphatic tissue) 5. Cartilage 6. Bone
Nerve Tissue	1. Tissue of central nervous system 2. Tissue of peripheral nervous system
Muscle Tissue	1. Smooth involuntary (as in wall of intestines) 2. Striated voluntary (as in skeletal muscle) 3. Striated involuntary (heart muscle)

lungs, liver, bones, skin, tongue; and organs are combined in characteristic ways to form *organisms,* such as the human body.

Let us consider the tongue as an organ. The tongue is made up of a combination of epithelial tissue, muscle tissue, and nerve tissue, all of which are interdependent in the functioning of the organ (Fig. 1–2). Epithelial tissue comprises the surface of the tongue and serves as a protective covering; and within the tongue is another type of epithelial tissue in the form of several sizable salivary glands. Beneath the surface epithelium is connective tissue which supplies both support and nourishment; and beneath this connective tissue layer are strong muscles which produce movement of the organ. Nerves of the tongue supply both motor and sensory functions.

Another organ of the human body is the skin. Skin is made up of a combination of epithelial tissue, connective tissue, and nerves. The skin covers and protects other body organs, such as bones and muscles. Bones support the body, and muscles move the bones and other organs under the direction of the nervous system which supplies the impulses. The entire organism is nourished by blood pumped through the pipe line of the blood vessels by the cardiac muscle, which is the chief tissue of the heart.

Epithelial Tissue

Epithelial tissue is distributed widely throughout the body and has many different kinds of structure. It occurs as a covering or lining tissue making up both the surface layer of the skin and the surface layer of the mucous membranes which line body cavities such as the mouth, the stomach, and the intestines. Epithelial tissue also gives rise to several organs during embryonic development. Of epithelial origin in the developing embryo are highly specialized cells of such organs as the pancreas, the liver, the thyroid gland, and the salivary glands. Also in certain locations in the upper and lower jaws epithelial tissue becomes differentiated into structures called the *enamel organs* which, located deep in the jaw, produce the enamel of developing teeth (Chapter 3).

The various kinds of epithelial tissues are similar to one another in that they

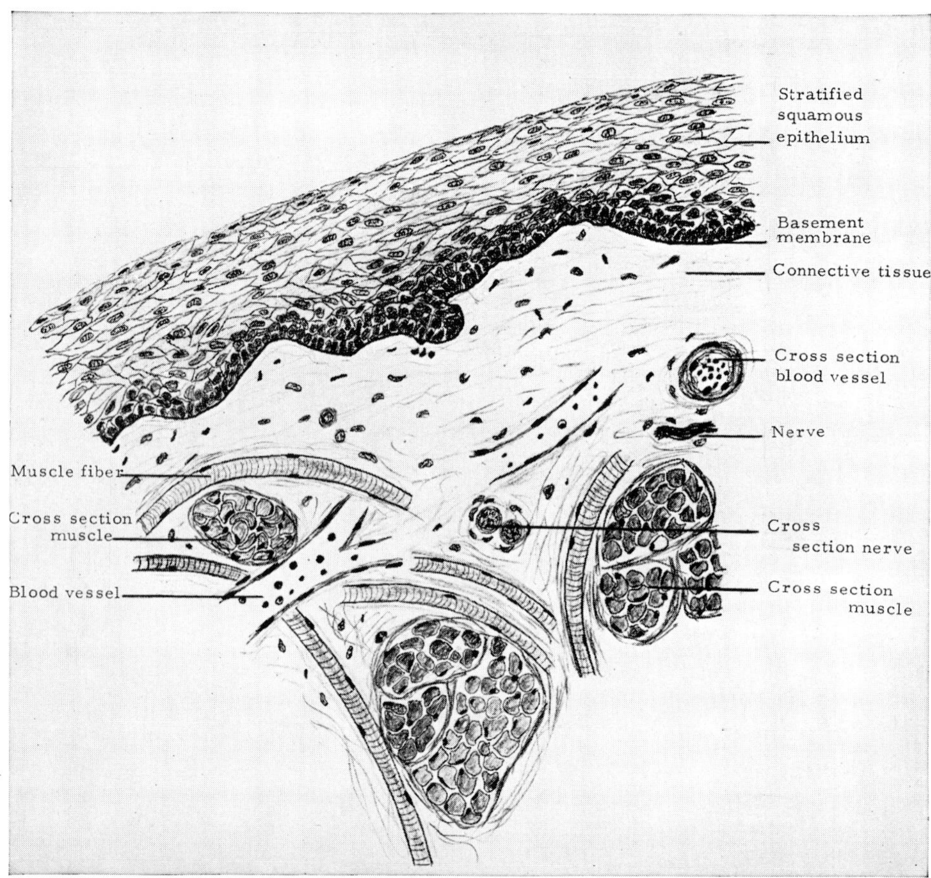

Fig. 1–2. Diagrammatic drawing of a section of tissue taken from the under side of the human tongue. This section illustrates the way in which tissues are combined.

have a proportionally large number of cells and very little intercellular substance. They are dissimilar in many ways, their structure in different locations in the body being fortunately adapted to the functions which they perform.

All lining and glandular epithelial tissues rest on a connective tissue. Interposed between the epithelial and connective tissues is a structure called the *basement membrane* (Fig. 1–3). Viewed under a light microscope the basement membrane appears as a single layer. Electron microscopic views of this layer reveal that it is actually composed of two layers. These layers are called *laminae;* specifically, *basal lamina* and *reticular lamina.* The basal lamina is secreted by the adjacent epithelial cells; the reticular lamina is produced by cells of the connective tissue. The laminae are composed of fibers and ground substance. The basal lamina is mostly comprised of ground substance, and the reticular lamina is more fibrous.

The basement membrane serves several functions: supports and cushions the epithelium; connects the epithelium to the connective tissue; acts as a filtration barrier for both the epithelium and the connective tissue.

For purposes of description histologists have classified epithelial tissues into two major groups and several subgroups:

1. Surface cells of covering and lining membranes

   a. Simple { Squamous, Cuboidal, Columnar }

   b. Pseudostratified columnar

   c. Stratified { Squamous, Cuboidal, Columnar, Transitional }

2. Glandular Tissue
   a. Endocrine glands, e.g., thyroid
   b. Exocrine glands, e.g., salivary glands
   c. Mixed endocrine and exocrine, e.g., liver, pancreas

Surface Epithelia

Epithelial cells of covering and lining membranes are not all alike in shape and arrangement. The *shape* of epithelial cell is described by the words squamous, cuboidal, and columnar; and the *arrangement* of epithelial cells is described by the words simple, stratified, and pseudostratified. The word *squamous* means scale-like, or flat; and *squamous epithelial cells* are flat cells. *Cuboidal epithelials cells* are roughly cube-shaped; and *columnar epithelial cells* are tall and narrow. When the arrangement of epithelial cells is in a single layer the tissue is said to be *simple epithelium*. When epithelial cells are arranged in several layers the tissue is called *stratified epithelium* (stratified = in layers). The word *pseudostratified* is applied to an arrangement of columnar epithelial cells in which the cells appear to be stratified but are actually in a single layer (pseudo = false).

All *simple epithelium* is delicate in structure. Simple epithelium is found only

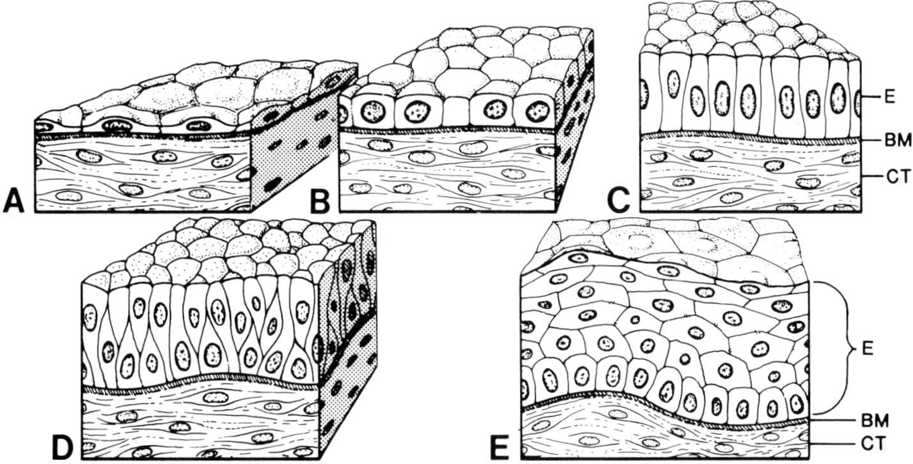

Fig. 1–3. Diagrammatic drawings of some different types of lining epithelia. A, Simple squamous epithelium. B, Simple cubodial epithelium. C, Simple columnar epithelium. D, Pseudostratified columnar epithelium. E, Stratified squamous epithelium. The epithelium (E) is connected to the underlying connective tissue (CT) by a basement membrane (BM).

in those areas of the body which are subjected to a little or no friction in functional use. *Simple squamous epithelium* (a single layer of flat epithelial cells) is found lining the inside of the walls of blood vessels (Fig. 1–3A). *Simple cuboidal epithelium* (a single layer of cuboidal epithelial cells) is found in the covering epithelium of the ovary (Fig. 1–3B). *Simple columnar epithelium* (a single layer of columnar epithelial cells) lines the cervix of the uterus (Fig. 1–3C).

Pseudostratified columnar epithelium (Fig. 1–3D) makes up the epithelial part of the mucous membrane which lines the upper respiratory tract: the maxillary sinuses, the nasal cavity, and the trachea. This epithelium is actually composed of a single layer of columnar epithelial cells; but because in some of the cells the nucleus is located near the base of the cell, while in other cells the nucleus is located nearer the outer end, this epithelium has the appearance of being made up of two of three layers of cells. In the upper respiratory tract the pseudostratified columnar epithelium is supplied with *cilia* and with *goblet cells.* Cilia are minute, hair-like projections which cover the surface ends of the columnar cells and act as dust catchers, or filters, for the air breathed in through the nose. Goblet cells are modified epithelial cells which are interspersed among the other columnar cells and which secrete substances that keep the tissue surface of the nose and sinuses moist.

Stratified epithelium consists of cells which are similar in shape to cells of simple epithelium, but which are arranged so that they are from 2 or 3 to many layers deep. *Stratified cuboidal epithelium* and *stratified columnar epithelium* occur as the lining of some of the larger ducts of glands, such as the large ducts of the major salivary glands. The stratified epithelial cells which line the urinary bladder change in shape from round to flat, depending on whether the bladder is empty or full, and this epithelium is therefore described as *stratified transitional epithelium.* Stratified epithelium is more resistant to hard use than the simple types of epithelium. By far the most sturdy of all kinds of epithelia is *stratified squamous epithelium* which is found covering all surfaces of the body which are routinely subjected to considerable wear and tear.

Statified squamous epithelium (Figs. 1–2, 1–3E) makes up both the surface of the skin and the surface of the mucous membrane of the oral cavity. In both of these locations the epithelium is composed of many layers of cells and, as is true with all epithelia, it rest on a fine structure called the *basement membrane* which separates the epithelial tissue from its underlying connective tissue. The epithelial cells of the deepest layer, called *basal cells,* are not flat in shape but are somewhat cuboidal and often show cell division. As these basal cells multiply, some cells are gradually moved toward the outside surface, becoming flatter as they approach the surface and finally becoming dead cells. In some areas of the oral cavity the flat, dead epithelial cells on the surface are sloughed off as they are replaced from below. In other areas of the oral cavity, and on the skin, these dead surface cells are not quickly sloughed off. Instead they may lose their nuclei and their cell boundaries and become converted into a tough, resistant surface layer which is called the *keratinized layer* (Fig. 1–4). This keratinized layer, of course, gradually wears off and is replaced from beneath as a result of continued cell division in the basal cell layer. The most heavily keratinized epithelium of the body is found on the palms of the hands and on the soles of the feet (Fig. 1–5), particularly if these areas have been subjected to hard use and are calloused.

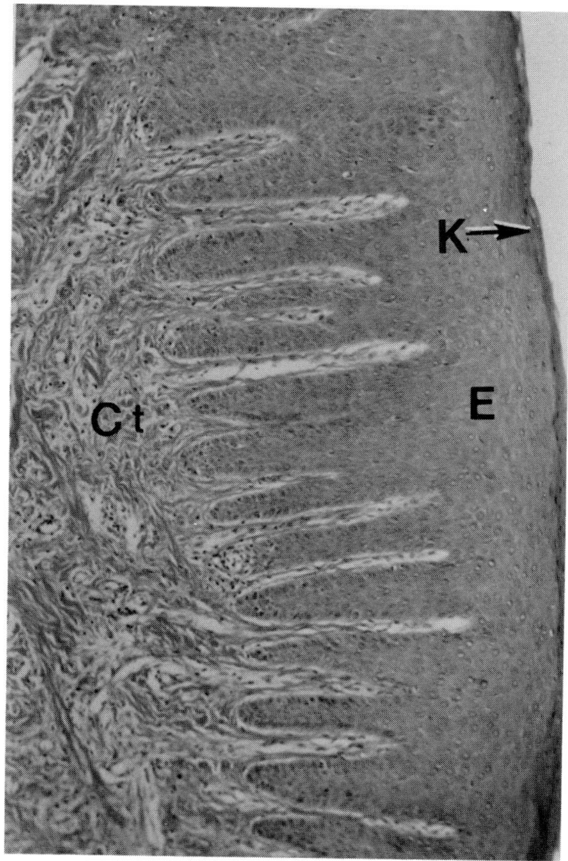

Fig. 1–4. Histologic section of the human gingiva part of the oral mucous membrane showing the thin keratin (K) layer of the stratified squamous epithelium (E). Note the fibrous nature of the connective tissue (Ct) and its interdigitation with the epithelium.

More about nonkeratinized and keratinized epithelium will be learned in the study of the oral mucosa (Chapter 10).

Covering and lining epithelial tissues do not contain blood vessels; they receive nourishment via the blood vessels contained in the connective tissue which surrounds or underlies them.

Glandular Tissue

Glands are secreting organs that produce a specific product or secretion. The main tissue of glands is *epithelial* tissue. It is the epithelial cells of this tissue that are specialized to produce the secretions.

Glands can be classified several different ways. There will be no attempt here to deal with all the different ways. Those which are more commonly used will by discussed in general terms. The interested student should consult any of the many fine general histology textbooks.

During development all glands arise as an invagination of covering or lining epithelium into the underlying connective tissue. The epithelium, at first, is a solid mass of cells. These epithelial cells continue to proliferate and migrate,

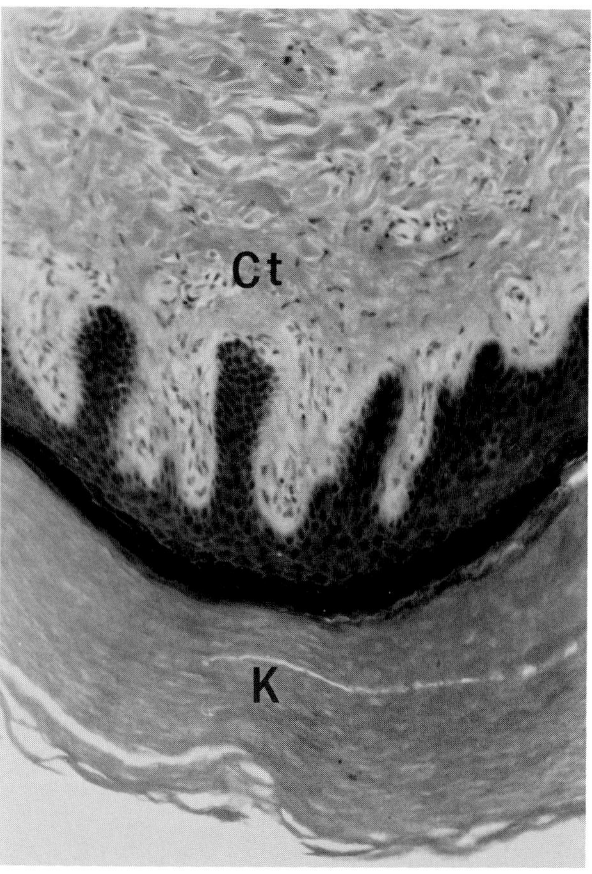

Fig. 1–5. Histologic section of the sole of a human foot showing the heavily keratinized (K) surface layer of the epithelium and the underlying connective tissue (Ct). Compare this section of skin to the section of oral mucous seen in Figure 1–4.

and become the grandular epithelium that will give rise to all epithelial portions of the gland.

The surface connection may remain intact, thus retaining a union between the secretory epithelial cells and the *free* surface (surface of skin, of oral cavity, and etc.). Eventually the epithelium hollows out throughout its length, providing a transport duct system for the secretions. This type of of gland is classified as a *duct* gland. Since the secretion of this type of gland is discharged onto the surface from which it developed, it is also classified as an *exocrine* gland (gland of external secretion).

The continuous invaginated glandular epithelium of some developing glands may lose the connection with the free surface; the secretory epithelial cells become isolated from the original site of origin. Since this type of gland loses the transport system to a free surface, it is called a *ductless* gland. The secretions of this type of gland diffuse into the nearby blood and lymph vessels, thus it discharges its products internally and so is also called an *endocrine* gland.

The glands can be classified according to the kind of secretion they produce. Endocrine (ductless) glands secrete *hormones.* A hormone is a discrete chemical substance that is secreted into blood and lymph vessels. It has a specific effect on the activities of other cells and organs.

The kind of secretion produced by exocrine glands may be *serous, mucous,* or a combination of *serous* and *mucous.* The secretory cells of these glands are named according to the type of secretion they produce, e.g., *serous* or *mucous* cells. If a particular gland is composed of only serous cells, it is referred to as a *pure* serous gland; if a gland is composed of only mucous cells, it is referred to as a *pure* mucous gland. Some glands have both serous and mucous cells making up their secretory portions; these glands are called *mixed.* Their products will be a *sero-mucous* secretion.

In summary, some glands are classified as *duct, exocrine, serous, mucous,* or *mixed* (salivary glands are in this group—see Chapter 10). Other glands are classified as *ductless,* or *endocrine;* their secretions are called *hormones.*

Connective Tissue

The tissues which have been classified together as connective tissue differ from epithelial tissues basically in that they are made up of a relatively larger amount of intercellular substance and relatively fewer cells. In spite of this characteristic which connective tissues have in common they differ so greatly in form and in function that at first glance they sometimes appear to be unrelated. Connective tissue (fibrous) underlies the epithelium of the skin and the epithelium of the oral mucosa and also makes up tendons and ligaments. Connective tissue (areolar) attaches skin to muscle. Connective tissue (fat) stores food. Connective tissue (hemopoietic) forms blood. Connective tissue (cartilage) gives

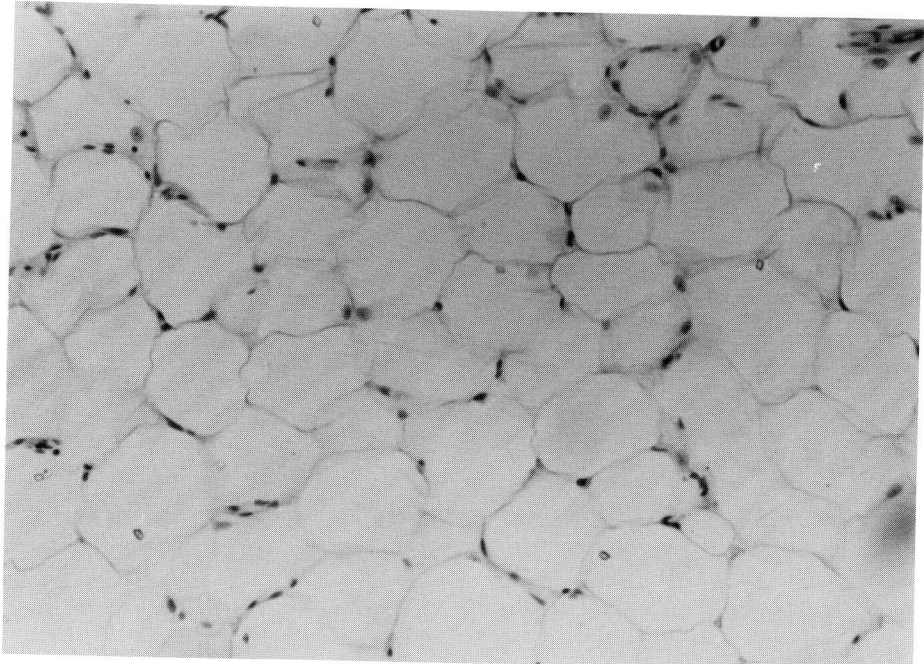

Fig. 1–6. Histologic section of a fatty type of connective tissue. Fat is stored in the ringed areas. Fat nuclei are pushed to the periphery of the rings; at this magnification the cell nuclei resemble dots.

support and permits skeletal growth. Connective tissue (bone) supports the body.

Fibrous connective tissue is found throughout the body. In its most dense form it makes up tendons and ligaments. In a less dense form it is the connective tissue which underlies the epithelial part of skin and of mucous membranes (Figs. 1–5, 1–6). Like other tissue, fibrous connective tissue is made up of cells and intercellular substance, and the intercellular substance is of two kinds: fibrillar and amorphous ground substance. The fibrillar component of the intercellular substance is the predominant element.

The fibers of fibrous connective tissue are produced by cells called *fibroblasts* (blast = germ, builder). The individual fibers are made up of minute fibrils. Special staining techniques used on histologic sections reveal that the fibers are not all alike, some being *collagenous fibers* and others *elastic fibers.* These fibers are distributed in different proportions in different kinds of fibrous connective tissue.

Suspended along with the fibers in the all-encompassing amorphous (ground) substance are the various kinds of cells of the fibrous connective tissue. Proportionally the most numerous type of cell is the *fibroblast.* Special tissue preparation will show also the presence of other types of cells, some of which are capable of becoming defense cells when the tissue suffers injury or bacterial infection.

Areolar connective tissue is seen during any gross dissection of a mammal where skin is attached to muscles, muscles to muscles, or where internal organs are held together by membranes of connective tissue. These tissue membranes, called *fascia,* are made up of areolar connective tissue and fat tissue. The areolar connective tissue is composed of a relatively small number of cells and a very loose and thin network of fibrous intercellular substance, all held together by a large amount of ground substance.

Fat tissue (Fig. 1–6) is distributed throughout the body among the soft tissues and in the marrow cavities of bones, and is found more or less generously concentrated in certain parts of the body beneath the skin. It is composed of specialized connective tissue cells, called *fat cells,* which are held together by fibrous intercellular substance. Fat cells are capable of storing fat. They may become so filled with fat that the cytoplasm is pressed into a thin layer around the periphery of the cell, and the nucleus is crowded against the side of the cell.

Hemopoietic tissue (hemo = blood; poietic = to make) not only produces blood cells which are added to the circulating blood, but removes worn out blood cells from the blood stream. In the adult, hemopoietic tissue occurs in two different forms: as *red bone marrow* and as *lymphatic tissue.* In the human fetus, red bone marrow is found in nearly all of the bones; but in the adult, the marrow in many of the bones has become converted to so-called *yellow bone marrow* which is largely fat. Certain bones, however, such as the vault of the skull, the ribs, the sternum, the bodies of vertebrae, retain the red bone marrow throughout adult life. Yellow bone marrow in other bones can be converted into hemopoietic red marrow in circumstances of emergency.

Red bone marrow consists of a fibrillar meshwork of intercellular substance throughout which are scattered many cells that have the potentiality of differentiating into several kinds of blood cells. Red bone marrow produces *red bone cells (erythrocytes)* and certain kinds of *white blood cells (granular leukoytes),* which

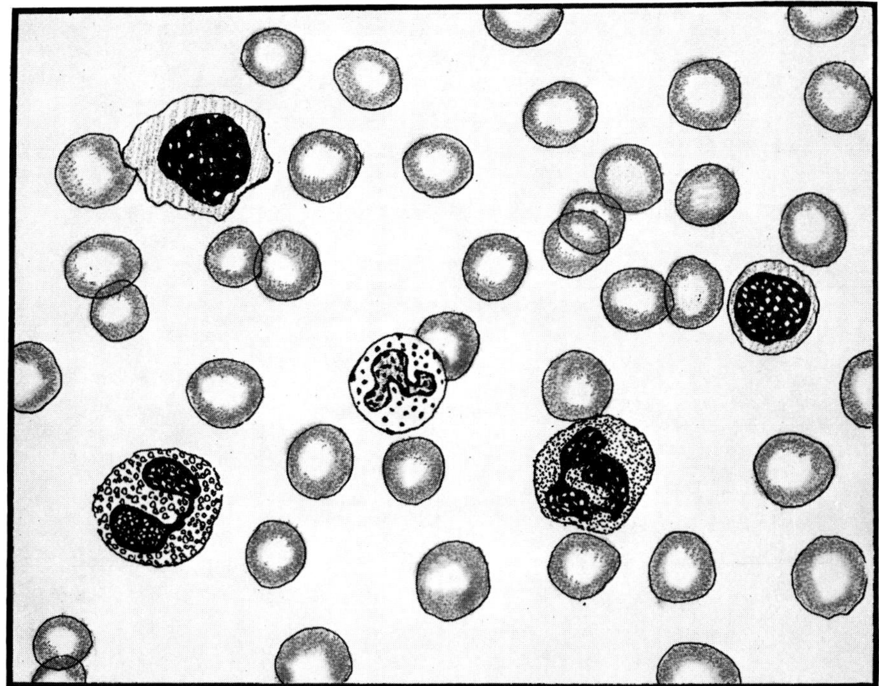

Fig. 1–7. Diagrammatic illustration of a human blood smear showing *erythrocytes* (red blood cells) and *leukocytes* (white blood cells). The more numerous red blood cells are small biconcave disks about 8 microns in diameter having neither a nucleus nor cytoplasmic granules. The five larger cells are different types of white blood cells: they have nuclei, and some have granules in the cytoplasm. The *nongranular leukocytes* are the *large lymphocyte* (upper left) and the *small lymphocyte* (upper right). They have round-shaped nuclei. The three white blood cells below are *granular leukocytes.* They have multilobed nuclei and conspicuous cytoplasmic granules. Left to right, these cells are an *eosinophilic leukocyte, a basophilic leukocyte,* and a *neutrophilic leukocyte.*

are white blood cells that have granules in the cytoplasm *(eosinophilic leukocytes, basophilic leukocytes,* and *neutrophilic leukocytes)* (Fig. 1–7).

Lymphatic tissue is composed of fibrillar intercellular substance and scattered undifferentiated cells. Some of these undifferentiated cells are capable of becoming differentiated into certain kinds of white blood cells, chiefly *lymphocytes.* Conspicuous areas of lymphatic tissue are seen in several places around the oral cavity: the palatine tonsils, which are located between the oral cavity and the pharynx; and the lingual tonsils, which are located on the posterior part of the dorsum of the tongue. Lymphatic tissue is found also in other parts of the body.

In *cartilage* (Fig. 1–8) the most conspicuous component of the tissue is the ground substance type of intercellular substance, which in gross examination resembles a firm gel. Fibers, which may be made visible by special histologic preparation of tissue sections, are scattered throughout the ground substance. The cells of cartilage, called *chondrocytes,* occupy spaces, called *lacunae,* in the intercellular substance. Nutrients are transmitted to the cells through the intercellular substance. Cartilage exists as a nonmineralized tissue.

A large part of the skeleton of the human fetus is first constructed in cartilage, which seems to act as a pattern for the developing bone tissue. The arm and leg bones, for example, are first formed in cartilage, which is resorbed as bone

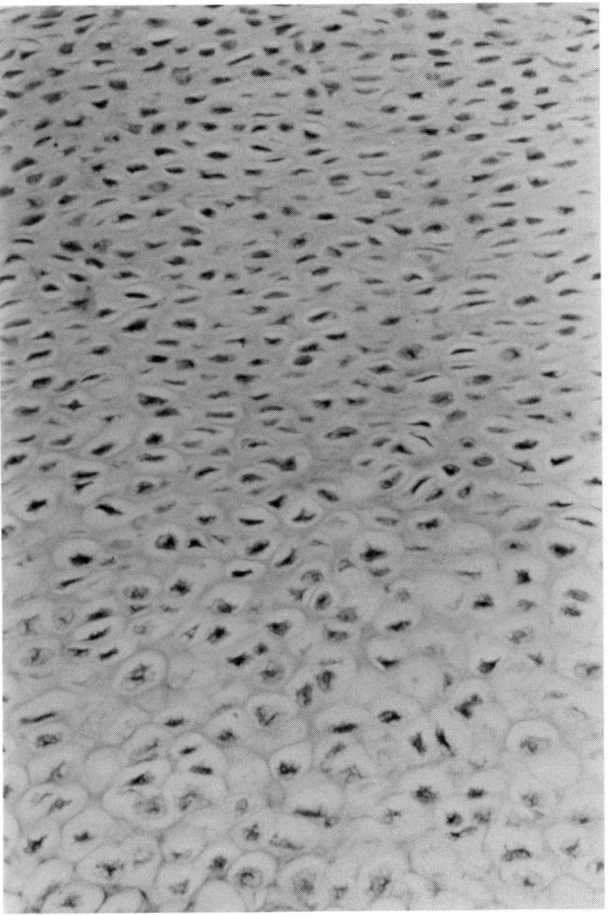

Fig. 1–8. Histologic section of a type of cartilage. The cells *(chondrocytes)* are in *lacunae*. The variation in size of the chondrocytes indicates stages of growth within the cartilage skeleton.

tissue develops to replace it (Fig. 9–9). While bone replaces most cartilage in the human skeleton at an early stage, cartilage persists in some places for years. At the ends of the long bones the presence of cartilage throughout childhood and adolescence permits growth in the length of the bones. In adults cartilage comprises parts of the nose, larynx, trachea, and ear. Cartilage tissue contains no nerves or blood vessels.

Bone is mineralized connective tissue. Bone contains a large amount of dense fibrous intercellular substance. The fibrils which make up the fibrous intercellular substance are of course surrounded by ground substance. In the ground substance mineral salts are deposited in solution as the bone is developing. As the bone matures, these mineral salts crystallize out of solution and the bone becomes a mineralized tissue. The cells of bone, called *osteocytes,* occupy spaces known as *lacunae* in the hard intercellular substance. More will be learned in Chapter 9 about the microscopic picture of bone tissue.

Nerve Tissue

Nerve tissue, which comprises the total nervous system, is made up nerve cells and a tissue which supports them. Nerve cells are called *neurons,* and they are like other cells in that they have a nucleus and a cytoplasm. However, they are highly specialized, that is, different from other cells, in that they have to a high degree the properties of reacting to stimuli (irritability) and of transmitting waves of excitation from the point where the stimulus is applied (conductivity). These waves of excitation, or *nerve impulses* as they are called, are transmitted through the cytoplasm of the neuron which is peculiarly adapted to this function.

The nervous system consists of two chief divisions: the *central nerous system* (the brain and spinal cord) and the *peripheral nervous system* (nerves associated with the various other organs of the body). The gross appearance and the histologic structure of the nerve tissue in these two divisions are very different. The tissue of the central nervous system is extremely soft due to the absence of connective tissue as a supporting tissue for the nerve cells. In the central nervous system the nerve cells are supported by a delicate and fragile tissue called *neuroglia* (literally, nerve glue). The brain and spinal cord are made up to two distinct types of this soft nerve tissue called *gray matter* and *white matter* which differ greatly in histologic structure.

In contrast to the nerve tissue of the central nervous system the nerves of the peripheral nervous system are tough. This firm quality is derived from the considerable amount of connective tissue which covers and supports the bundles of nerve fibers. A microscopic examination of a cross section of a nerve shows it to be circular in shape and covered by a connective tissue wrapping, or *sheath.*

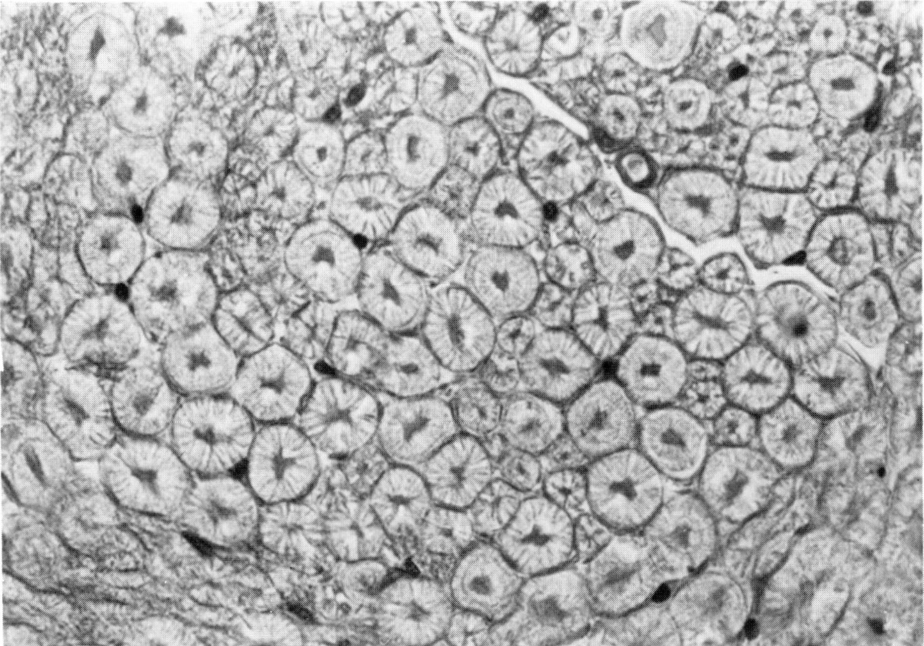

Fig. 1–9. Cross section of a myelinated peripheral nerve whose shrunken fibrils appear as dark spots, surrounded by a myelin sheath.

Inside this sheath are several bundles of *nerve fibers*, each bundle being surrounded by another connective tissue sheath. Each nerve fiber inside the bundles is encased in its individual connective tissue sheath, and often between this sheath and the individual fiber is a layer of substance of a fatty nature called a *myelin sheath* (Fig. 1–9). Each nerve fiber in this nerve is actually a long, thin, stretched-out part of the cytoplasm of a neuron. The body of the neuron, which contains the nucleus, lies deep in the body of the individual.

Nerve cells do not multiply with the growth of the human body. A person is born with all the neurons he will ever possess. However, if a fiber in the peripheral nervous system is cut, repair may eventually take place: the end of the fiber which has been cut off will degenerate, and the part of the fiber still attached to the body of the neuron may after a time grow out to the length of the original fiber. In the central nervous system, on the other hand, damage is permanent. There is no regeneration following damage to the brain or spinal cord.

Muscle Tissue

Muscle tissue is composed of muscle cells which are supported by connective tissue. Muscle cells are in all cases much longer than they are wide, and for this reason an individual muscle cell is called a muscle fiber. Muscle fibers have to a greater degree than other cells the property of contraction.

Microscopic examination of muscle tissue from various parts of the body shows a difference in the appearance of the cytoplasm of muscle fibers. In muscle tissue from some areas, for example from the intestine, the cytoplasm of the muscle fibers appears relatively clear. In muscle tissue from other areas, such as from the arm or the heart, the cytoplasm of the muscle fibers has cross striations. This difference in the appearance of the cytoplasm of different muscle fibers led histologists to classify muscle tissue as *smooth muscle tissue* (where the cytoplasm of the fibers is not cross striated), and *striated muscle tissue* (where the cytoplasm of the fibers is cross striated).

This division of muscle tissue into two types was not quite adequate, however. Smooth muscle is *involuntary muscle*—that is, the contraction of its fibers, is not under the control of the will of the individual. For instance, the peristaltic movements of the intestine, which contains smooth muscle in its walls, are not willfully controlled. On the other hand, striated muscle is for the most part *voluntary muscle* because the contractions of the muscle fibers may be consciously controlled by the individual. One moves an arm or a leg as one wishes. However, there is an exception. The fibers of the heart muscle, although striated like the fibers of the muscles of the arm, are not consciously controlled by the individual. Therefore cardiac muscle has been described as belonging to a class by itself and is called *striated involuntary muscle* in contrast to skeletal muscle which is referred to as *striated voluntary muscle.*

Thus we arrive at a classification for muscle tissue consisting of three categories: *smooth muscle, striated voluntary muscle,* and *striated involuntary muscle* (Fig. 1–10).

Smooth muscle tissue is found in such places as in the walls of the intestines, in the walls of the blood vessels, and at the roots of hairs where its contraction produces an erection of the hair. The individual muscle fibers (cells) of smooth muscle tissue are shaped somewhat like a cigar and have a centrally located nucleus. In length they may vary from 1/1000 mm in the small blood vessels to

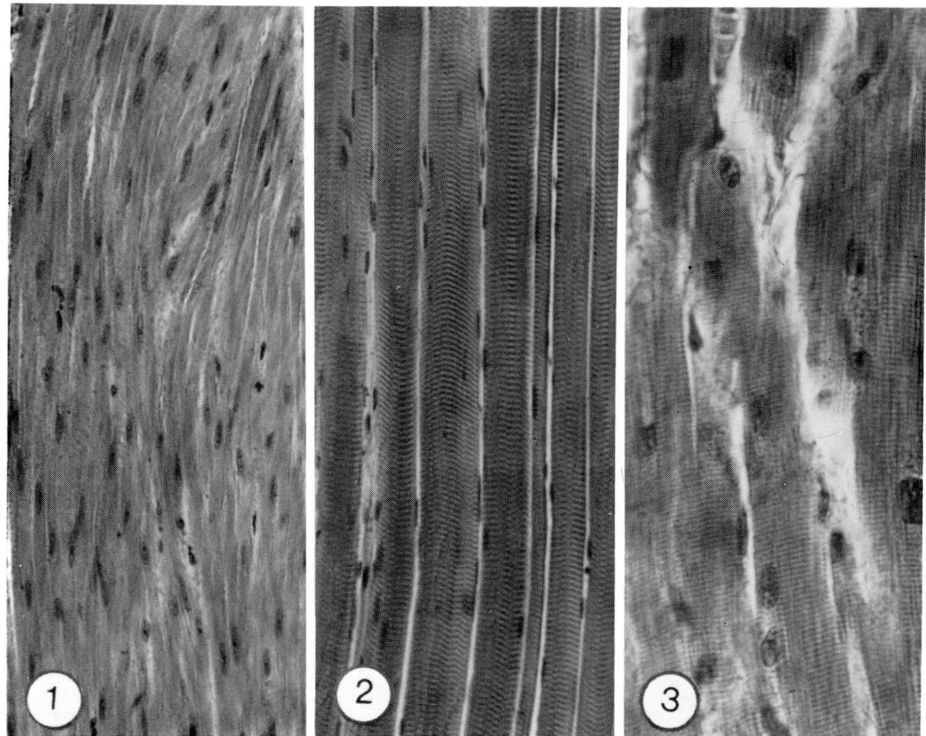

Fig. 1–10. Section of (1) smooth muscle, (2) striated voluntary muscle, and (3) striated involuntary muscle (cardiac).

½ mm in the pregnant uterus. The fibers are supported by associated connective tissue.

Striated voluntary muscle is known also as *skeletal muscle.* As well as the obvious inclusion in this class of such muscles as those which move the arms and legs, skeletal muscles also include those in and about the oral cavity: muscles of the tongue, of the lips and cheeks, of the soft palate. The muscle fibers of skeletal muscle differ in a number of ways from those of smooth muscle. Most conspicuous of course is the difference in the appearance of the cytoplasm, which shows microscopic cross striations (Fig. 1–10). Also, the nuclei in skeletal muscle fibers are pushed to one side of the fibers instead of lying in the center, and there is more than one nucleus in a fiber. Skeletal muscle fibers are relatively long, varying from 1 to 40 mm, and they are supported by connective tissue which not only covers individual fibers, but binds the fibers into bundles. This supporting connective tissue is well supplied with blood vessels and nerves.

Striated involuntary muscle is confined to the heart and is known as *cardiac muscle.* In microscopic appearance it resembles skeletal muscle in that the cytoplasm of the muscle fibers has microscopic cross striations (Fig. 1–10). Its appearance differs from that of skeletal muscle in the arrangement of the fibers. Whereas skeletal muscle fibers exist as individual fibers with several nuclei, cardiac muscle fibers branch and come together so that they form a sort of network which comprises the heart muscle. This network is supported by surrounding connective tissue which contains nerves and a rich supply of blood vessels.

Muscles are the organs responsible for both the voluntary and the involuntary movement of all of the various parts of the body. They act in response to impulses received from the nervous system. They are surrounded by, supported by, and nourished by the different kinds of connective tissue: the fibrous, areolar, and adipose; the bone and cartilage; and the blood.

ORAL HISTOLOGY

Of particular importance in Dentistry are the tissues of the oral cavity. The entire practice of Dentistry and Dental Hygiene is based on a knowledge of the structure, arrangement, and reactions of oral tissues. Instructions given to a patient by the dentist and the dental hygienist concerning the correct method of brushing the teeth are based on a knowledge of oral histology. A dentist prepares a tooth for a filling with careful attention to the nature and arrangement of the tissues comprising the tooth; and he constructs an artificial denture with regard for the structure of the tissues of the palate, of the alveolar ridge, and of the oral vestibule. The pathosis which occurs in the the tissues around a tooth when calculus is present can be understood only in the light of a knowledge of tissue structure and tissue reaction; and the tissue repair which follows removal of the calculus is explainable in the same terms. Other diseases of the soft tissues of the mouth are recognized and treated only as normal tissue structure is known. The nearly universal disease of the hard tooth tissues, dental caries, must be described in terms of the microscopic structure of the tissues beneath the lining, the tissues of the tongue, the periodontium, the tooth, and the tissues from which a tooth develops. This book includes also a study of the process of tooth development.

Location of Oral Tissues

The relative locations of some of the oral tissues may be seen in the diagram of a section through a human mandible in the region of the second premolar tooth (Fig. 9–1). The *tooth* is attached by fibers of the *periodontal ligament* to the *lamina dura* which comprises the tooth socket. The outside surface of the mandible consists of *cortical plate* inside of which is *trabecular bone* and bone marrow. The lining of the inside of the cheek, the gingiva, and the covering of the *tongue* are mucous membrane. Under the tongue are located *salivary glands* and several *muscles.*

Tissue of a Tooth

The tissues which make up tooth are the enamel, the dentin, the cementum, and the pulp. Figures 1–11, 1–12, and 1–13 are diagrams of teeth which have been cut approximately through the middle in a faciolingual direction. *Tooth enamel* comprises the surface of the crown of the tooth and *cementum* comprises the surface of the tooth root. *Dentin,* which lies beneath the enamel of the crown and beneath the cementum of the root, makes up the bulk of the hard tissue of the tooth. The *tooth pulp* is the only nonmineralized tissue of the tooth. It occupies the *pulp chamber* in the crown of the tooth and continues through the *root canals* to its union with the periodontal ligament at the *apical foramen.*

The line of union between the dentin and the enamel is the *dentinoenamel*

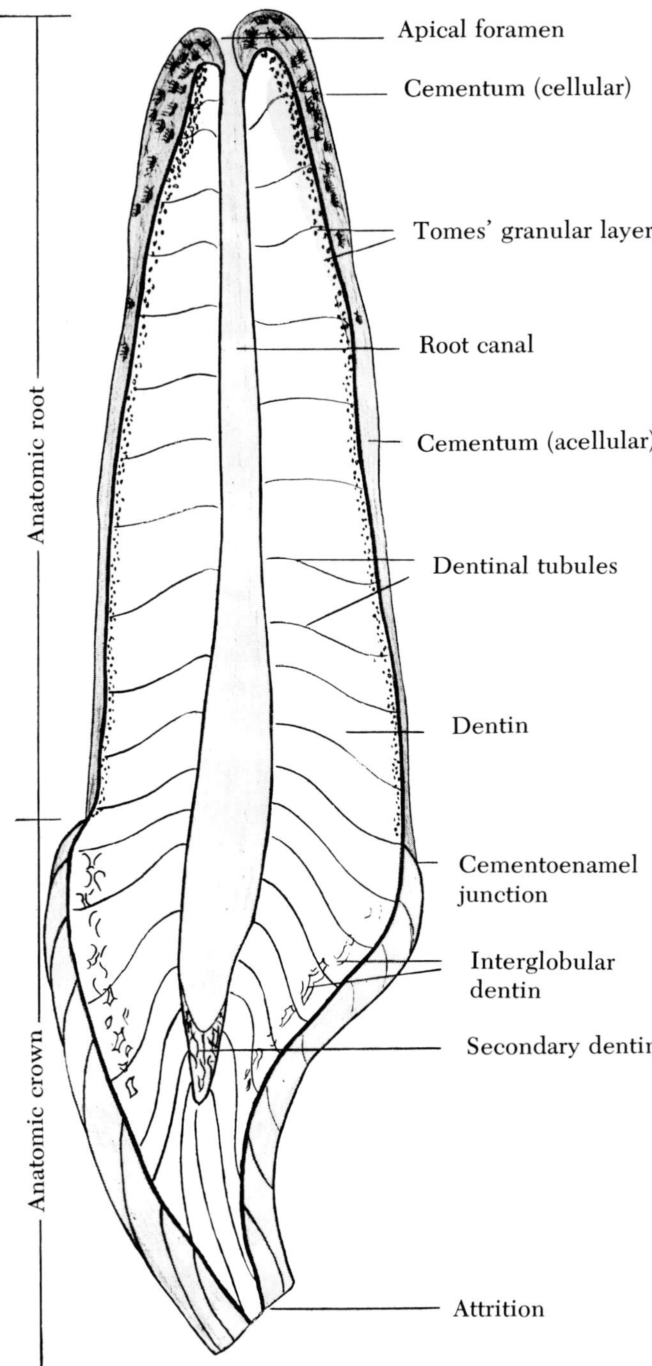

Fig. 1–11. Diagrammatic drawing of a longitudinal faciolingual section of a maxillary incisor. The cementum lacunae in this and in the following diagrams of tooth sections are somewhat exaggerated in size.

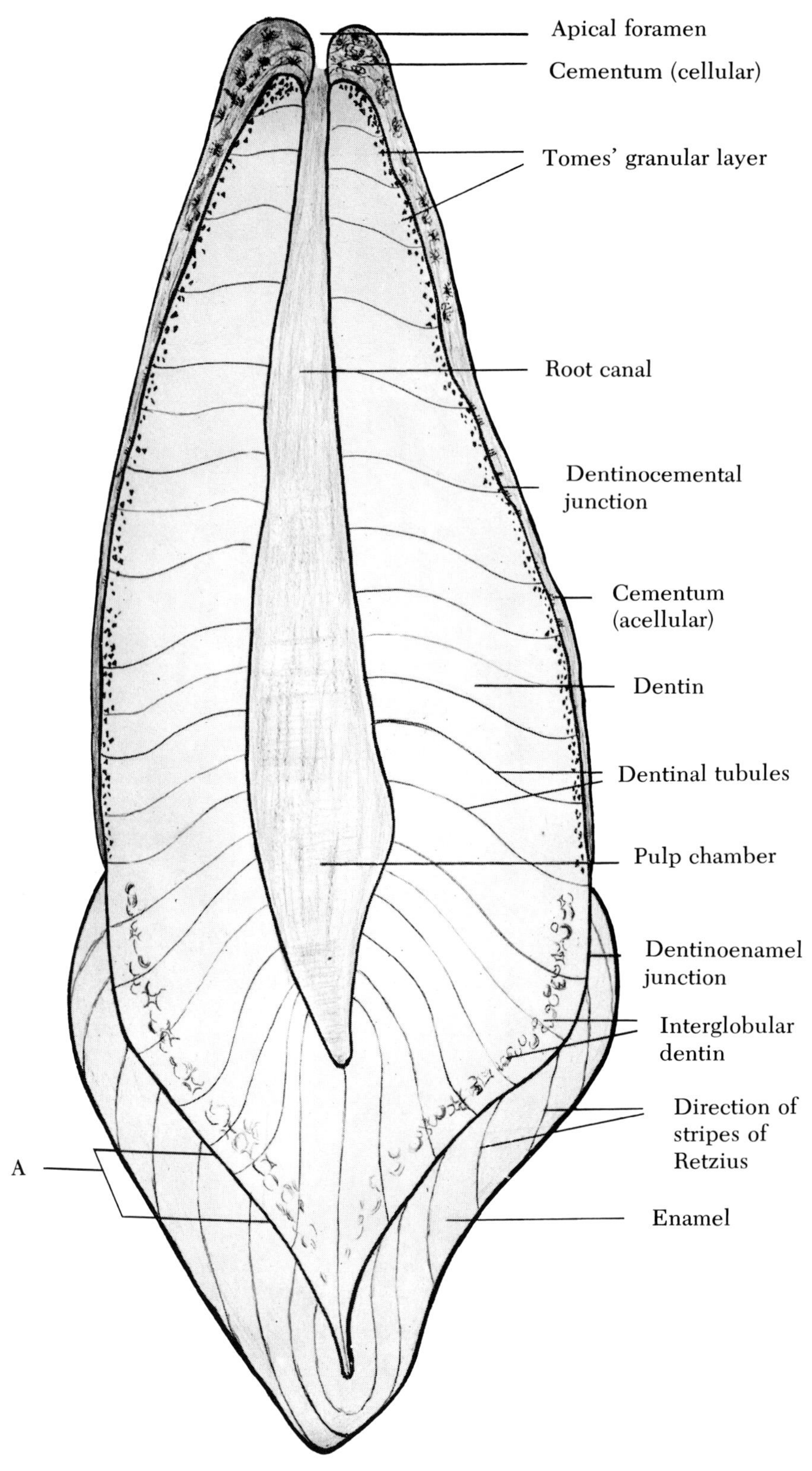

Fig. 1–12. Diagrammatic drawing of a longitudinal faciolingual section of a maxillary canine. The area marked A indicates a location in the enamel similar to that shown in Figure 4–16.

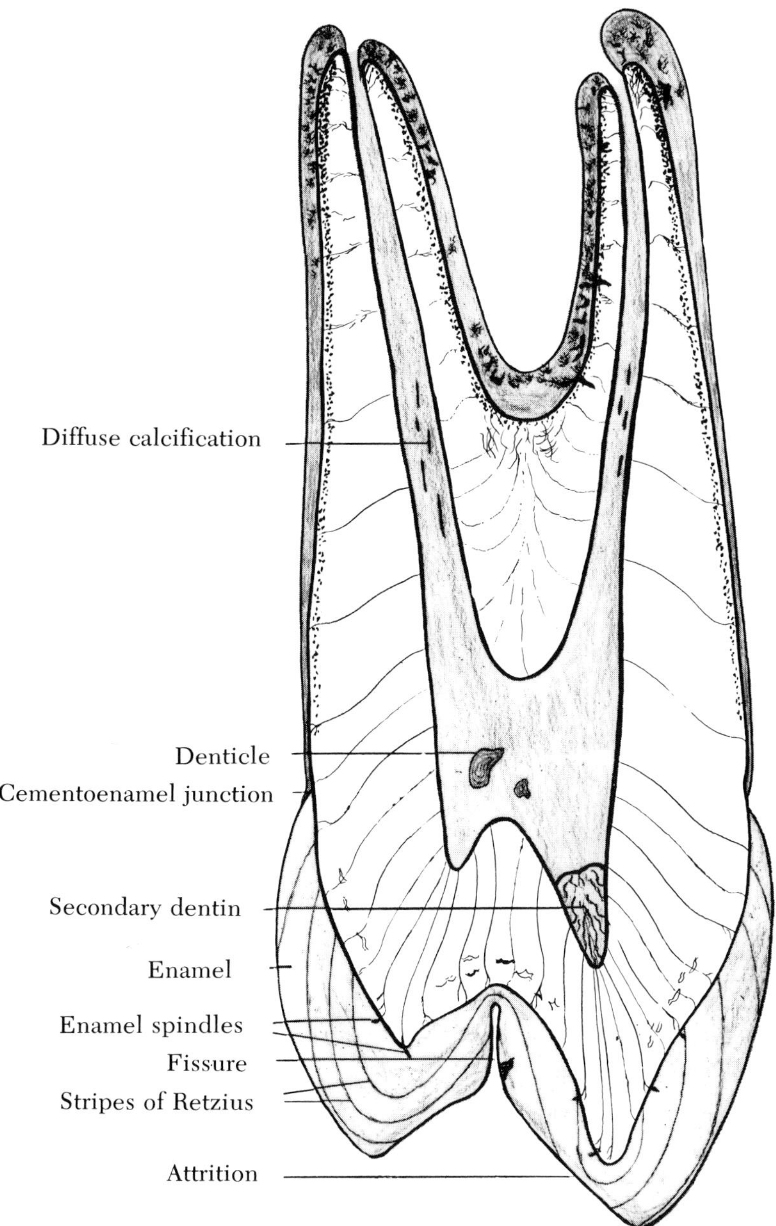

Fig. 1–13. Diagrammatic drawing of a longitudinal faciolingual section of a maxillary first premolar. See *Frontispiece* for a photograph of a similar tooth and compare the structure indicated in the diagrammatic drawing with the same structures seen in the photograph of the actual tooth section.

junction. The line of union between the dentin and the cementum is the *dentinocemental junction*. The line of union between the cementum and the enamel is the *cementoenamel junction*. These are frequent points of reference in descriptions of a tooth.

Chapter 2

EMBRYONIC DEVELOPMENT OF THE FACE AND ORAL CAVITY

1/13/93

THE HUMAN BODY

The Beginning of a Human Body

Beginning of life for an individual human being is the moment the sperm unites with the ovum and forms a fertilized egg. The fertilized egg is called a *zygote* (from the Greek *zygotus,* meaning "yoked together"). This egg divides into two cells, each of these into two more, and the resulting cells divide again and again. At first there is only a mass of but slightly differentiated cells; then begins a shaping—a shaping that eventually results in the formation of a tiny tubular embryo that foreshadows the plan of the adult human body.

An adult body is essentially a thick-walled tube. Or perhaps it can be better described as two tubes, a larger outer one (outside body wall) and a small inner one (digestive tract), between which is a space (body cavity) that contains the internal organs: heart, lungs, liver. The mouth is the *cephalic* (head) opening of the inner tube, and the anus, is the *caudal* (tail) opening.

Similarly in the tiny embryo, the tube which is the outside body wall encases a smaller tube, the *primitive digestive tract,* or *primitive gut,* which at this time is closed at both ends because the mouth and anus have not yet formed. In early stages of development, before the internal organs are formed, cells located between the outer body wall and the primitive digestive tract make the wall of the tubular embryo relatively thick.

In fact, the embryo wall is made up of three layers: *ectoderm* (ecto = outside; derm = skin); *mesoderm* (meso = middle); *endoderm* (endo = inside). Collectively, these layers are called *primary embryonic layers,* or *primary germ layers,* and each is destined to form certain organs, or parts of organs, of the adult body. For example, ectoderm will give rise not only to the epithelium covering the outside of the body, but to the epithelium lining the oral cavity, nasal cavity, and sinuses, and to the enamel of the teeth, and to the nervous system. For the most part, from mesoderm will be derived the skeletal system, muscles, blood and lymph cells and vessels, kidneys, and some other internal organs. And from endoderm will come the epithelial lining of the pharynx, stomach, and intestines, and of the lungs, bladder, vagina, and uretha.

From these three primary embryonic layers the manner of formation of the facial and oral structures, will become clear as we study the embryonic development of the face and oral cavity, and later the development of the teeth.

Definition of Growth and Development

Growth may be defined as an increase in weight and spatial dimensions that an organism or organ goes through. The organism or organ gets heavier and takes up space. For growth to occur, three things must happen: (1) increase in number of cells, (2) increase in size of cells, and (3) increase in the product of the cells.

Development is an organism or organ going toward *maturity.* While the organism or organ is growing it is *maturing* (becoming older). By comparing the changes of the human face (head), as depicted by the models in Figure 2–1, it is easy to understand *growth* and *development.*

The Size of a Human Fetus

At the end of the third week after fertilization the embryo is about 3 mm long. In later stages of development the size usually is given in terms of crown-rump length. By the end of the eighth week the crown-rump length is about 23 mm and the embryo has acquired a form recognizable as a human being (Fig. 2–2). At the end of three months the fetus* has a crown-rump length of about 61 mm, and at four months about 116 mm.

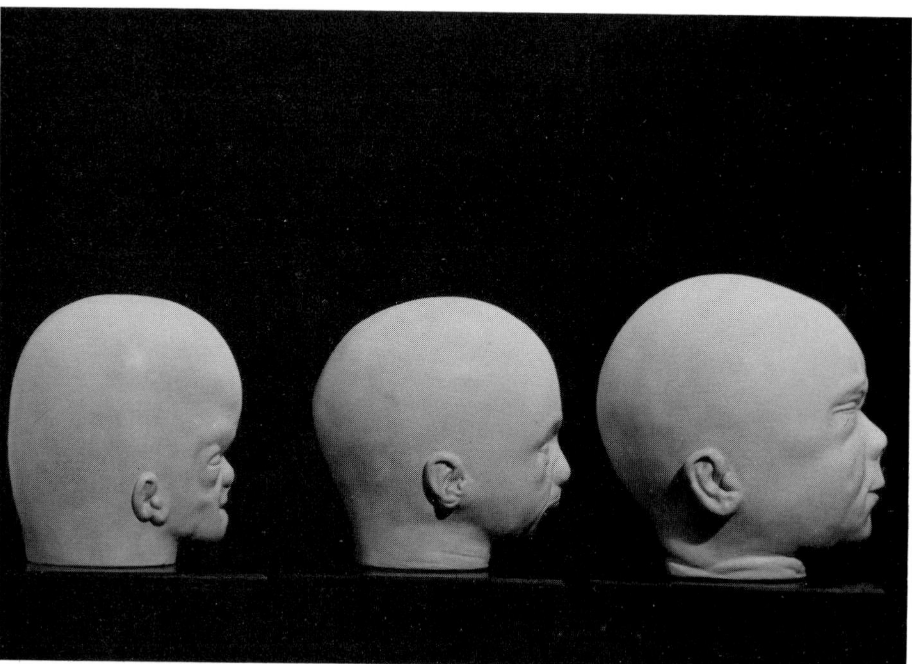

Fig. 2–1. Lateral view of models illustrating growth and development of the human head (face). The approximate ages represented are, from the left: Ten weeks in utero; four months in utero; and birth.

*The unborn child is called an *embryo* until the end of the eighth week, after which time it is called a *fetus*.

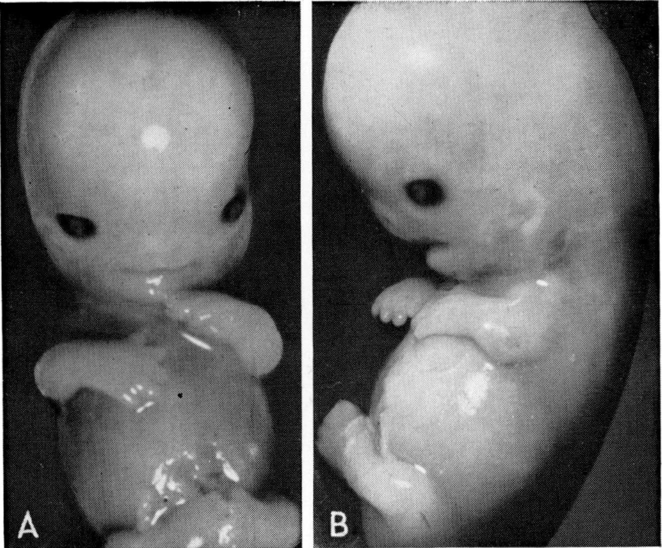

Fig. 2–2. A and B. A human embryo 25 mm long-eight to nine weeks old. The head is large, making up nearly half of the body length. Compared to the size of the brain, the face appears small. The eyes are widespread; the ears are close to the neck. The nose is nearly flat. Notice the small size of the lower jaw. Inside of the mouth of an embryo of this age the lateral palatine processes are in a vertical position and the tongue is tall and narrow and nearly touches the lower border fo the nasal septum (Fig. 2–10A).

THE DEVELOPMENT OF THE FACE

The Establishment of the Primitive Mouth

Throughout embryonic development the cephalic end of the embryo evolves in advance of the caudal end. The faces starts to develop during the third week in utero with the beginning of the formation of the mouth, and by the end of third week the *stomodeum* (primitive mouth)* has been established. Through growth and development the stomodeum becomes the oral and nasal cavities. This will be understood when you study the development of the palate. The stomodeum forms in this manner:

On the ventral side of the cephalic end of the embryo there occurs an invagination, an apparent pushing in, of the ectoderm. This depression is the *stomodeum* (Figs. 2–3, 2–4). At the deepest part of this invagination the ectoderm is in contact with the endoderm of the *foregut* (the cephalic part of the primitive digestive tract). There is no intervening mesoderm. This combined ectoderm and endoderm is the *buccopharyngeal membrane.* (Examine Figure 2–3 carefully.) It is located approximately in the region where the palatine tonsils will later appear, and it separates the primitive mouth from the foregut. The location of the buccopharyngeal membrane indicates that the stomodeum is lined with ectoderm, and that the primitive digestive tract caudal to the stomodeum is lined with endoderm.

During the fourth week in utero the buccopharyngeal membrane ruptures, and there is thus established communication between the stomodeum and the primitive digestive tract.

Shortly befor the rupture of this membrane, about the end of the third week,

Pronouced stō mō dē′ um.

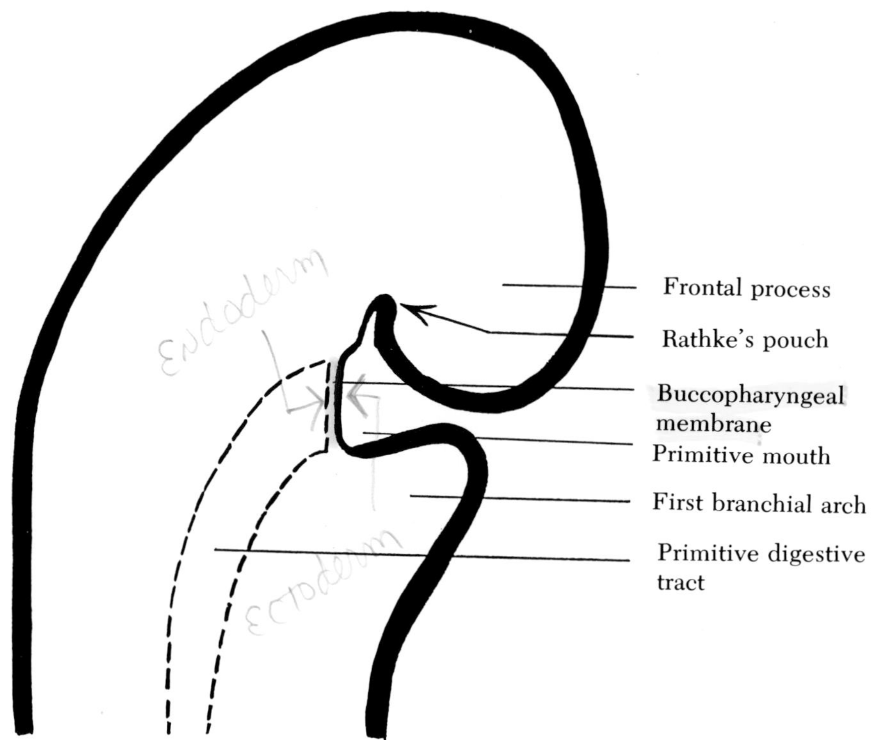

Fig. 2–3. A diagrammatic illustration of a median sagittal section through the head of a human embryo at the end of the third week in utero. About 3mm.

begins the formation of a structure not usually thought of as being associated with the oval cavity—the *anterior lobe of the hypophysis*. The hypophysis, or pituitary gland, is a gland of internal secretion located in the sella turcica of the sphenoid bone. It is attached to the brain. Its development starts as a small evagination of the stomodeal ectoderm (Fig. 2– 3) in the roof of the primitive mouth just in front of the buccopharyngeal membrane. The pit formed by this evagination, known as *Rathke's pouch*, deepens toward the developing brain, and the cells of this pouch, derived from stomodeal ectoderm, develop into the anterior lobe of the hypophysis. The connection with the stomodeum is soon lost. The posterior lobe of the hypophysis has a different origin; it is derived from the brain.

Now on the outside of the head, above and below the stomodeum opening, enlargements appear which will give rise to the face and to the various parts of the oral and nasal cavities.

Above the stomodeum the recently developed forebrain causes a large bulge (Figs. 2–4; 2–5). The ectoderm and mesenchyme that make up the surface of this bulge develop into an embryonic structure called the *frontal process* which will give rise to the upper part of the face, the nasal septum, and the anterior part of the roof of the mouth.

Below the stomodeum, in the region of the future neck, are formed five paired *branchial arches* ordinarily designated as branchial arches, I, II, III, IV, and V (Figs. 2–6; 2–7). In the development of the face and oral cavity only the first

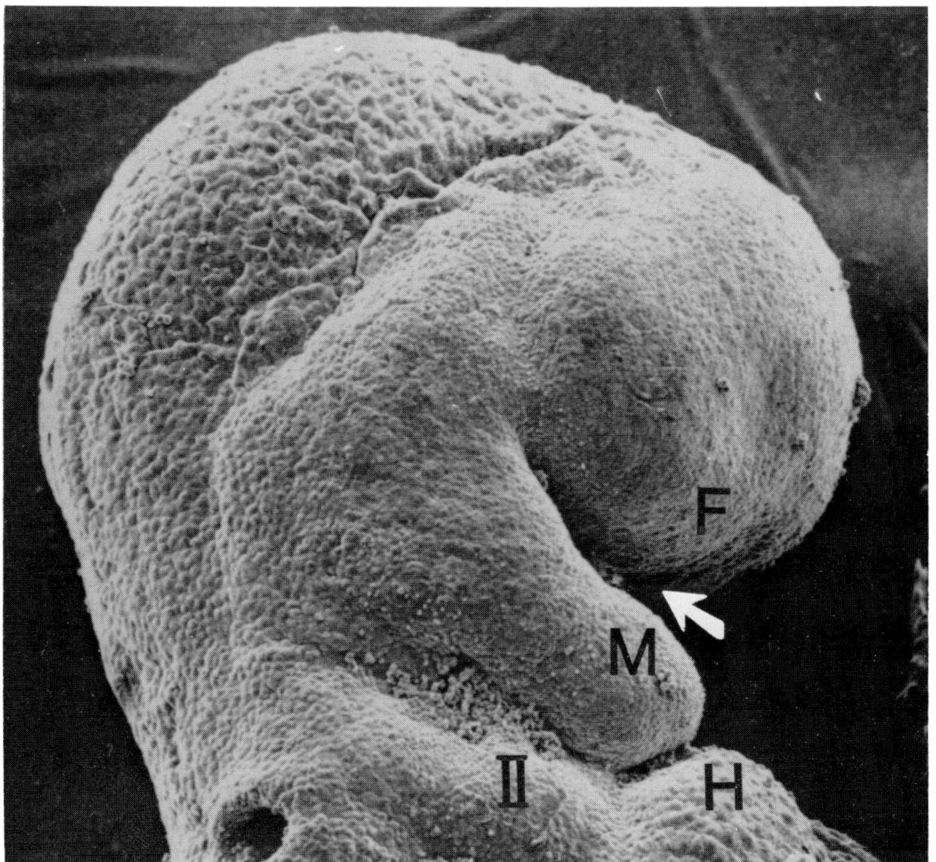

Fig. 2–4. Scanning electron micrograph of a nine-day-old mouse fetus. This is a lateral view. At this early stage the frontal process (F) and the mandibular arch (M) are prominent. The arrow points into the stomodeum. *II* is the second branchial arch, and *H* is the developing heart. (Courtesy Dr. Ruth Paulson, Collage of Dentistry, The Ohio State University.)

three arches play a part: branchial arch I develops into the mandible and a large part of the maxilla, and branchial arches II and III join the first branchial arch in the development of the tongue.

And so by the end of the fourth week in utero the picture is this: The stomodeum has been established and the buccopharyngeal membrane has ruptured. Above the stomodeum is the frontal process, and immediately below it is the first branchial arch (Figs. 2–4; 2–5). Excepting the base of the tongue, which is formed from branchial arches II and III, all of the face and all parts of the oral and nasal cavities will now develop from these two *primary embryonic structures*— the *frontal process* and the *first branchial arch*.

Early Development of the Face

The development of the face centers about the mouth. After the establishment of the stomodeum, the frontal process, and the branchial arches, the next thing that happens is the budding of a round process on either end of the first branchial arch. These buds grow upward and medially (toward the center) at the right and left sides of the primitive mouth. They are the *maxillary processes* (Figs. 2–6;

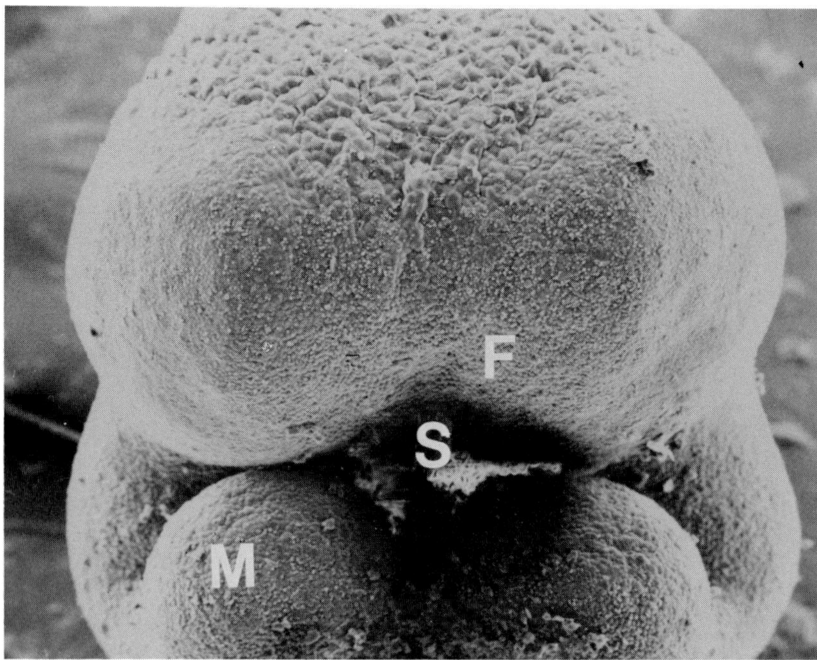

Fig. 2–5. Scanning electron micrograph of a nine-day mouse fetus. The stomodeum (S) is bounded above by the frontal process (F) and below by the mandibular arch (M) which has not yet merged at the midline. Compare to lateral view seen in Figure 2–4.

2–7; 2–8). After their appearance the remaining portion of the first branchial arch is called the *mandibular arch* (Figs. 2–6; 2–8). Eventually the maxillary processes will give rise to the upper part of the cheeks, the sides of the upper lip, and most of the palate (Fig. 2–9). The mandibular arch will form the lower part of the cheeks, the lower jaw, and part of the tongue.

After the maxillary processes have formed, growth of the lower part of the face is retarded and the upper part of the face starts a rapid development. On the lower border of the frontal process appears a pair of depressions, the right and left *olfactory pits,* which are the future openings into the nose (Figs. 2–7; 2–8). The olfactory pits divide the lower part of the frontal process into three parts—a center portion called the *medial nasal process* and two lateral portions called the *right and left lateral nasal processes.* The lateral nasal processes become the sides of the nose and the median nasal process forms the center and tip of the nose (Fig. 2–9). Later, an ingrowth from the median nasal process (the center of the nose) into the stomodeum forms the nasal septum (the division between the right and left nasal chambers).

At its lower border, the median nasal process now grows in length and produces a pair of bulges called the *globular process.* The globular process is not separated into two parts, but remains as a single median structure which grows downward so that it extends below the olfactory pits and lies between the right and left maxillary processes. It forms the center of the upper lip *(the philtrum)* (Fig. 2–9) and during the formation of the interior of the mouth it gives rise to the anterior part of the palate, the premaxillary area *(primary palate).*

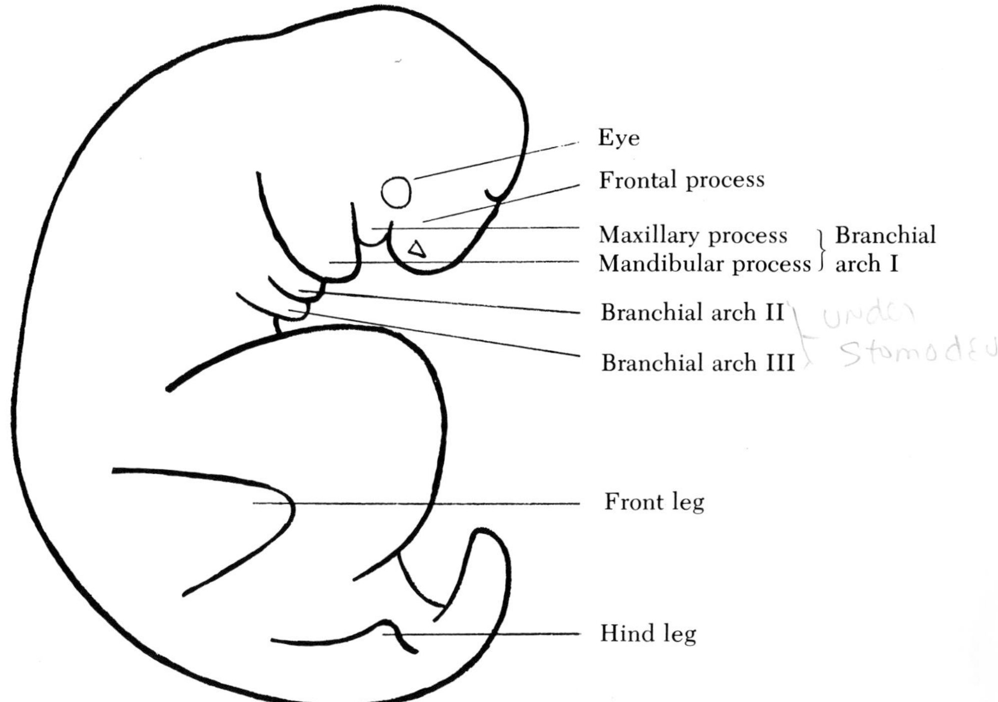

Fig. 2–6. A drawing of a lateral view of a pig embryo. This is similar to human development at about six weeks in utero. Branchial arches IV and V are visible here.

Later Development of the Face

In the course of facial development there is considerable *differential growth:* that is, some parts grow faster than other parts. These differences in the rate of growth result in marked progressive changes in the relative size and position of the various structures. Because of the rapid growth of surrounding areas, the slower growing median nasal process becomes relatively more narrow, and the nasal openings relatively closer together. The eyes, which appeared first on the sides of the head (Fig. 2–2), due to differential growth come to be located on the front of the head, while the ears change in position from the neck region to the sides of the head. For a time the relatively slow growth of the mandiblular arch results in a lag in the development of the lower part of the face. The mandible of a two-month-old embryo (Fig. 2–2) is small in proportion to the upper part of the face.

Along with the development of the various embryonic structures there is a coming together of certain of the processes. The only openings that remain in the fully formed face are the openings of the mouth and of the two nostrils, all other divisions between embryonic parts having merged.

The right and left maxillary processes, which bud from the superolateral borders of the first branchial arch (Fig. 2–7) grow forward and merge with the right and left sides of the globular process. Thus the globular process forms the center of the upper lip, and the maxillary processes form the sides of the upper lip (Fig. 2–9). The upper lip is completed by the end of the second month in utero.

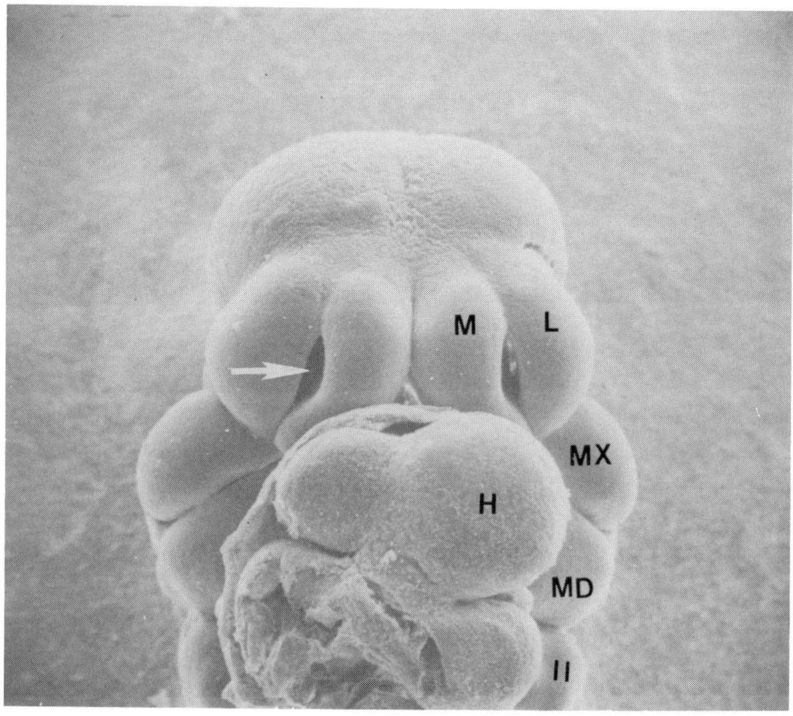

Fig. 2–7. Scanning electron micrograph of a ten-day mouse fetus seen from the front. The nasal pits (arrow) are surrounded by the median nasal (M) and lateral nasal (L) processes. The cervical region is formed by the maxillary processes (MX), the mandibular processes (MD), and the second branchial arches (II). The forming heart (H) covers the stomodeal opening. (Courtesy Dr. Ruth Paulson, College of Dentistry, The Ohio State University.)

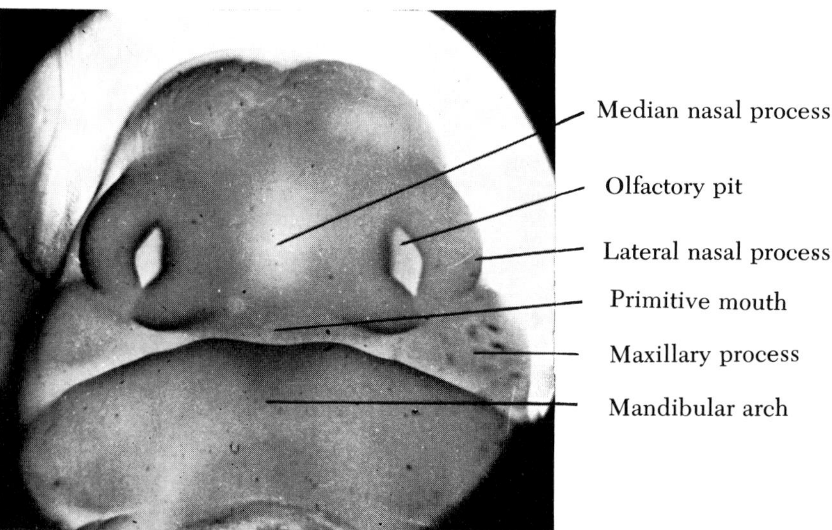

Fig. 2–8. A photograph of the face of a pig embryo of about 12 mm. At this stage of development the pig face and the human face are very much alike.

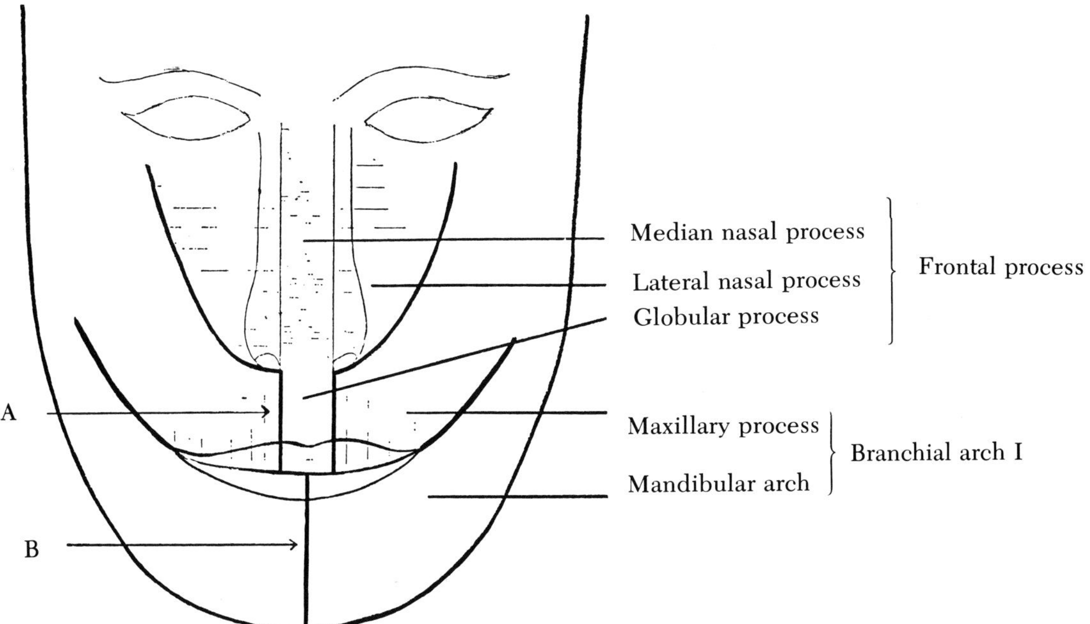

Fig. 2–9. Diagram of an adult human face showing the derivations of its parts form the frontal process and the first branchial arch. A and B indicate the locations where clefts sometimes occur in the upper lip and in the lower jaw.

A partial or complete failure of merging of a maxillary process with the globular process results in a condition known as *cleft lip* (Fig. 2–9). Cleft lip may be either unilateral or bilateral: that is, it may involve a failure of merging of the globular process either with the right or with the left maxillary process, or with both the right and the left maxillary processes. If a cleft of the lip occurs, it will be apparent by the end of the second month in utero, since that is the time that the formation of the lip is ordinarily completed.

Closure also occurs at the corners of the mouth between the maxillary processes and the mandibular arch. This decreases the breadth of the oral opening. In this instance, there is a filling in by mesenchyme of the angle formed at the junction of the mandibular arch with the right and left maxillary processes. In the adult a line of yellowing spots frequently seen extending laterally along the inside of the cheek from either corner of the mouth is said to be evidence of embryonic merging. These small yellowish elevations, called *Fordyce's-spots,* are sebaceous glands. Sebaceous glands are expected, of course, only on the outside of the body, but are thought to have become entrapped here in the cheek at the time of closure between the right and left maxillary processes with the right and left ends of the mandibular arch and to persist in the adult oral mucosa.

A failure of mesenchymal "flow" at the corners of the mouth of the maxillary processes and the mandibular arch leaves a cleft which results in an exceptionally large mouth opening. This anomaly (deviation from the usual) is known as *macrostomia.**

*Interesting paper: Powell, W.J, and H.P. Jenkins: Transverse Facial Clefts. Plast. Reconstr. Surg., 42(5):454, 1968. (Note: The condition called *transverse facial cleft* in this paper is in this textbook called *macrostomia.*)

microstomia = too small of mouth due to overflow of mesochine during development.

Early in the life of the embryo there is a filling of the deep depression originally present between the right and left sides of the mandibular arch at the midline. In the adult mandible evidence of the early existence of this depression may persist as a deep dimple in the chin. A failure of proper filling of this depression in the development of the embryo may result in a *median cleft* of the lower jaw (Fig. 2–9). This kind of cleft is rare.

Also rare is a cleft extending from the upper lip to the eye, called an *oblique facial cleft*. Apparently it is due to the failure of swellings of the maxillary process and the lateral nasal process to merge. The manner of the development of this defect is at present not clear.

Summary of the Development of the Face

The beginning of face development is seen in the human embryo during the third week in utero when an invagination of the ectoderm forms the *stomodeum*. Above the stomodeum is the *frontal process*, and below the stomodeum is the *first branchial arch*. Buddings on the superolateral border at either end of the first branchial arch form the *maxillary processes*, and the first branchial arch is thus divided into (1) two *maxillary processes* and (2) a *mandibular arch*. Invaginations on either side of the lower border of the frontal process, the *olfactory pits*, divide the frontal process into the *median nasal process* and *right* and *left lateral nasal processes*. The lateral nasal processes become the sides of the nose. The right and left maxillary processes grow medially from the corners of the primitive mouth and beneath the nose they merge with the globular process to form the upper lip. At the corners of the primitive mouth a filling in at the angles of the maxillary processes and the mandibular arch reduces the size of the broad oral opening. Early in development the midline depression in the mandibular arch disappears. *Differential growth* results in, among other things, a movement of the ears from the neck to the sides of the head. By the end of the second month in utero most of these developments have taken place. The mandible is still relatively underdeveloped.

Clefts which sometimes occur in the face as a result of faulty development include cleft lip, cleft chin, oblique facial cleft, and clefts at the corners of the mouth.

THE DEVELOPMENT OF THE ORAL CAVITY AND NASAL CAVITY

The Development of the Palate and Nasal Septum

The palate (the roof of the mouth) shows marked development near the end of the second month in utero. It arises from three sources: from the *right* and the *left maxillary processes* and from the *globular process*. It forms this way: Inside the stomodeum, near the end of the second month, appear three ingrowths. One is from the inner surface of the right maxillary process, one is from the inner surface of the left maxillary process, and one is from the inner surface of the globular process (Fig. 2–10). The ingrowths into the stomodeum from the the inside of the maxillary processes are called the *right* and *left lateral palatine processes*. An ingrowth from the globular process originates first at the bar of tissue inside the stomodeum between and a little beneath the right and left olfactory pits. This is about the place where the globular process arises from the median nasal process. Further ingrowth into the stomodeum develops into the

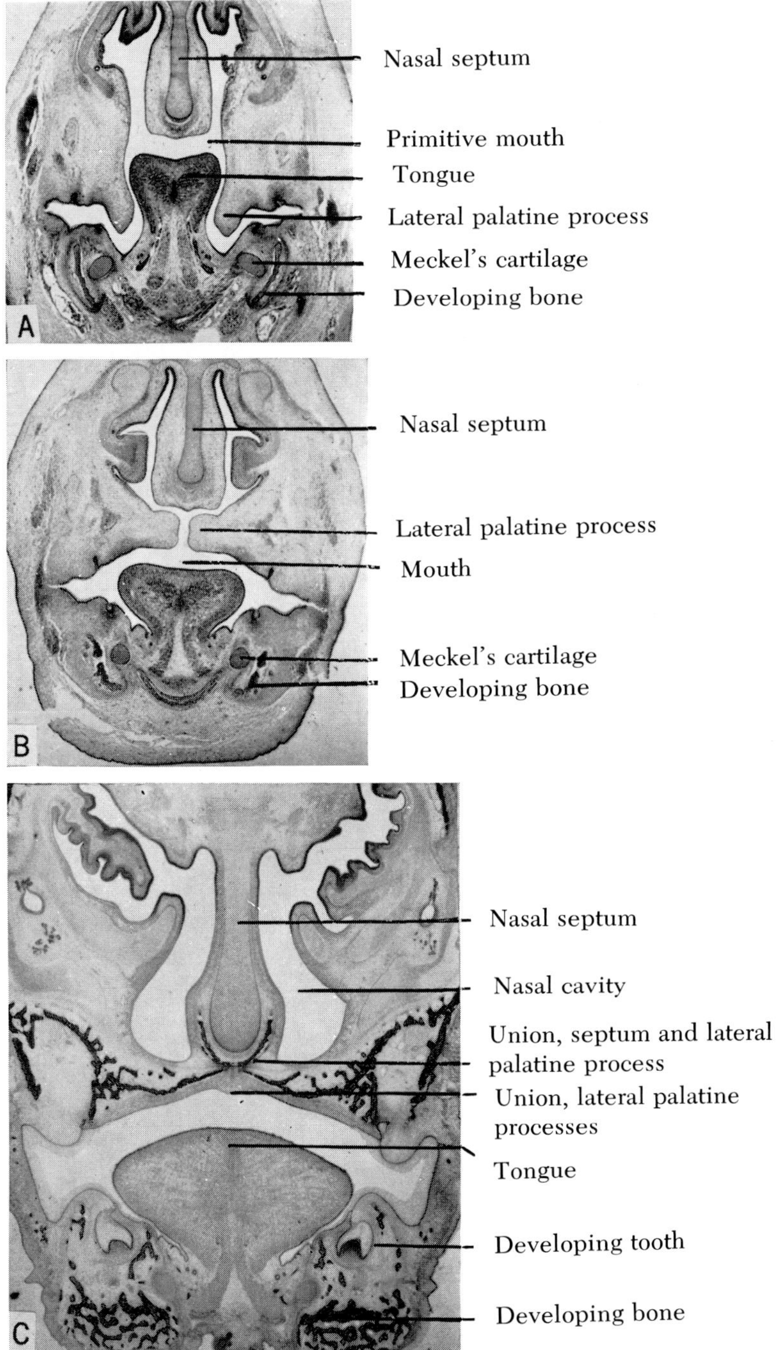

Fig. 2–10. Frontal sections through the heads of 3 pigs showing progressive stages in development of the palate. This is similar to human palatal development. A. The vertical position of the lateral palatine processes and the position of the tongue which nearly touches the lower border of the nasal septum are similar to the condition in an eight-week-old human embryo (Fig. 2–2). B. The lowering and broadening of the tongue, the horizontal position of the palatine processes, and their lack of union at the midline are similar to the condition in a nine-week-old human embryo. C. In a human fetus of twelve weeks, as in this pig fetus, the palatine processes have fused with each other and with the lower border of the nasal septum. The oral cavity and the nasal cavity are now separated by the roof of the mouth.

premaxillary area of the upper jaw (primary palate). The eventual union of the two lateral palatine processes with each other and with the premaxillary area (Fig. 2–12) will close the Y-shaped opening in the roof of the mouth.

In the course of union, or fusion, of these palatal structures the developing tongue becomes strangely involved. The tongue begins to develop at the end of the first month in utero. By the end of the second month, when the lateral palatine processes appear, the tongue is a comparatively large organ which extends upward in this primitive cavity until its upper surface nearly touches the lower border of the nasal septum. At first the newly developing right and left lateral palatine processes grow not horizonally, but rather they grow downward to the right and left of the elevated tongue (Fig. 2–10A).

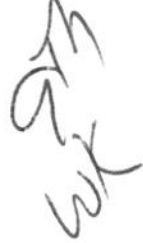

The determinant of the subsequent lifting of these processes to a horizontal position (Fig. 2–10B) has been the subject of much careful study. A frequent explanation is that as a result of enlargement of the mandible and a change in the degree of flexion of the fetus head, the tongue drops to the floor of the stomodeum; and when the tongue is thus removed from the path of the growing lateral palatine processes, the processes are straightened to a horizontal position by a sort of hinge movement, the causative force being, perhaps, rapid cell division at their lateral borders.

Changes in position from vertical to horizontal of the lateral palatine processes

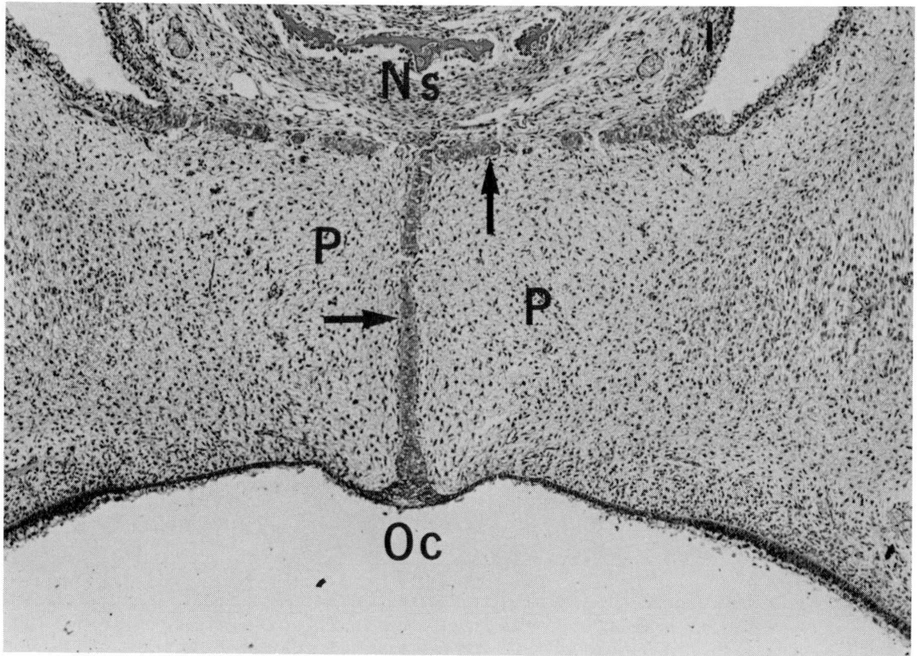

Fig. 2–11. Higher magnification of the epithelial fusion (arrows) of the palatine processes (P) with each other and the nasal septum (Ns). Note the delicate cellular detail of the palatine processes; these are mostly mesenchymal cells. Oral cavity (Oc).

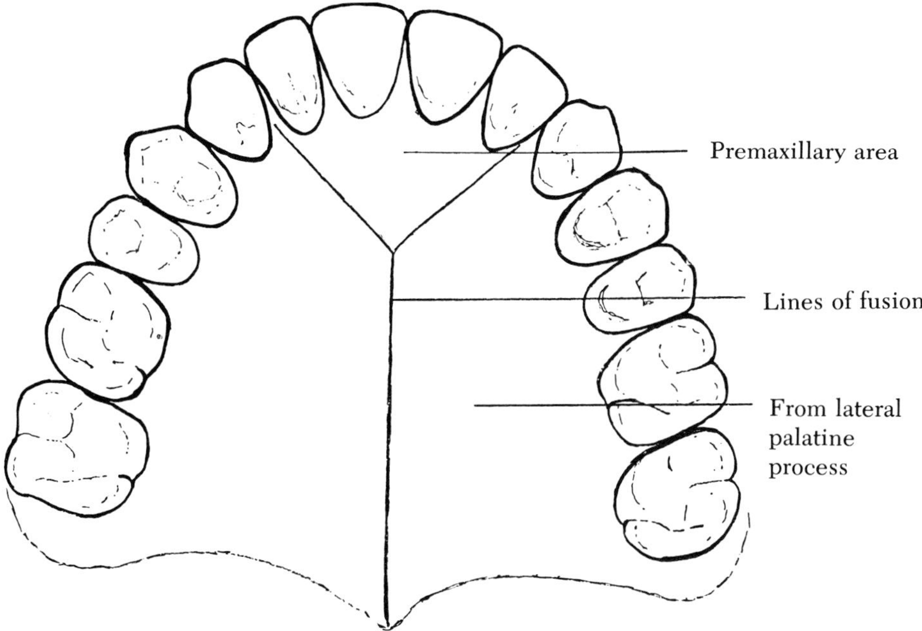

Fig. 2–12. Drawing of the oral surface of a human palate. The Y-shaped lines of embryonic fusion are indicated.

occur rapidly. In the mouse embryo this elevation has been found to take only a few hours, and apparently it is correspondingly rapid in the human embryo.*

Having attained a horizontal position early in the third month, the lateral palatine processes grow medially, toward each other (Fig. 2–10B), and the developing premaxillary area grows posteriorly. The palatine processes meet at the midline and fuse with each other and with the lower border of the nasal septum (Figs. 2–10C; 2–11); and at their anterior borders they meet and fuse with the posterior border of the premaxillary growth (Fig. 2–12). The structure thus formed is at once the roof of the oral cavity and floor of the nasal cavity: the stomodeum has been divided into a lower chamber and an upper chamber.

The critical period for movement and complete closure of the lateral palatine processes and the premaxillary part of the palate lies between eight and twelve weeks in utero. The fusions of the roof of the mouth are normally completed by the end of twelve weeks in utero.

The palatal fusions, at the time they occur, are fusions of soft tissue, not of bone. Small areas of forming bone tissue are first seen in the developing palate during the eighth week in utero, when the lateral palatine processes are still in a vertical position. By the end of the third month, when the embryonic palatal structures are completely fused, there is considerable bone tissue in the area, but the bones of the right and left sides of the hard palate are not together at

*Interesting papers:

1. Greene, R.M., and D.M. Kochhar: Palatal Closure in the Mouse As Demonstrated in Frozen Sections. Am. J. Anat. *137*:(4):477, 1973.
2. Walker, BE: Palate Morphogenesis in the Rabbit. Arch. Oral Biol., *16*:275, 1971.
3. Kraus B.: Prenatal Growth and Morphology of the Human Bony Palate. J. Dent. Res., *39*(6):1177, 1960.

the midline. A separation of the *bones* of the right and left sides of the roof of the mouth still exists at the end of the fourth month *in utero*.

During the time the roof of the mouth is forming, the nasal cavity becomes divided into a right and a left chamber by the *nasal septum*. This septum develops chiefly as a growth into the stomodeum from the inside of the median nasal process. When the right and left lateral palatine processes fuse with each other in the midline of the palate, they fuse also with the inferior border of the nasal septum (Figs. 2–10C; 2–11).

As is true in any location where fusions of embryonic processes occur, in the lines of palatal fusions groups of epithelial cells, called *epithelial rests*, may become entrapped. These misplaced rudiments of epithelium are the origin of cysts that sometimes are found in the palatal area.

Just as a failure of proper merging of one or both maxillary processes with the globular process results in a cleft of the upper lip, a failure of the lateral palatine processes to fuse with each other or with the premaxillary area results in a *cleft of the palate* (Fig. 2–13). If the cleft palate occurs, it will be apparent by the end of the third month in utero, since this is the time that the palatal fusions are ordinarily completed.

Cleft palate may be slight or extensive. It may involve only the uvula,* in which case it does not affect oral function. It may involve the soft palate, or a small part of the hard palate, or both the soft and hard palates. Cleft palate

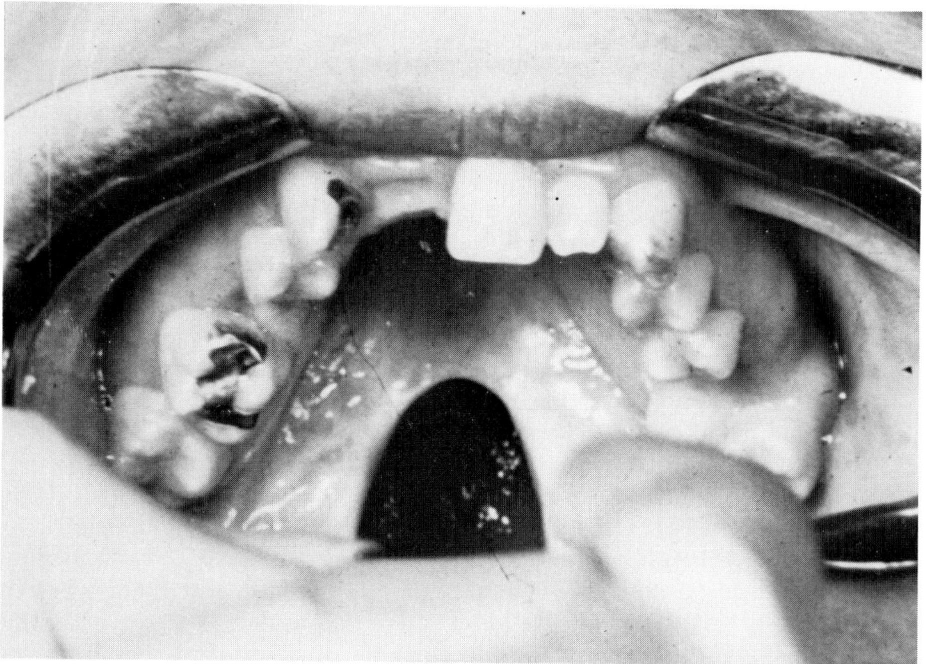

Fig. 2–13. Example of an incomplete cleft of the palate. Here, the lateral palatine processes fused with the premaxillary area, but failed to fuse with each other.

*The pendulum of soft tissue hanging down toward the base of the tongue from the center of the posterior border of the soft palate. Examine someone's mouth and see this structure.

sometimes involves the alveolar ridge on one or both sides of the midline—that is, cleft of the alveolar ridge may be either unilateral or bilateral (Fig. 2–12). Often such a cleft is located between the maxillary lateral incisor and the canine teeth. Sometimes the lateral incisor is missing. In any kind of severe intraoral cleft the maxillary teeth may be incomplete in number, and often they are greatly displaced. Any severe cleft of the palate produces a crippling opening between the oral and nasal cavities. This opening is a serious handicap to the individual in both speaking and eating. Cleft palate may occur with or without the presence of a cleft lip.

A review of the literature on cleft lip and cleft palate in human beings* has revealed substantial evidence in support of the following conclusions:

Nearly 6,000 new cases of cleft lip and cleft palate occur each year in the United States.

Cleft lip, with or without associated cleft palate, is more common in boys than in girls (65:35 ratio).

Cleft palate is more common in girls than in boys (60:40 ratio).

Considering all types of cleft, boys are more frequently affected than girls (58:42 ratio).

Clefts of the lip occur more frequently on the left side than on the right. Over 61% of unilateral clefts of the lip occur on the left side.

A *possible* explanation for the greater frequency of palatal clefts in girls than in boys was deduced from a study of 46 human embryos.† There seems to be a time lag in females compared to males in the change in position of the palatal processes from vertical to horizontal, and this may render females suceptible for a longer period of time to conditions which could interfere with palatal closure.

Strong indication exists that genetic factors can determine the occurrence of cleft palate. It has been found that in 20 to 30% of affected children there is some family history of clefts, but a definite hereditary pattern has not been determined. Also, clefts have been induced in unborn rats and mice by events that occur *during the time of normal palatal closure,* such as the administration at this precise time of cortisone or of excessive vitamin A (or a number of other things) to the pregnant female. This information obtained from animal studies cannot, of course, be applied directly to human development.

The Development of the Tongue

Anatomically the tongue has a *body* (the anterior part) and a *root* (the posterior part). The body extends from the tongue tip to the *terminal sulcus,* which is the V-shaped groove on the top surface just behind a V-shaped row of circumvallate papillae (Fig. 10–7). (Examine someone's tongue as far back as you can see and find this row of papillae.) The root of the tongue lies behind the terminal sulcus. The tongue has been aptly described as a sac of mucous membrane filled with voluntary muscle.

When the embryo is four weeks old the tongue begins to develop from the anterior wall of the primitive throat, and protrudes upward and anteriorly. Embryologically it develops from the region of the first three branchial arches.

*Greene, J.C.: Epidemiology of Cleft Lip, Cleft Palate. Public Health Rep., *78*:589, 1963.
†Burdi, A.R., and R.G., Silvey: Sexual Differences of the Human Palatal Shelves. Cleft Palate J., *6*(1):1, 1969.

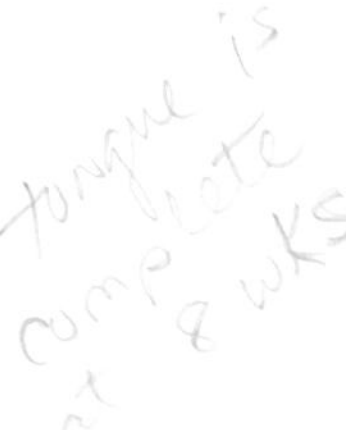

To picture its development, imagine yourself standing in the throat of a human embryo at the beginning of the second month and facing forward. Before your eyes near the center line on the inner surface of the mandibular arch are recently formed *lingual swellings* which will unite and become a single structure, the body of the tongue. Behind these, in the center line between the second and third branchial arches, involving the inner ends of these arches, is a swelling which will become the base of the tongue. These swellings from the three branchial arches unite into the single organ which by the end of the second month in utero will have acquired a recognizable form and will extend upward and forward toward the opening of the mouth.

In the fully formed tongue behind the circumvallate papillae at the tip of the V-shaped line (Fig. 10–7) is a small depression, the *foramen caecum,* which marks the point of embryonic origin of the *thyroid gland.* At about seventeen days in utero in the midline between the first and second branchial arches, the gland originates as a small proliferation of epithelium. As it develops, it descends to its final position in the neck, remaining attached to the tongue during its migration by a narrow *thyroglossal duct.* The duct eventually disappears, but the place of origin of the thyroid gland is marked on the tongue by the presence of the foramen caecum.

A rare deformity is a bifurcation of the body of the tongue. When this anomaly occurs it is probably because the lingual swellings of the first branchial arch failed to merge. Other possible anomalies are too large a tongue (macroglossia), too small a tongue (microglossia), and absence of a tongue (aglossia).

Summary of the Development of the Oral and Nasal Cavities

The *premaxillary region* of the *palate* develops from the *globular process,* a downward growth of the *median nasal process* which is the center part of the original *frontal process.* The sides of the palate are formed by the *lateral palatine processes.* These arise from the *maxillary processes,* which are buds from the ends of the *first branchial arch.* These three structures, the premaxillary area and the right and the left palatine processes, fuse in the roof of the mouth in a Y-shaped pattern (Fig. 2–12). From the part of the frontal process that forms the center of the nose (the *median nasal process*), the *nasal septum* grows back and downward, and its inferior border fuses with the right and left palatine processes as they fuse with each other at the center of the palate (Fig. 2–11).

The *tongue* develops as growths from the mid-anterior region on the inner surface of the *first three branchial arches:* The body of the tongue from the first branchial arch; the base from the second and third.

Clefts which sometimes occur inside the mouth as a result of faulty development include partial or complete clefts of the palatal structures, and cleft of the tongue.

SUMMARY OF THE DEVELOPMENT OF THE FACE AND ORAL CAVITY

A summary of the derivations of the structures of the face and oral cavity is presented in the following outline:

I. From the *Frontal Process* are derived:
   1. Median nasal process, which gives rise to:
      a. Center and tip of nose
      b. Nasal septum

c. Globular process, which gives rise to:
(1) Philtrum of upper lip
(2) Premaxillary area of the palate
2. Lateral nasal processes, which form:
a. Sides of nose
b. Infraobital areas
II. From *Branchial Arch I* are derived:
1. Mandibular arch, which gives rise to:
a. Lower jaw
b. Lower parts of face
c. Anterior part of tongue
2. Maxillary processes, which give rise to:
a. Lateral palatine processes (i.e., all of palate and maxillary alveolar arch excepting the premaxillary area)
b. Upper part of cheeks
c. Sides of upper lip
III. From *Branchial Arches II and III* are derived portions of the posterior part of the tongue.

All of the face and most of the structures of the oral cavity develop from two primary embyronic structures: the *frontal process* and the *first branchial arch.* The tongue alone adds to its origin the second and third branchial arches.

OTHER INTERESTING READINGS

Bohn, A.: Dental Anomalies in Harelip and Cleft Palate. Acta Odontol. Scand., *21*:Supp. 38, 1963. (Good Bibliography.)

Farbman, A.R.: Electron Microscope Study of Palate Fusion in Mouse Embryos. Dev. Biol., *18*:93, 1968. (Describes technique of specimen preparation.)

Fraser, F.C.: Cleft Lip and Cleft Palate. Science, *158*(3808):1603, 1967. (This is a review article and very worth reading.)

Fraser, F.C.: The Genetics of Cleft Lip and Cleft Palate. Am J. Hum. Genet., *22*:336, 1970 (Good bibliography.)

Fukuhara, T.: New Method and Approach to the Genetics of Cleft Lip and Cleft Palate. J. Dent. Res., *44*(1):259, 1965. (Extensive bibliography.)

Humphrey, T.: Development of Oral and Facial Motor Mechanism in Human Fetuses and Their Relation to Craniofacial Growth. J. Dent. Res. *50*(6):Part I, 1428, 1971.

Latham, R.A.: Role of the Tongue in the Pathogenesis of the Pierre Robin Type of Cleft Palate: Report on a 17-week Human Fetus. (Abstract). J. Dent. Res., *44*(6):Part I, 1159, 1965.

Moller, P.: Cleft Lip and Cleft Palate in Iceland. Arch. Oral Biol., *10*:407, 1965.

Mott, W.J., P.D. Toto, and D.C. Hilgers: Labeling Index and Cellular Density in Palatine Shelves of Cleft-Palate Mice. J. Dent. Res. *48*(2):263, 1969.

Provenza, D.V., and Seibel, W.: *Oral Histology—Inheritance and Development*, 2nd ed, Philadelphia, Lea & Febiger, 1986.

Ross R.B., and Johnston, M.C.: Cleft Lip and Palate, Baltimore, Willians & Wilkins, 1972.

Walker, Bruce E.: Palate Morphology and Fetal Movements in Mice After DPH. J. Dent. Res. *58*(7):1740, 1979.

Wragg, L.E., V.M. Diewert, and M. Klein: Spatial Relations in the Oral Cavity and the Mechanism of Secondary Palate Closure in the Rat. Arch. Oral Biol., *17*(4):638, 1972.

Chapter 3

TOOTH DEVELOPMENT

Before the human embryo is three weeks old the stomodeum is established. At the anterior end of the embryo the ectoderm has invaginated to meet the endoderm, thus forming the primitive mouth and the buccopharyngeal membrane (Fig. 2–3). This membrane is located in approximately the position the palatine tonsils will later occupy. The primitive mouth is lined with ectoderm, beneath which is mesenchyme.* The ectoderm gives rise to the oral epithelium, and the mesenchyme becomes the underlying connective tissue.

THE BEGINNING OF TOOTH DEVELOPMENT

Odontogenesis is the name given to the origin and tissue formation of the teeth (Fig. 3–1).

Not all teeth start development at the same time. The earliest sign of tooth development in the human embryo is found in the anterior mandibular region when the embryo is five to six weeks old. Soon after this, evidence of tooth development appears in the anterior maxillary region, and the process progresses posteriorly in both jaws.

A tooth is formed from ectoderm, one of the three germ layers, and from *ectomesenchyme.* The ectomesenchyme tissue is the name given to head mesenchyme (embryonic connective tissue). Ectomesenchyme is derived from *neural crest cells.* These cells arise along the lateral margins of the *neural plate* of an embryo and migrate into the head region. The neural plate arises from the ectoderm layer, and thus the name *ectomesenchyme.* The term *mesenchyme* will be used here with the understanding that the head mesenchyme is not from mesoderm germ layer, as is true for the rest of the body.

Development begins with the formation of the *primary dental lamina* (Figs. 3–1A; 3–2; 3–3). The primary dental lamina is a narrow band of thickened oral epithelium (ectoderm) which extends along what will become the occlusal borders of the mandible and maxillae on a line where the teeth will later appear. This dental lamina grows from the surface into the underlying mesenchyme. Concurrently with the development of primary dental lamina, at ten places in the mandibular arch and at ten places in the maxillary arch some cells of the dental lamina multiply at a rate faster than the surrounding cells, and ten little knobs of epithelial cells are formed on the dental lamina in each jaw. These little knobs of epithelial cells grow deeper into the underlying mesenchyme (Fig. 3–4). Each of these knob-shaped structures is an early *enamel organ* (also called *dental organ*) and is the beginning of the *tooth germ* of a primary tooth.

*Mesenchyme (pronounced *mĕs' ĕn kīm*) is an embryonic connective tissue. The adjective is mesenchymal (*mĕs ĕn' kĭm al*).

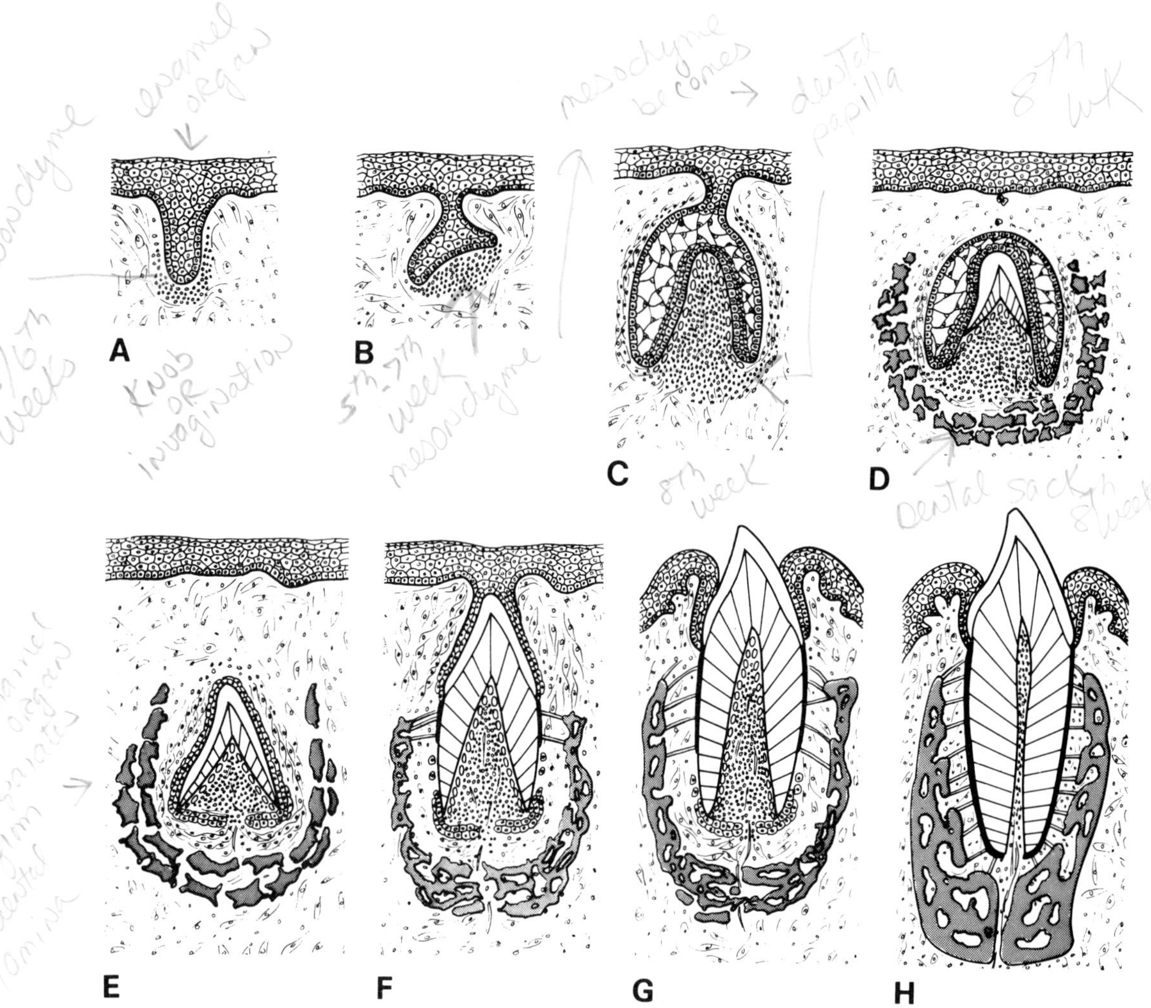

Fig. 3–1. Diagram of the growth and development of a tooth. A. *Dental lamina* stage—invagination of oral epithelium into underlying connective tissue (mesenchyme). B. Early *enamel organ* stage—budding of the epithelium of the dental lamina. C. *Tooth germ* stage—*enamel organ, dental papilla, dental sac.* D. Initiation of dentin and enamel formation within tooth germ. E. *Reduced enamel organ* and root sheath stage. F. Active eruption stage—break-up of root sheath and start of cementum formation. G. Emergence and *attachment epithelium* stage—reduced enamel epithelium becomes attachment epithelium and tooth enters oral cavity. H. Occlusal plane stage—tooth in functional position.

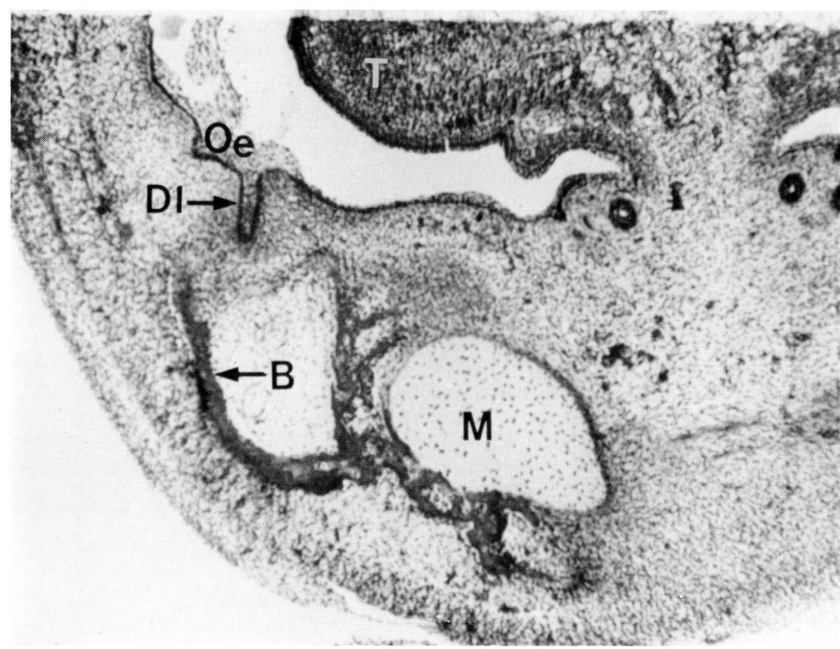

Fig. 3–2. Photomicrograph of one half of the lower jaw of an eight week human embryo, frontal view. The primary dental lamina (Dl) invaginates from the oral epithelium (Oe) into the underlying mesenchyme. Here, the dental lamina appears as a finger-like process, actually it is a continuous band of epithelium which extends along the occlusal boarder of the jaw. B, bone of forming mandible; M, Meckel's cartilage; T, tongue. See Figure 3–3.

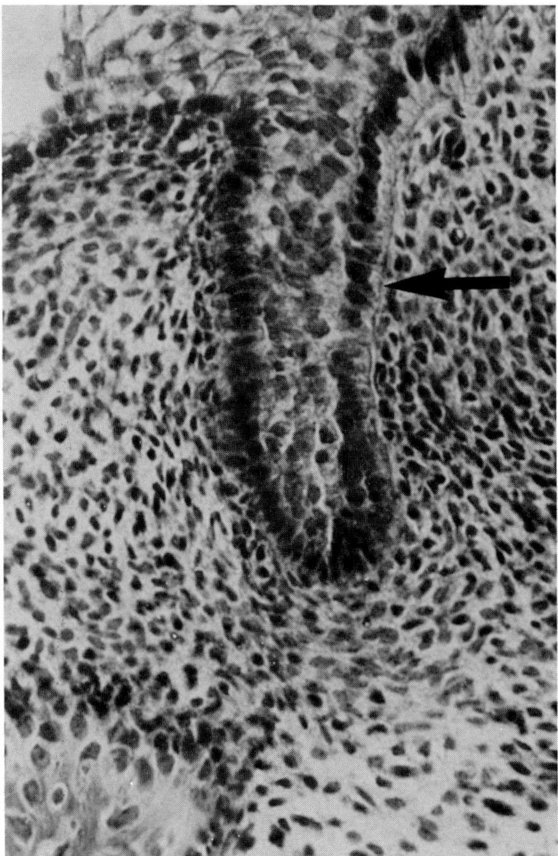

Fig. 3–3. Higher magnification of a primary dental lamina. The finger-like lamina (epithelium) is connected to the surrounding mesenchyme (connective tissue) by a basement membrane. (arrow). Compare to Figure 3–1A.

The development of each individual tooth starts with the formation of a *tooth germ*. Now a tooth germ is derived form two embryonic tissues: the part which develops from the dental lamina is derived from ectoderm, and the remaining parts are derived from the mesenchyme which underlies this ectoderm.

The *enamel organ* is the first part of the tooth germ to form. It develops from the *dental lamina* as a growth of oral epithelium into the underlying connective tissue (Fig. 3–4). As it enlarges, the enamel organ acquires the shape of a cap (Fig. 3–5). By the eighth week in utero this cap formation is seen in the enamel organs of the deciduous incisor tooth germs. The connective tissue inside the cap undergoes a change and becomes the *dental papilla*. The connective tissue beneath the dental papilla becomes fibrous and encircles the papilla and part of the enamel organ forming what is called the *dental sac* (Figs. 3–1C; 3–6). The enamel organ for a time remains connected, by means of the dental lamina, with the epithelium lining the stomodeum (Figs. 3–4; 3–5).

In summary, a *tooth germ* is comprised of three parts: (1) *enamel organ;* (2) *dental papilla;* (3) *dental sac*. The enamel organ is composed of epithelial cells which arise from the ectoderm germ layer; the dental papilla and the dental sac are connective tissues which arise from mesenchyme.

THE TOOTH GERM

As the tooth germ grows, the cap-shaped enamel organ changes form and becomes somewhat bell-shaped, and four layers are distiguishable (Figs. 3–7; 3–8; 3–9):

The *outer enamel epithelium* is the outside layer of the enamel organ, and is composed of low cuboidal cells.

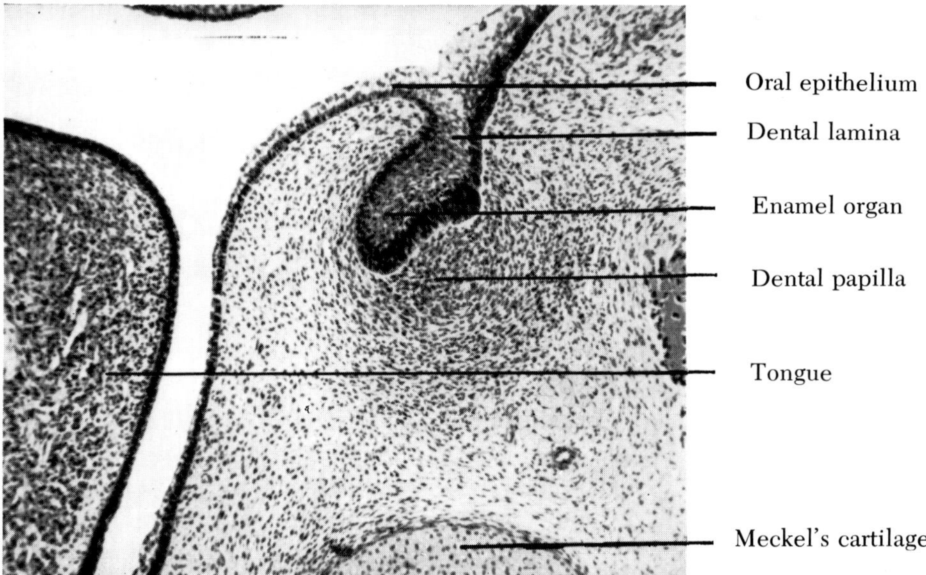

Fig. 3–4. Photomicrograph of a faciolingual section of a pig mandible showing the beginning of tooth development. The oral epithelium appears to be growing into the underlying mesenchyme. The enamel organ is forming, but has not yet attained its final shape. The dental papilla is becoming organized from the cells of the mesenchyme.

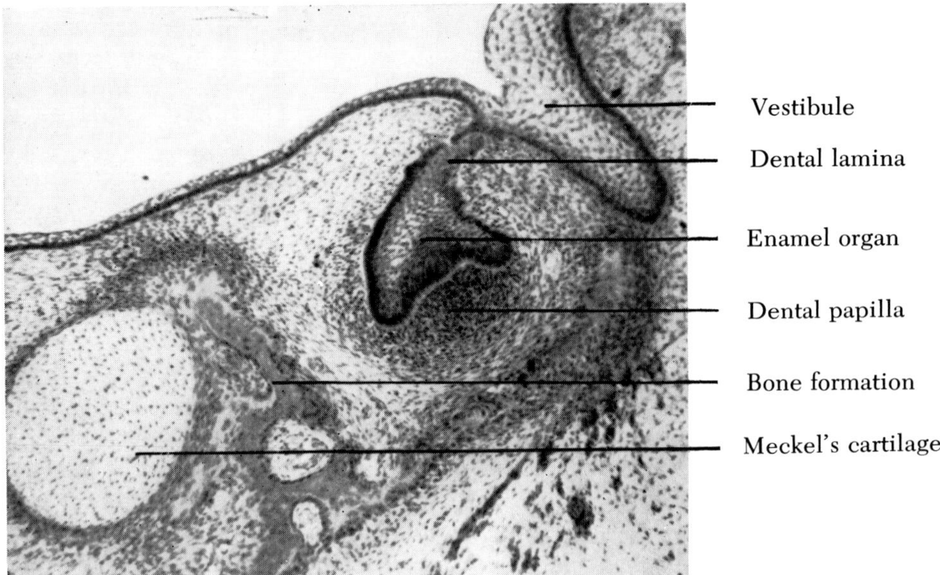

Fig. 3–5. Photomicrograph of a frontal section of a pig mandible showing a tooth germ in a stage of development slightly more advanced than the one in the Figure 3–4. The tongue is not visible in this section, but Meckel's cartilage is just lateral to the center line of the jaw. The center line is at the left of the picture. Notice the areas of forming bone of the mandible. The oral vestibule is forming lateral to the developing tooth germ.

The *stellate reticulum* is the layer immediately inside the outer enamel epithelium and is composed of a very loose network of epithelial cells.

The *stratum intermedium* is a layer of closely packed, flat epithelial cells inside the stellate reticulum.

The *inner enamel epithelium* lines the inside of the enamel organ. It is a single layer of cuboidal cells. This layer of cells is separated form the dental papilla by a *basement membrane* (Figs. 3–3; 3–6; 3–9).

The growing tooth germ changes form rapidly at first, but by the time the four layers of the enamel organ are well defined the shape of the basement membrane has become fixed. When the final shape of the basement membrane is established it marks the line which will become the dentinoenamel junction of the finished tooth (Fig. 3–10).

Further cell differentiation in the tooth germ occurs along either side of the basement membrane. First the cuboidal cells which make up the inner enamel epithelium elongate into columnar cells called *ameloblasts**. Formation of the ameloblasts is followed by a change in the peripheral cells of the dental papilla which also take a columnar form and become *odontoblasts*. The ameloblast and odontoblast layers are separated from each other by the basement membrane.

In embryonic development many things are occurring, of course, at the same time. As the early tooth germs are developing they become surrounded by islands of bone which eventually coalesce and form the mandible (or maxillae). Figure 3–11 is a mesiodistal section cut through the center of the maxillary primary incisor tooth germs. The tooth germs, having formed earlier, are be-

---

*Pronounced *am ĕl' ō blăst.*

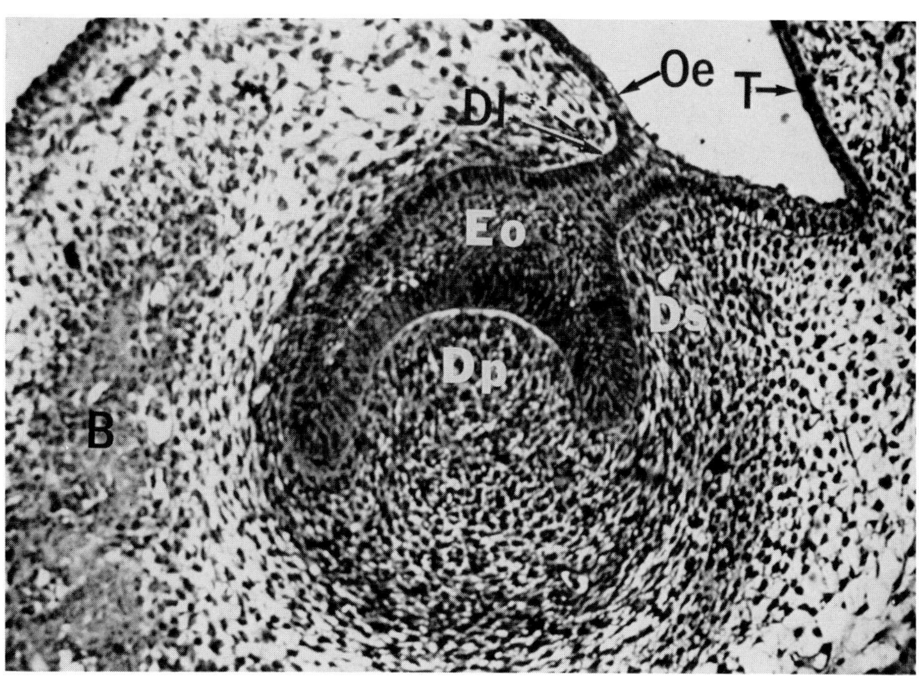

Fig. 3–6. Higher magnification of an early primary tooth germ. The cap shaped enamel organ (Eo) is enclosing the mesenchymal cells of the dental papilla (Dp); the mesenchymal cells around the dental organ and dental papilla are forming the dental sac (Ds). The epithelial enamel organ is connected to oral epithelium (Oe) by way of the dental lamina (Dl). Tongue (T). Forming mandible (B).

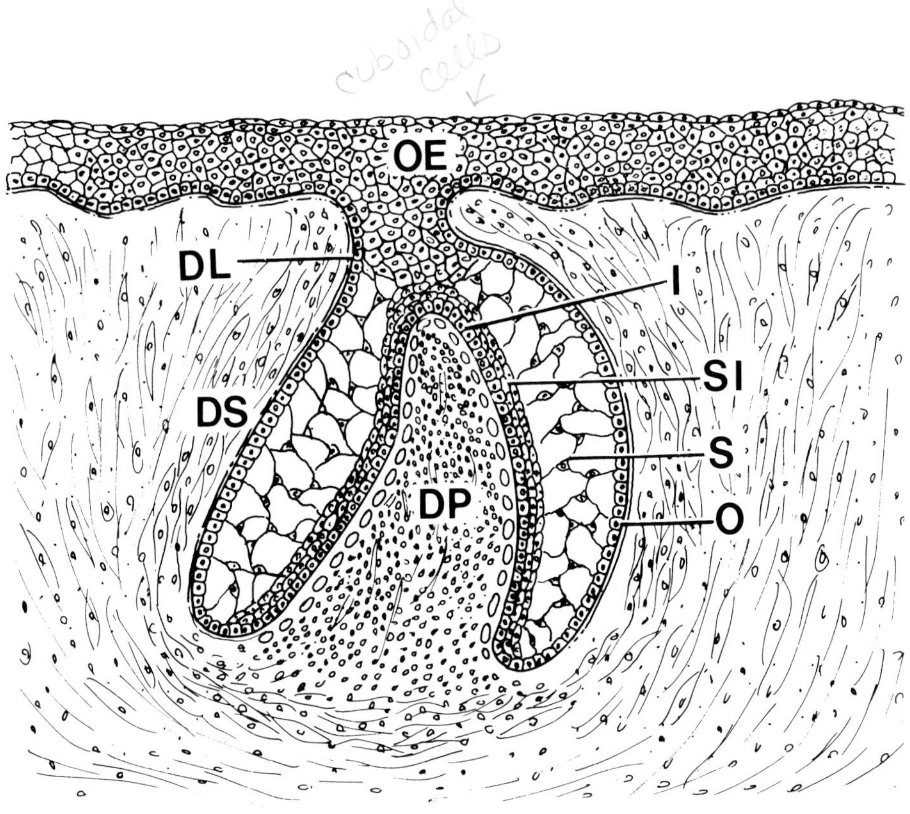

Fig. 3–7. Diagram of a tooth germ. The four epithelial cell layers of the enamel organ are seen—*inner* (I), *stratum intermedium* (SI), *stellate reticulum* (S), outer (O). The *dental papilla* (DP) is enclosed in the dental organ, and the *dental sac* (DS) surrounds the dental organ and is continuous with the dental papilla. The dental lamina (DL) is connected to the oral epithelium (OE). Compare to photomicrographs seen in Figures 3–8 and 3–9.

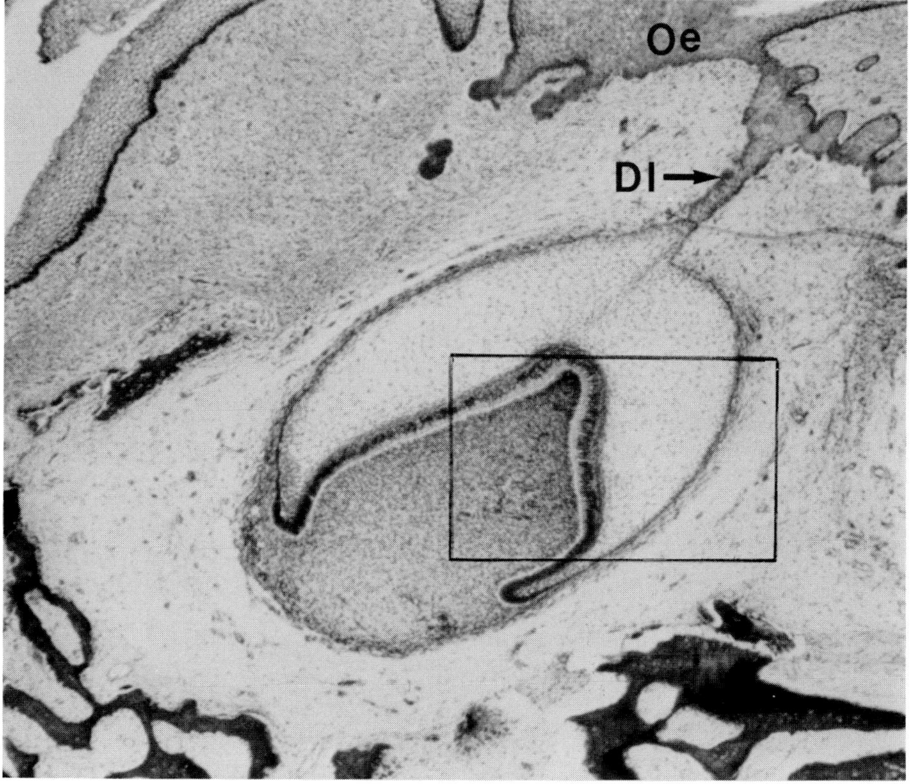

Fig. 3–8. Photomicrograph of a human primary tooth germ. Compare to Figure 3–7. For higher magnification of box area see Figure 3–9. Note that the dental organ part of the tooth germ is still attached to the oral epithelium (Oe) by way of the dental lamina (Dl).

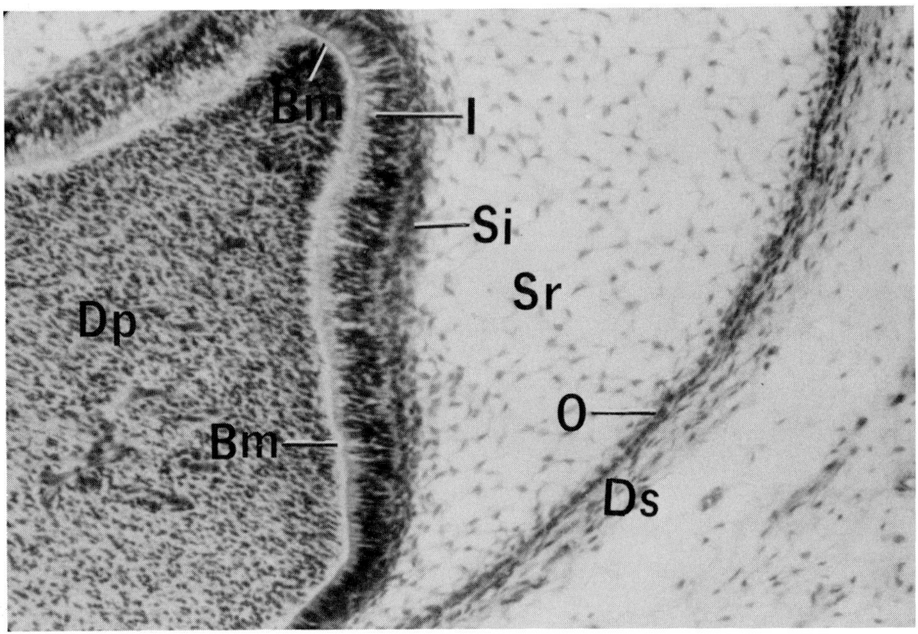

Fig. 3–9. High magnification of box area in Figure 1–8. *Dental papilla* (Dp); basement membrane (Bm); four epithelial layers of the *enamel organ—inner* (I), *stratum intermedium* (Si), *stellate reticulum* (Sr), *outer* (O); *dental sac* (Ds).

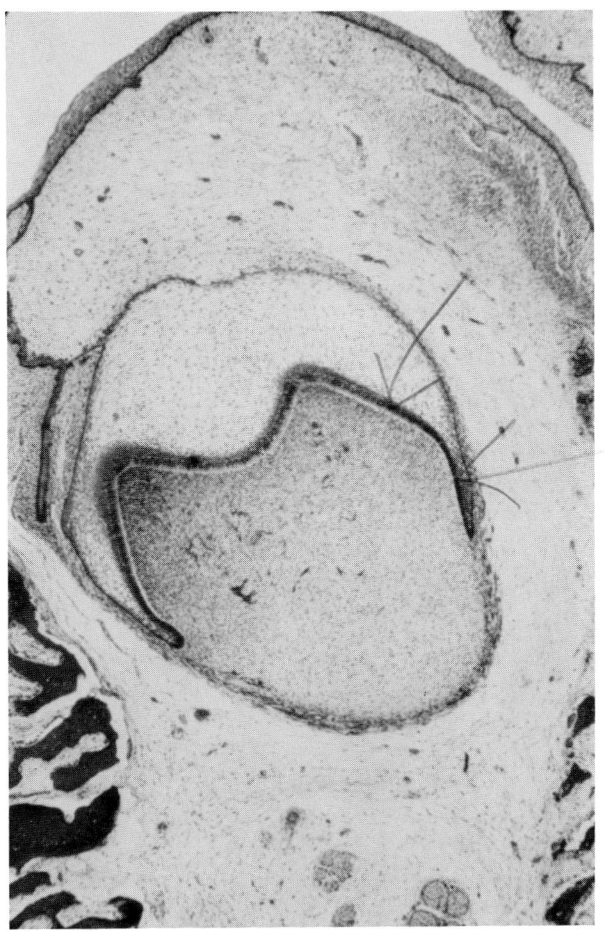

Fig. 3–10. Photomicrograph of human primary molar tooth germ. The junction between the enamel organ and the dental papilla is formed by a basement membrane. It determines the outline and position of the dentioenamel junction. Compare this junction outline to that of the anterior tooth germ seen in Figure 3–8.

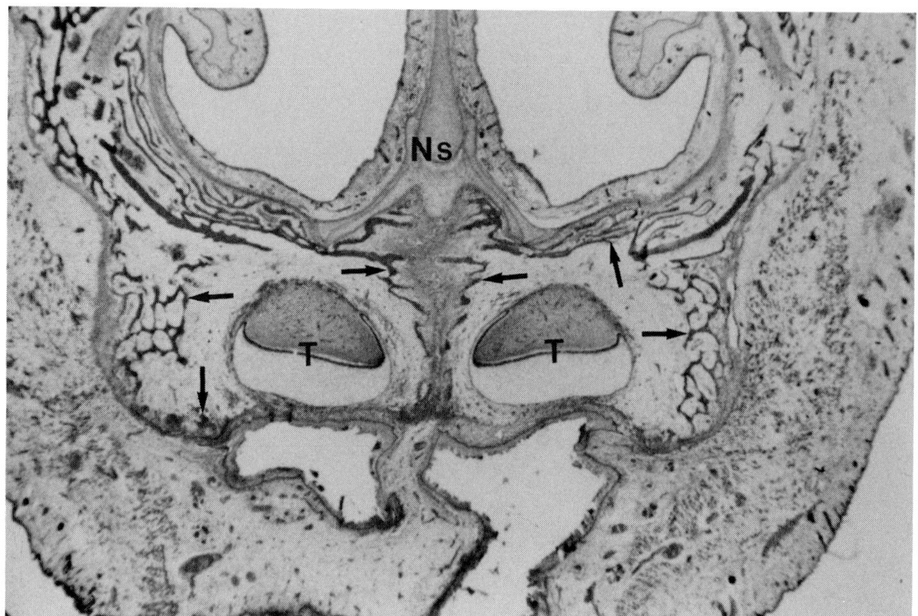

Fig. 3–11. Photomicrograph showing the relation of the maxillary primary central incisor tooth germs (T) to the surrounding forming bone of the maxillae (arrows). Notice the relation of the developing teeth to the nasal cavity, the spaces on each side of the nasal septum (Ns).

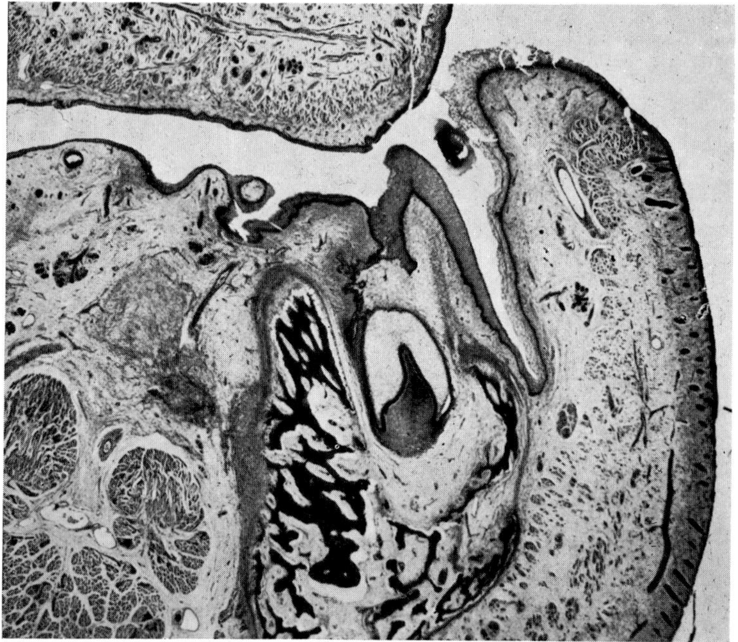

Fig. 3–12. Sagittal section of the lower jaw of the human fetus. The lower lip is on the right and the tongue is above. A developing incisor tooth is becoming partially surrounded by the developing bone of the mandible.

coming enclosed in the forming bone of the maxillary bones. In Figure 3–12 the same bone growth is seen in a fetal human mandible.

By the time a primary tooth germ has reached the stage of development where ameloblasts and odontoblasts are becoming differentiated, other changes are taking place. Lingual to the enamel organ of the primary tooth germ the dental lamina is giving rise to the beginning of the enamel organ of the succeeding permanent tooth germ (Figs. 3–14; 3–15; 3–16). The permanent tooth germ will develop slowly as the primary tooth develops and goes into function. Also there occurs disintegration of the dental lamina that connects both enamel organs with the oral epithelium. The cells of the dental lamina break apart into small groups and either gradually disappear or remain as small epithelial cells. These groups of epithelial cells are called *glands* of *Serres* because they resemble glands, histologically. They are clinically significant in that they may be the source of epithelium for cysts.

The *succedaneous* enamel (dental) organs—permanent central and lateral incisors, canines, and first and second premolars—arise from the *secondary dental lamina* which arises from the *primary dental lamina* (Figs. 3–17; 3–18).

The primary dental lamina continues to invaginate from the oral epithelium posterior to the primary second molar and gives rise to the enamel organs of the permanent first, second and third molars. The permanent molars are not succedaneous teeth (they do not replace primary teeth). The last enamel organs to appear are those of the third molars; this occurs in about the fifth year of postnatal life. Since the third molars are the last to begin development they are, naturally, the last to appear in the oral cavity.

When ameloblasts and odontoblasts have differentiated along either side of the basement membrane in the tooth germ, formation of the hard tooth tissues begins. The earliest formation of the hard tooth tissues in the human fetus occurs during the fifth month in the primary incisors. Dentin formation starts just a little before enamel formation begins.

DENTIN FORMATION

Dentinogenesis is the name given to the origin and formation of dentin.

Dentin is the first mineralized tissue to appear in any developing tooth. It is composed of (1) a *fibrillar matrix* which mineralizes and (2) *odontoblastic processes* which remain unmineralized.

The first dentin is formed at the incisal or cusp area of a tooth, and formation progresses in a rootward direction (Figs. 3–19; 3–20). It may be accomplished somewhat in this manner:

The odontoblasts, which have differentiated from the mesenchymal cells of the dental papilla, form a single layer of columnar cells at the line of the dentinoenamel junction (Figs. 3–21; 3–22). They start moving inward—that is, they back up toward the center of the pulp. As the cells pull back, they behave as if several spots of their cytoplasm were attached to the basement membrane, causing the cytoplasm to stretch out into several narrow extensions (Fig. 3–23). As the pulpward migration of the body of the odontoblasts progresses, the several cytoplasmic extensions of each cell join to make a single dentinal process. The part of the odontoblasts containing the nucleus comes to lie some distance pulpward of the basement membrane (soon to be the dentinoenamel junction),

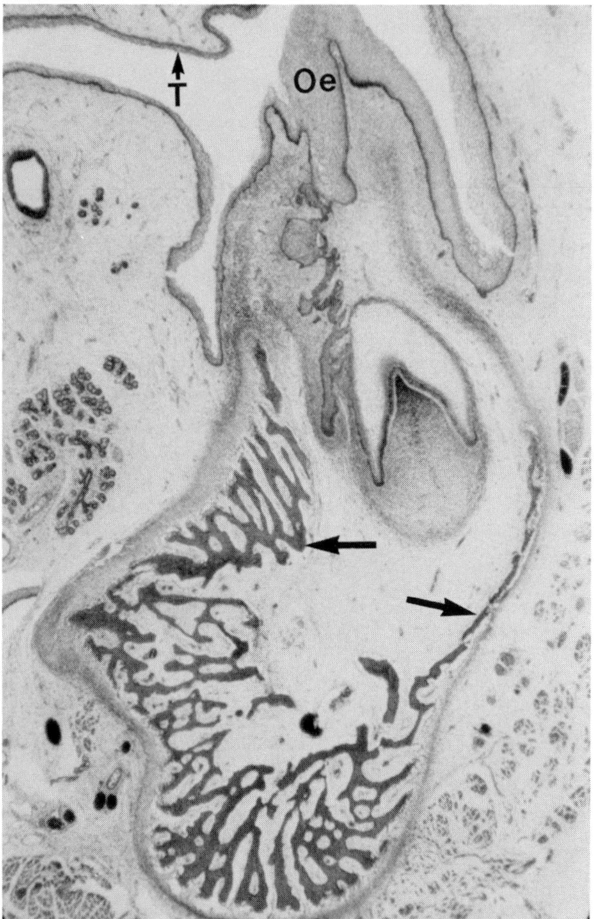

Fig. 3–13. Faciolingual section through a lower human primary canine tooth germ and the forming bone (arrows) of the mandible. Lingual is at left. Oral epithelium (Oe). Tongue (T).

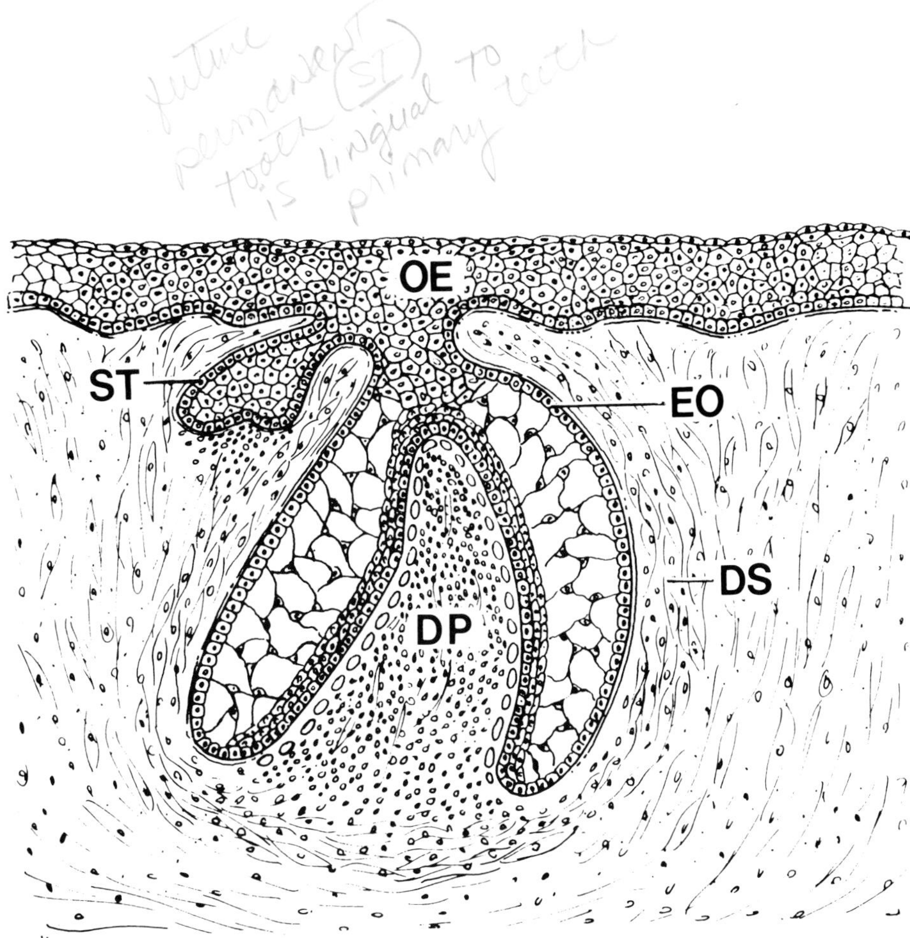

Fig. 3–14. Diagram showing the position of a developing succedaneous (permanent) tooth (ST) lingual to its primary tooth germ precursor. The three parts of the primary tooth germ—enamel organ (EO), dental papilla (DP), dental sac (DS)—are seen at an advanced stage. The primary enamel organ is still connected to the oral epithelium (OE).

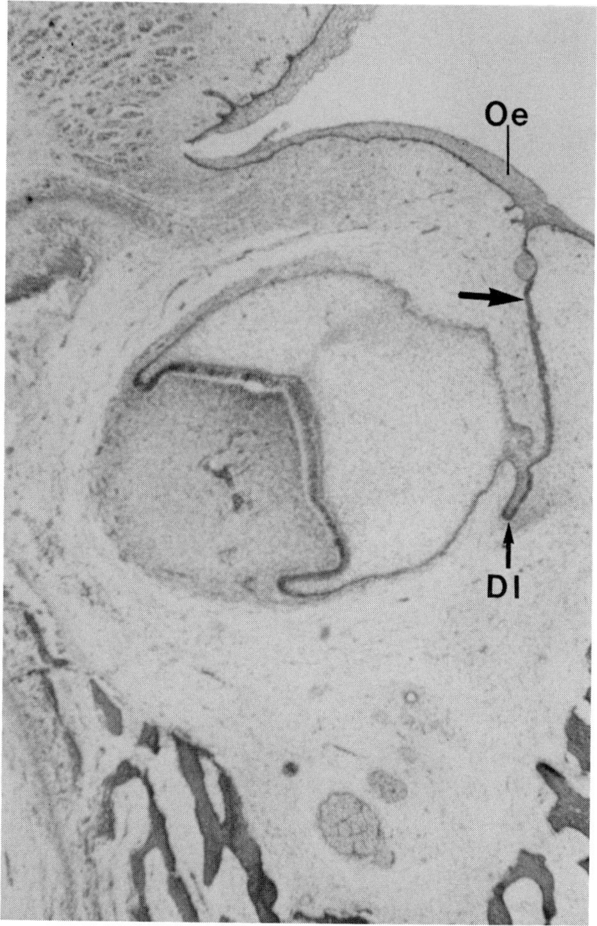

Fig. 3–15. Photomicrograph of a primary tooth germ showing the positions of the secondary dental lamina (Dl) from which the succedaneous enamel organ will arise. Notice that the primary dental lamina has reduced to a strain of epithelial cells (arrow) but is still connected to the oral epithelium (Oe). Lingual is at right.

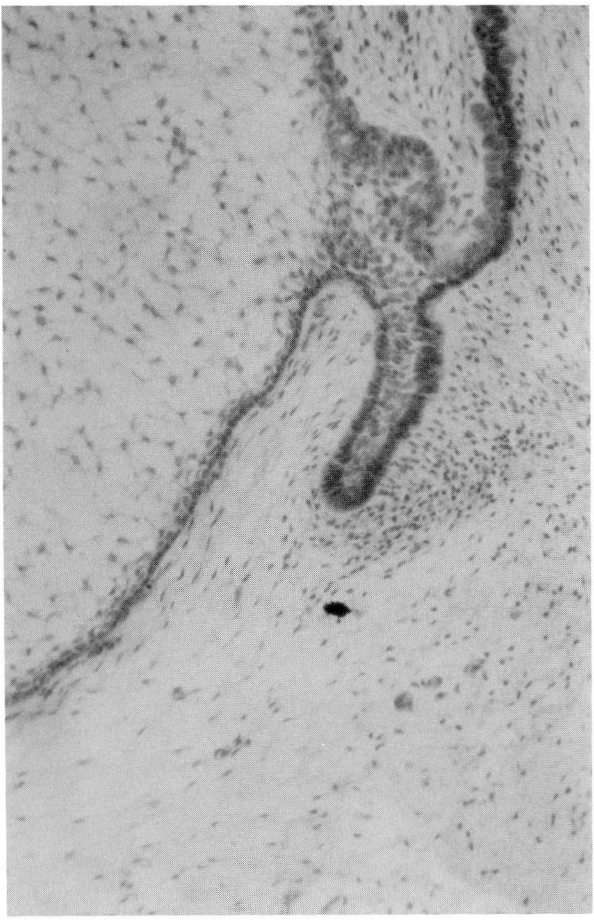

Fig. 3–16. Higher magnification of secondary dental lamina seen in Figure 3–15. Notice that the mesenchymal cells are beginning to concentrate about the epithelial lamina; these cells will give rise to the dental papilla and dental sac parts of the permanent tooth germ.

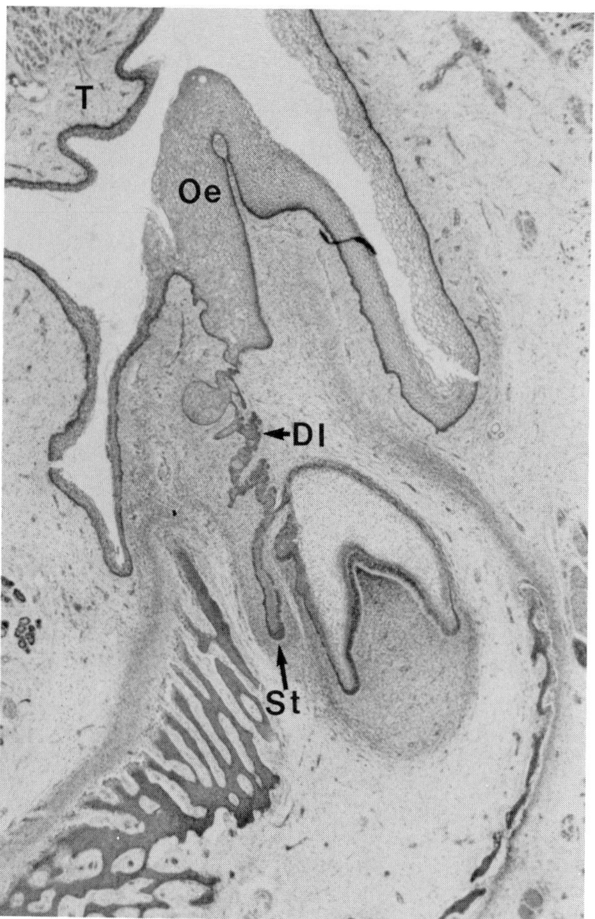

Fig. 3–17. Faciolingual section of a human primary canine tooth germ and its succedaneous tooth (St) developing lingually. Notice that the primary dental lamina (Dl) is still continuous with the oral epithelium (Oe); also note how the secondary dental lamina and developing dental organ extend from the primary dental lamina. Tongue (T).

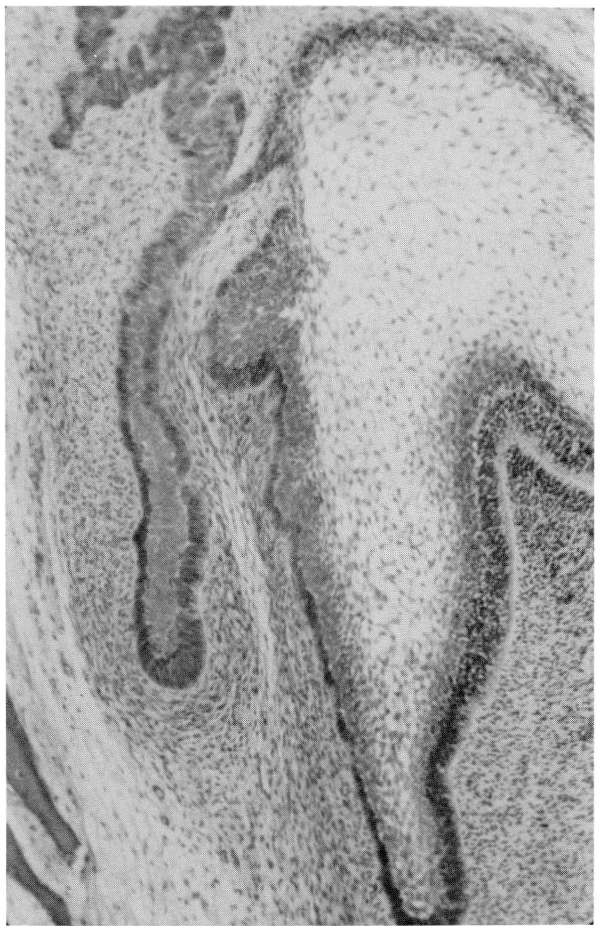

Fig. 3–18. Higher magnification of the early dental organ stage of the succeeding permanent tooth germ seen in Figure 3–17. Note the mesenchymal cells concentrating around the early enamel organ.

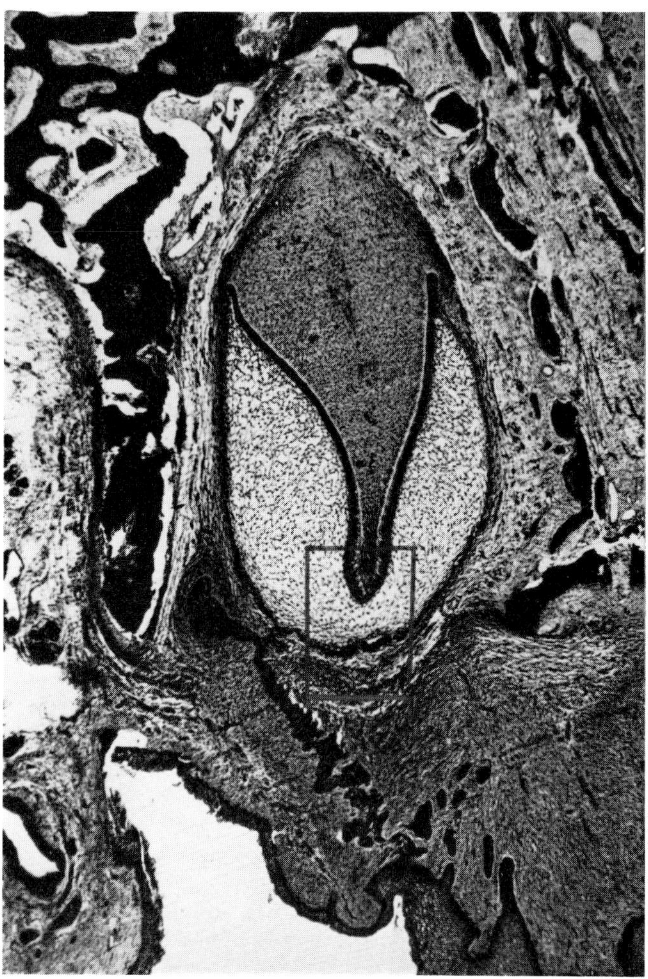

Fig. 3–19. Section of a developing human mandibular primary incisor. The first evidence of dentin formation is present at the most coronal part of the dental papilla. Boxed area, at the coronal end, is shown in detail in Figure 3–20.

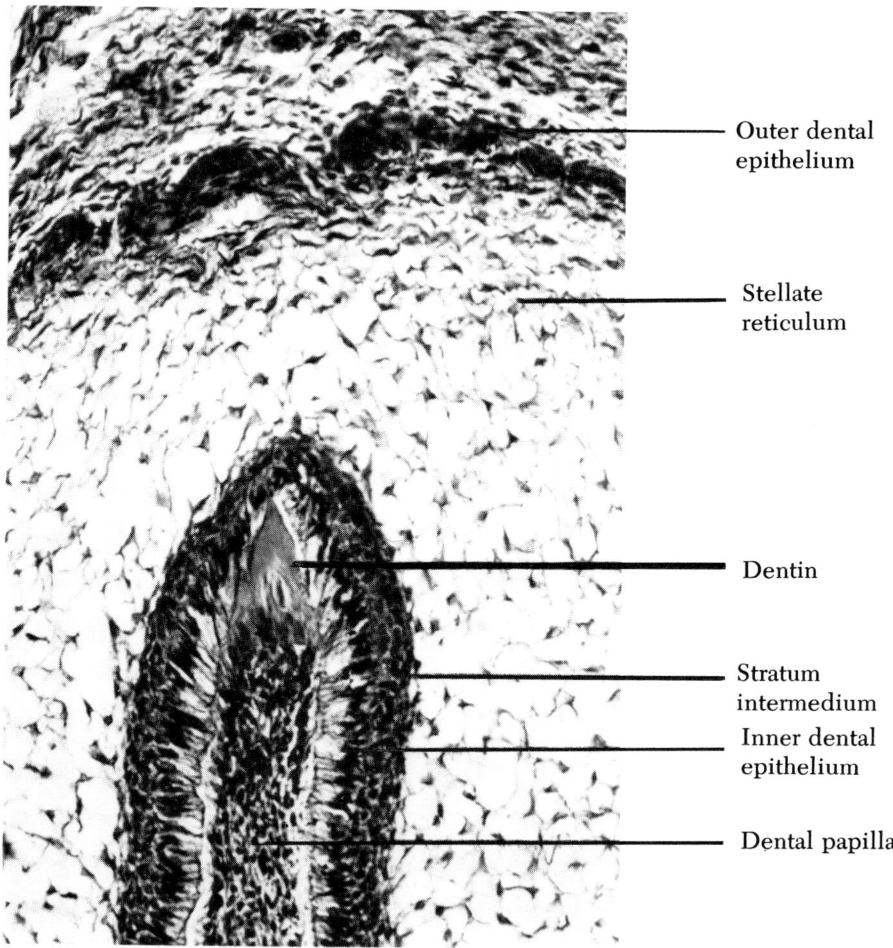

Fig. 3–20. Higher magnification of coronal most part of developing tooth shown in Figure 3–19. The first formed layer of dentin is seen at the coronal most end of the dental papilla.

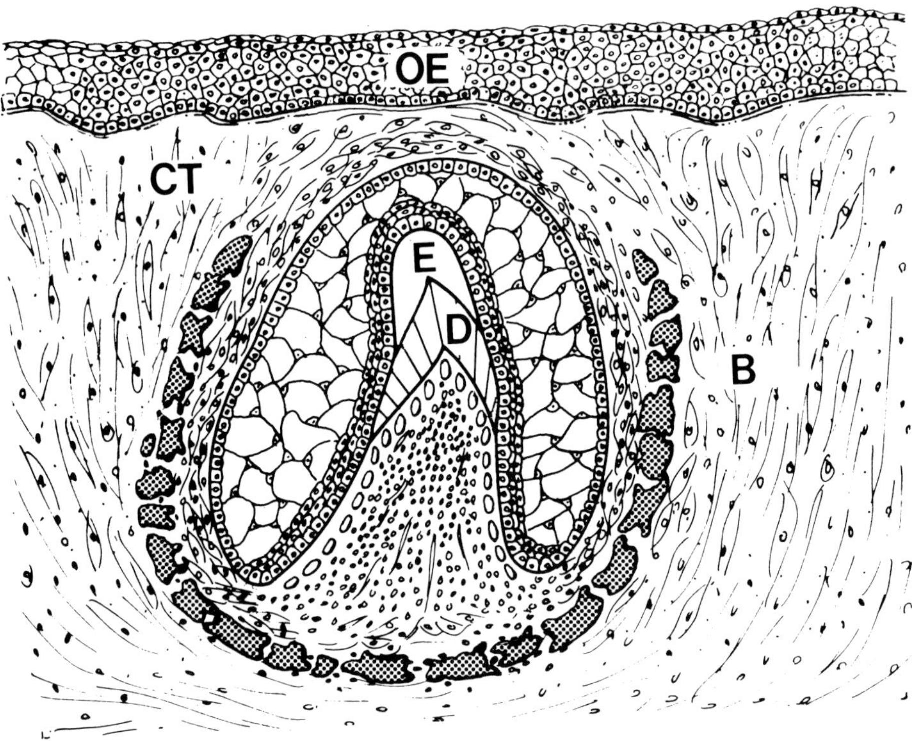

Fig. 3–21. Illustration of an advanced tooth germ with enamel (E) and dentin (D) present in the coronal most part. Ameloblast are present around the enamel whereas cervically, the inner epithelial cells have not yet differentiated into ameloblasts. The dental sac surrounds the enamel organ and is continuous with the dental papilla. Developing bone (B) of the jaw is present and the developing tooth is separated from the oral epithelium (OE) by connective tissue (CT). Compare to photomicrograph of Figure 3–22.

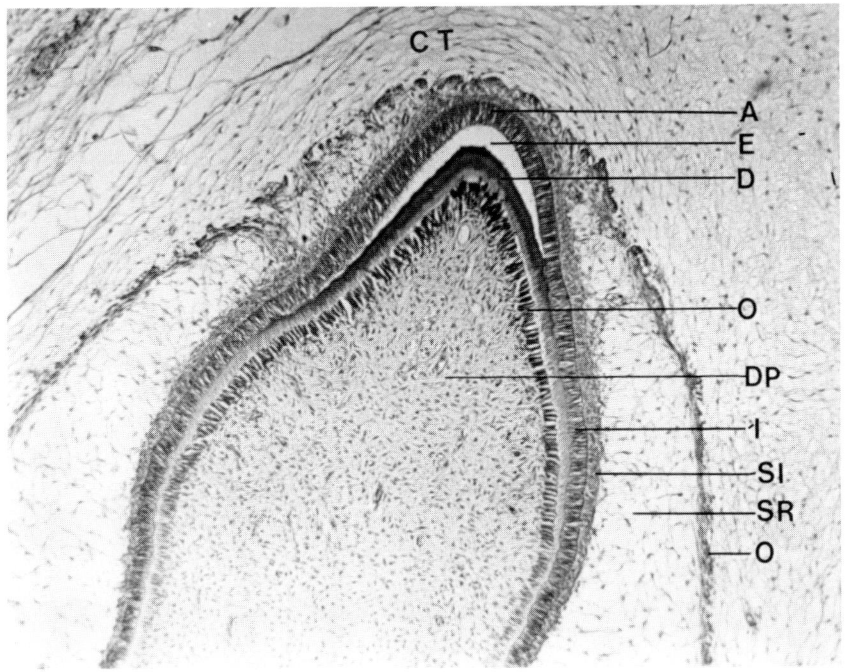

Fig. 3–22. Photomicrograph of an advanced tooth germ. The coronal most part of the tooth germ is more differentiated than the apical part. Coronally, ameloblasts (A) are seen, enamel (E) matrix has formed, along with the formation of dentin (D) and presence of odontoblasts (O) in the dental papilla (DP). Apically, the four epithelial cell layers are clearly seen: (I) inner, stratum intermedium (SI), stellate reticulum (SR), outer (O). Note the surrounding connective tissue (CT) and also note the absences of the dental lamina.

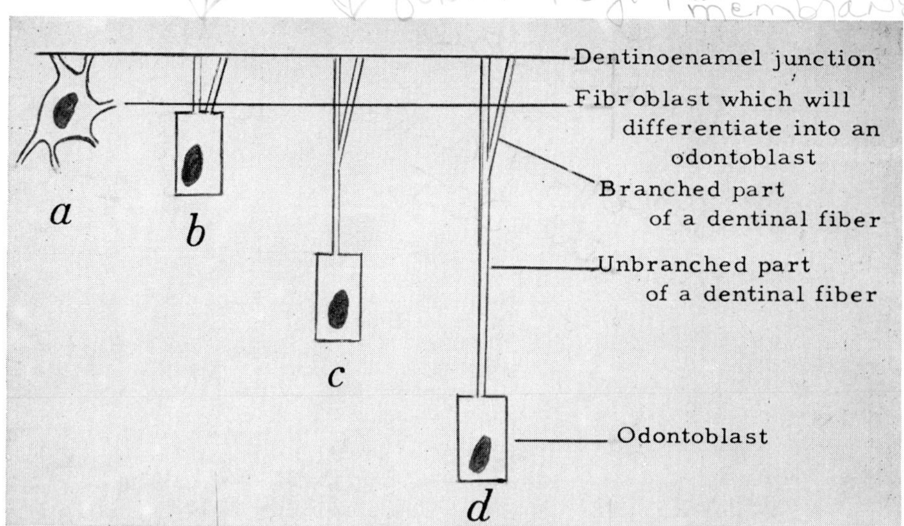

Fig. 3–23. Schematic diagram of the possible manner of formation of a dentinal fiber. (a) A pulp cell which will differentiate into a columnar odontoblast. (b) The odontoblast has moved away from the dentinoenamel junction, but part of its cytoplasm remains stretched behind in two places. (c) The odontoblast has moved farther inward, and its cytoplasmic processes have united. (d) The odontoblast has moved still farther inward, and a long cell process has been formed.

but the cells remain connected with their point of origin by the cytoplasmic extensions which are branched at their peripheral ends.

Now when the odontoblasts differentiated along the periphery of the dental papilla, there were formed among them heavy corkscrew-shaped collagen fibers called *Korff's fibers*. When the dentin formation begins with the odontoblasts moving inward, Korff's fibers remain in place (Fig. 3–24). With the bulky part of the odontoblast cells out of the way the thick Korff's fibers spread out, somewhat in the manner of a piece of rope becoming unwound and frayed. In this way Korff's fibers separate into tiny collagen fibrils which lie among the cytoplasmic extensions of the odontoblasts. These are the *fibrils* of the dentin matrix.* They are surrounded by the *ground substance of the dentin matrix*. Both the collagen fibers and the ground substance *(organic matrix)* are produced by the odontoblasts. The cytoplasmic extensions of the odontoblasts are the *odontoblastic processes*.

Dentin matrix mineralizes progressively as it is produced. The innermost layer of dentin matrix (next to the pulp) is the most recently formed, and in developing teeth it is not mineralized until a successive layer has been formed. This newest, nonmineralized dentin, is called *predentin* or *dentinoid* (Figs. 3–25; 3–26).

Dentin may be produced along the pulpal wall in a tooth of any age as long as the pulp is intact. Dentin formed in older teeth in response to attrition or caries is called *reparative dentin*. The tubules in reparative dentin are fewer and less regular in arrangement than those of the earlier dentin because, due to age

*Interesting paper: Whittaker, D.K., and D. Adams: Electron Microscope Studies on Von Korff's Fibers in the Human Developing Tooth. Anat. Rec., *174*(2):175, 1972.

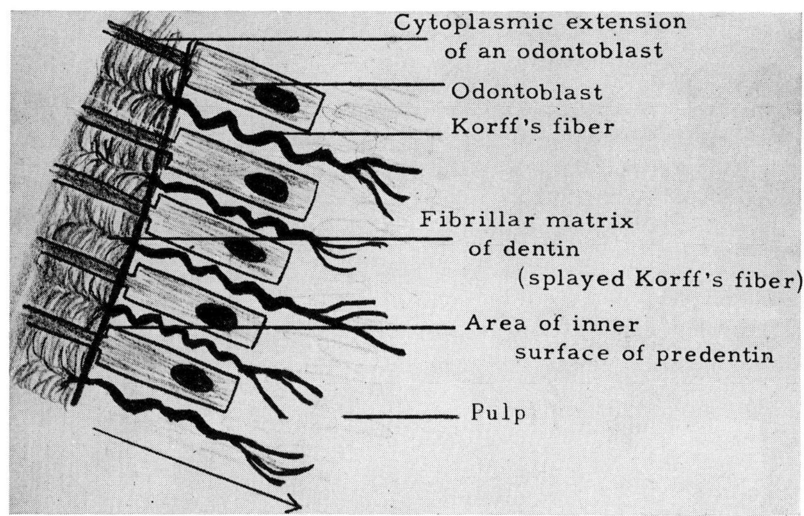

Fig. 3–24. Schematic diagram of odontoblast's and Korff's fibers. Much enlarged.

changes in the pulps of older teeth, there are fewer odontoblasts, and so fewer odontoblastic processes.

When dentin formation begins, the forming organ is called the *dental papilla*. After some amount of dentin has been produced the name of the dental papalla is changed and it is called the *dental pulp*.

ENAMEL FORMATION

Amelogenesis is the name given to the origin and formation of enamel.

Tooth enamel is a product of the enamel organ. The ameloblasts, which earlier in development were the inner enamel epithelial cells of the enamel organ, produce an organic enamel matrix in which mineral salts later crystallize out of solution, making enamel a hard tissue.*

Enamel matrix formation starts soon after the beginning of dentin formation. Enamel matrix formation begins at the dentin surface of the cusps (or incisal edge) and closely follows the progress of dentin formation. As the odontoblasts of the pulp move inward leaving a cell process and dentin matrix in the area they once occupied, the opposing ameloblasts move outward, leaving enamel matrix in their wake (Figs. 3–22; 3–25; 3–26; 3–27).

Enamel matrix is laid down in the form of enamel rods and interrod substance. The organic matrix is a product of ameloblasts. As ameloblasts move away from the dentinoenamel junction, they deposit drops of material which remain lined up behind the ameloblasts in such a way that they resemble a string of flattened

*Interesting papers: Frank R.M., and J. Nalbandian: Comparative Aspects of Development of Dental Hard Structures. J. Dent. Res., *42*(1):422, 1963.
Deutch, D., and Gedalia, I.: Chemically Distinct Stages in Developing Fetal Human Enamel. Arch. Oral Biol., *25*:635, 1980.
Deutsch, D., and Pe'er E.: Development of Enamel in Human Fetal Teeth. J. Dent. Res., *61*:1543, 1982.
Simimelink, J.W.: Mode of Enamel Matrix Section. J. Dent. Res., *61*:1483, 1982.

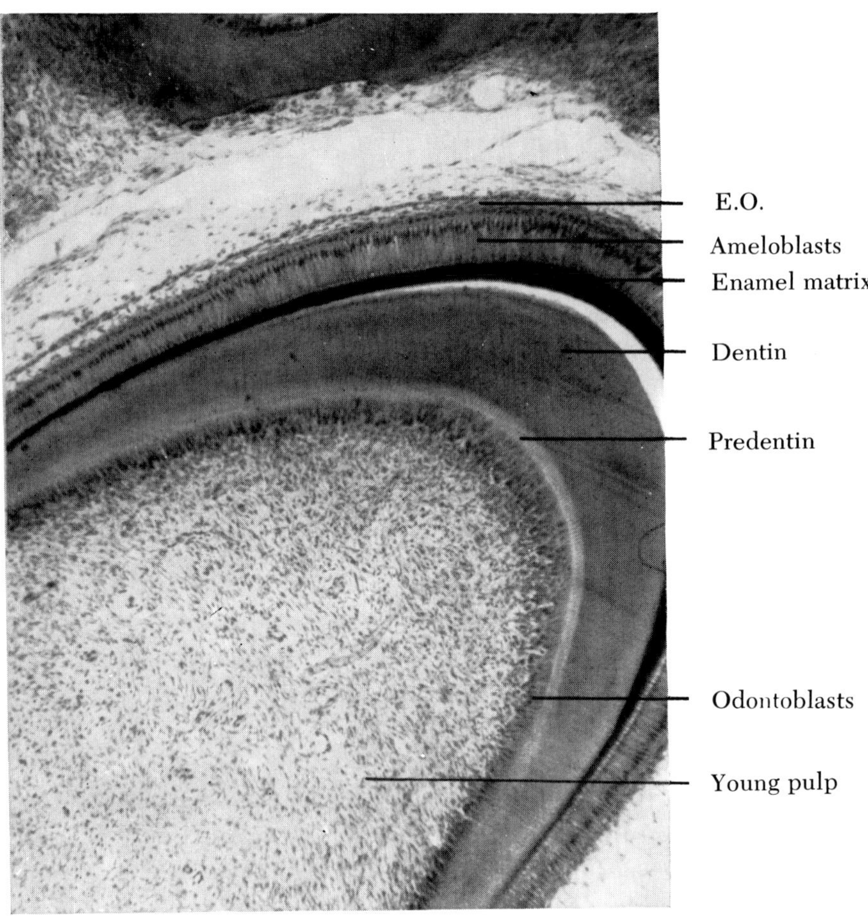

Fig. 3–25. Photomicrograph of a developing mandibular tooth of a kitten. This is a cusp tip. Odontoblasts lie around the periphery of the pulp. Outside of the odontoblasts is light-stained predentin, and then darker-stained dentin. The space between the dentin and the black-colored enamel matrix is an artifact. Outside of the enamel matrix are the tall, columnar ameloblasts with their nuclei located at their outer ends. Outside of the ameloblasts the outer three layers of the enamel organ (stratum intermedium, stellate reticulum, outer enamel epithelium), here marked E.O., have been reduced to a few layers of flat cells. When the enamel matrix is completely formed, the ameloblasts will become similarly flattened. The four indistinguishable layers are then collectively the *reduced enamel epithelium* (Fig. 3–28).

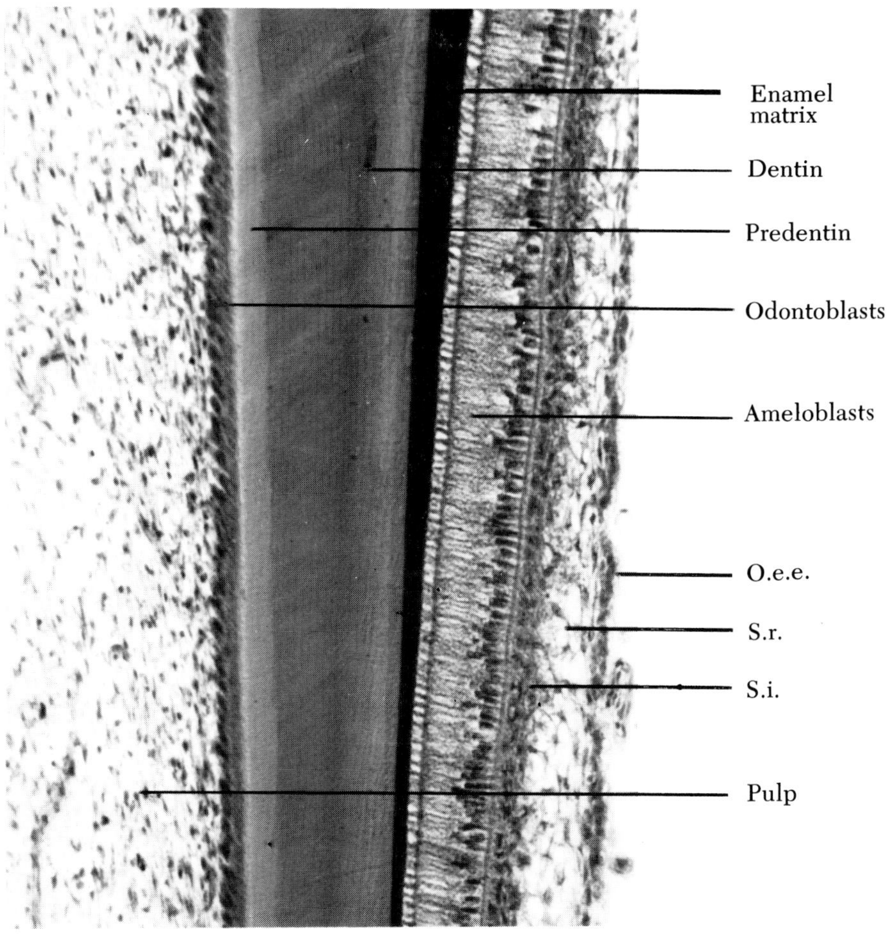

Fig. 3–26. Higher magnification of the cervical ameloblasts of a tooth at about the same development stage as the tooth seen in Figure 3–25. Note the regular arrangement of the tall columnar ameloblasts: Compare the ameloblasts to the smaller cell bodies of the odontoblasts. These cells move in opposite directions during the matrix formation stage. O.e.e.–outer enamel epithelial layer; S.i.–stratum intermedium layer; S.r.–stellate reticulum layer.

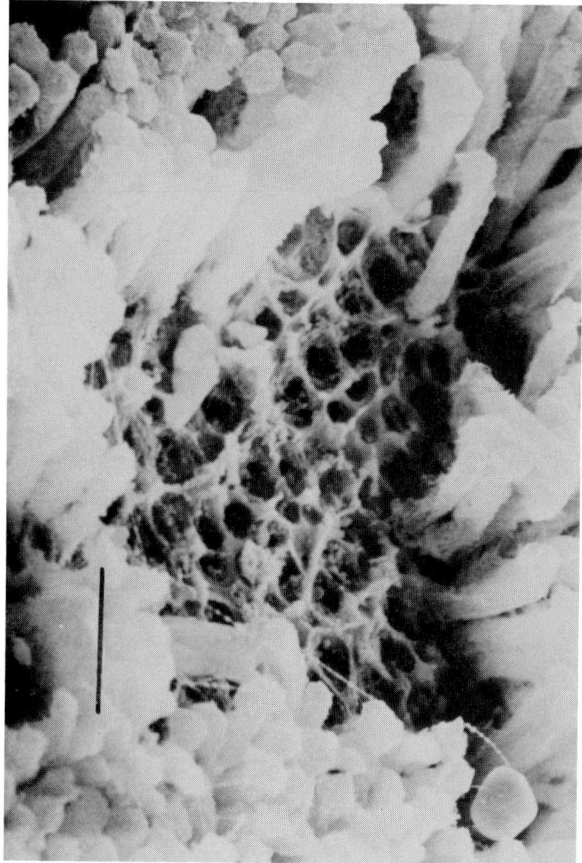

Fig. 3–27. This is an interesting scanning electron micrographic view of ameloblasts. Here, the ameloblasts are seen as white columnar cells. Their movement is toward you as they form the underlying enamel matrix. The honey-comb appearing matrix is seen in the center where the ameloblasts were lost during processing of the specimen. The marker represents 20 micrometers. (Courtesy of Dr. Dennis Foreman, Collage of Dentistry, The Ohio State University.)

beads in close union (Figs. 4–5; 4–16). It is believed that this drop formation produces the apparent segments, or units, of the enamel rods which are seen as cross striations in rods of mature teeth when such teeth are ground into thin sections and examined with the high power of the microscope. The interrod substance between the enamel rods is a product of the intercellular substance which lies between the ameloblasts. Current thinking is that the organic matrix of one enamel rod may be formed by more than one ameloblast. Whatever the case, there is no doubt that structures resembling rods exist in mature enamel, and that the organic matrix is secreted by the ameloblasts.

After the matrix has formed, the formation of enamel is completed when submicroscopic crystals of inorganic substances develop among and around the fibrils of the matrix of the rods and interrod substance. These crystals have distinct orientations: crystals in the center of the rods lie with their long axes parallel to the long axes of the rods; crystals between the rods—in the interrod substance—lie at an angle to the long axes of the rods. Tooth enamel, being about 96% mineral substance, is the hardest of all body tissues.

Some histologists believe that when the ameloblasts have completed the production of enamel matrix they produce a smooth coating over its surface. This coating mineralizes. It covers the entire surface of the tooth crown and is called the *primary enamel cuticle*. This coating is not visible in ground sections of tooth enamel, and so it is not shown in any of the illustrations in this book.*

The destiny of the enamel organ of the tooth germ is important. As the enamel matrix is being produced and the ameloblasts are moving from the dentinoenamel junction, the stellate reticulum of the enamel organ narrows and becomes indiscernible, and the enamel organ is reduced to a layer of ameloblasts plus a few layers of squamous epithelial cells which are the remains of the rest of the enamel organ (Figs. 3–1E; 3–26). When the ameloblasts have completed the formation of the matrix of the enamel rods, they change to flattened epithelial cells and blend indistinguishably with the remaining cells of the enamel organ. Thus the enamel organ, originally composed of ameloblasts, stratum intermedium, stellate reticulum, and outer enamel epithelium, has been reduced to a few layers of flattened cells covering the newly formed tooth crown. These combined layers of cells are called the *reduced enamel epithelium* (also called *reduced dental epithelium*) (Fig. 3–28).

The reduced enamel epithelium now produces nonmineralized enamel cuticle over the surface of the tooth crown. This is called the *secondary enamel cuticle* (also called *dental cuticle*). This cuticle may remain on the surface of the tooth after the tooth emerges into the oral cavity.

The reduced enamel epithelium surrounds the crown of the tooth until it emerges into the oral cavity (Fig. 3–28). After the tooth tip emerges, the part of the reduced enamel epithelium which remains surrounding the crown is henceforth referred to as the *epithelium of the gingival sulcus* and of the *attachment epithelium* (also called *junctional epithelium*). This epithelium in a newly erupted tooth is what remains of the original enamel organ of the tooth germ (Fig. 3–1).

---

*Interesting papers:
Listgarten, M.A.: Phase-contrast and Electron Microscopic Study of the Junction between Reduced Enamel Epithelium and Enamel in Unerupted Human Teeth. Arch. Oral Biol., *11*:999, 1966.
Listgarten, M.A.: A Mineralized Cuticular Structure with Connective Tissue Characteristics on the Crowns of Human Unerupted Teeth in Amelogenesis Imperfecta. Arch. Oral Biol., *12*:877, 1967.

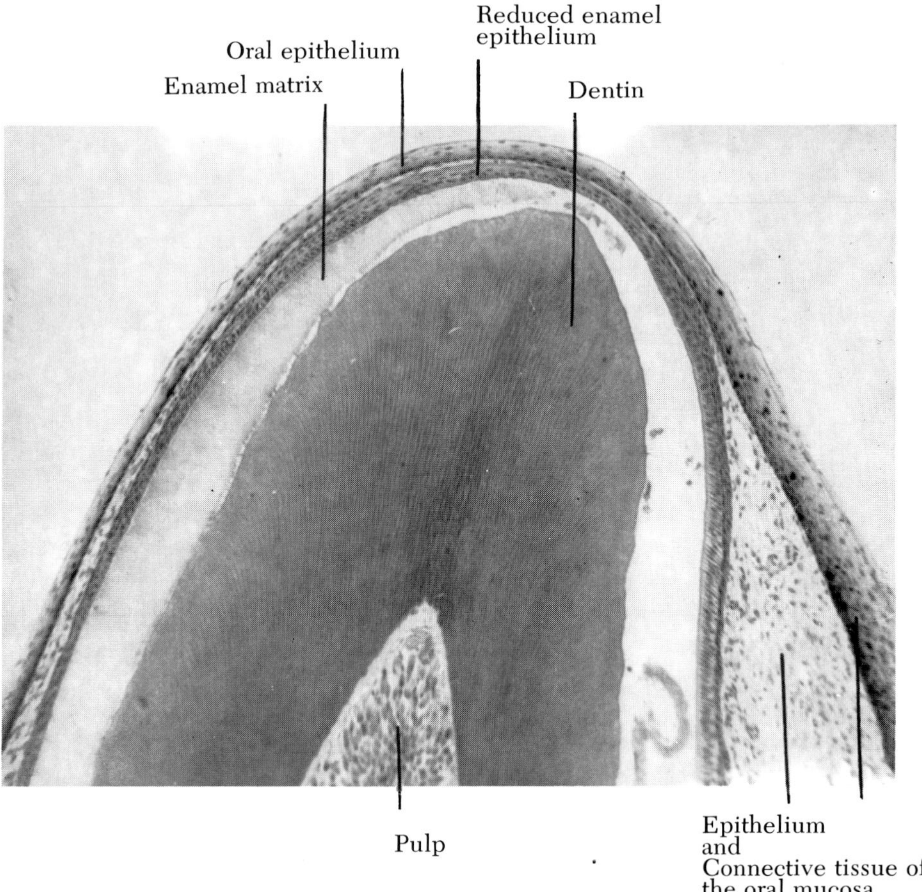

Fig. 3–28. Anterior tooth of a fetal pig. A little more occlusal movement and the tooth tip will break through into the oral cavity. Around the edge of the break-through the oral epithelium and the reduced enamel epithelium will become united and protectively seal in the connective tissue. With this incident of tooth emergence the name of the *reduced enamel epithelium* will change to attachment epithelium. The enamel matrix on the right of the picture was washed away in section preparation. At this stage calcification of enamel is well advanced. Notice the resemblance of this tooth to the kitten tooth in Figure 3–25.

ENAMEL SPINDLES

Enamel spindles originate in the early tooth germ before the cells that derive from ectoderm and mesenchyme have differentiated into ameloblasts and odontoblasts. Some of the cells that are to become odontoblasts have thin projections of cytoplasm crossing the line that will become the dentinoenamel junction and lying among the cells that will become ameloblasts. After cell differentiation the odontoblasts move inward as dentin matrix is formed, and as they move their cytoplasmic projections stretch out into what we call odontoblastic processes. But the ends of the processes remain among the ameloblasts. When enamel matrix forms and mineralizes, the ends of the odontoblast processes are the so-called *spindles*. In older teeth the spindle probably is only a space that once held odontoblast cytoplasm.

ROOT FORMATION

Formation of the dentin and of the enamel begins in the incisal or cuspal areas of the tooth and progresses cervically. Enamel formation stops at the termination of the enamel organ, which is the cervical border of the tooth crown. Dentin formation continues beyond this point, and the dentin of the root is formed (Fig. 3–1F, G). As the root dentin starts to form, the already formed tooth crown moves occlusally, although the tooth does not emerge into the oral cavity until a considerable portion of the root has been produced. If the tooth has but a single root, the dentin wall forms enclosing a single pulp canal. If the tooth is to be a multi-rooted tooth, the division of the pulp cavity into two pulp canals, each surrounded by a wall of dentin, is apparent soon after the completion of

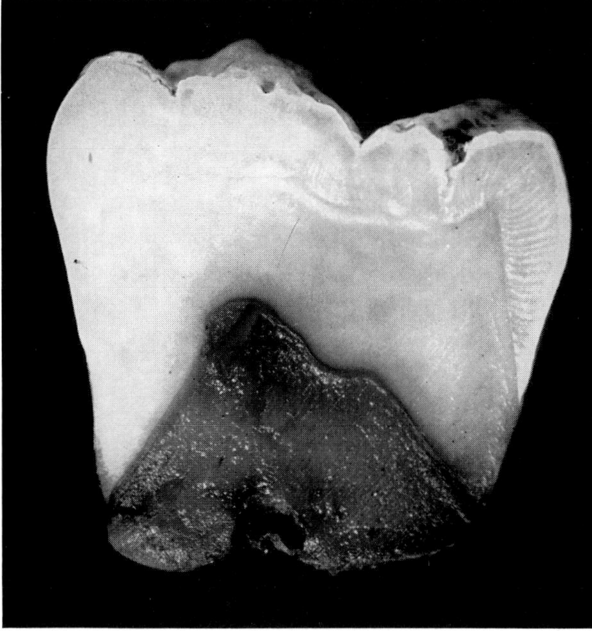

Fig. 3–29. Mandibular left third molar. Buccal side removed. The crown of this tooth is completed; the root has started to form. The lower border of the pulp chamber shows the beginning of a division into two root canals.

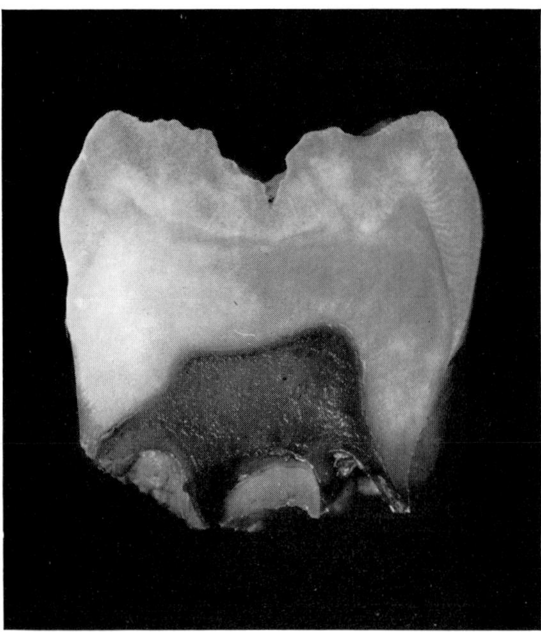

Fig. 3–30. Mandibular right third molar. Buccal side removed. The crown is completed. There is clearly the beginning of development of two roots.

the crown. Figure 3–29 is a photograph of a mandibular third molar from which the buccal wall is removed. The crown of this tooth is complete. Dentin has formed beyond the cervical border of the enamel, and a short root trunk is present. In the center of the lower edge of this young tooth pulp there is evidence of its division into two branches, one for the mesial root and one for the distal root. Figure 3–30 is a similar tooth, the roots of which are slightly more advanced in development. Here the root bifurcation is obvious. Owing to drying out of the specimen during preparation, the tooth pulp in each root shows some shrinkage at its lower border, making it erroneously appear, at first glance, that there may be four roots developing.

Figure 3–31 is a photograph of a mandibular third molar, the roots of which have attained perhaps three fourths of their final length. The root canals are broad and their apical openings are large.

Figure 3–32 is a photograph of the buccal surface of a mandibular third molar, the roots of which are perhaps about two thirds of their final length. The apical openings are large. In the process of studying extracted teeth students often mistake the short, square shape of such roots as an indication of partial root resorption. A permanent tooth with the apical third of its roots resorbed would have small root canals (because it probably would be an older tooth), and the root ends probably would not have this square shape.

Figure 3–33 is a tooth similar to the one shown in Figure 3–32. This picture was taken looking up into the open ends of the root canals. Notice the large size of the root canals and the thinness of the dentin wall.

Root length is not complete until one to four years after the tooth emerges into the oral cavity. A newly emerged tooth has a short root and a very large apical opening. As teeth become older the root length is completed, additional

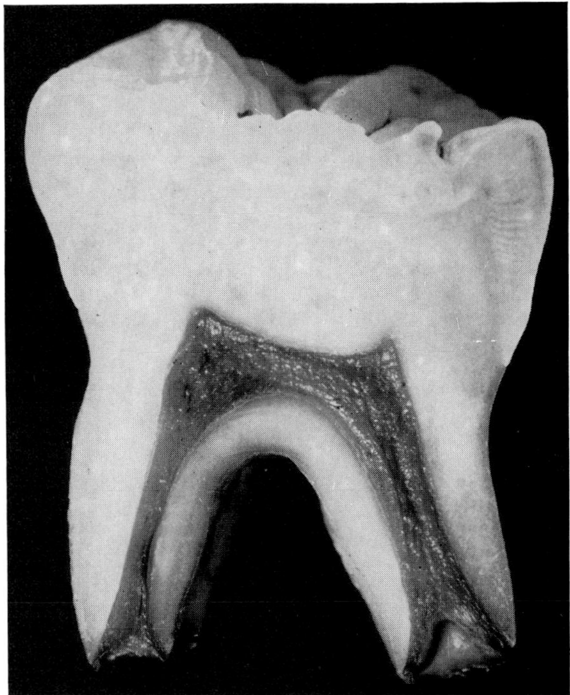

Fig. 3–31. Mandibular left third molar. Buccal side removed. The roots have attained about three fourths of their length. The root canals are broad, and the opening at the ends of the incompletely formed roots are large.

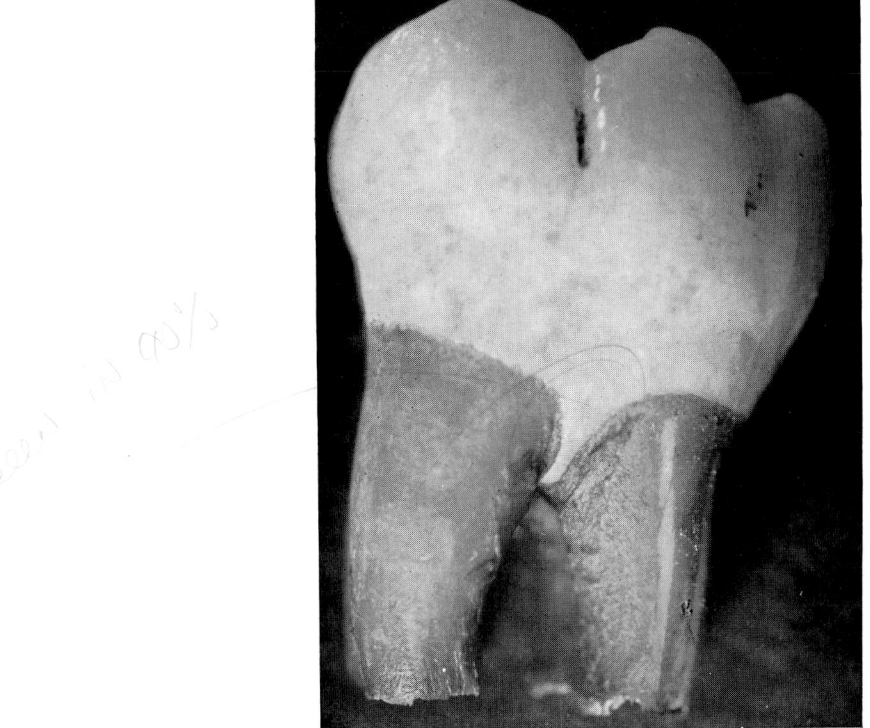

Fig. 3–32. Buccal surface of a left mandibular third molar. The roots have attained about two thirds of their length. The openings at the ends of the incompletely formed roots are large. In this tooth the enamel extends between the roots and meets the enamel on the lingual surface of the tooth.

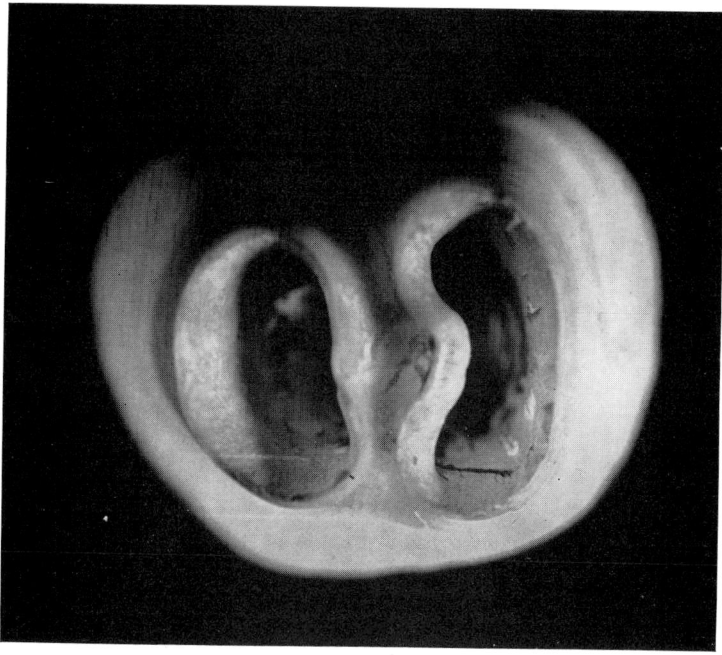

Fig. 3–33. A mandibular second molar. This picture was taken looking into the large opeinings at the ends of the incompletely formed roots.

dentin continues to form on the pulpal surface of the existing dentin until the root canal becomes narrow and the apical opening becomes small. The stage of development of the root—that is, the size of the root canal and of the apical foramen—is important to the dentist if accident or dental caries makes endodontic treatment necessary.

FORMATION OF PERIODONTAL LIGAMENT AND CEMENTUM

As dentin is forming apical to the cervical line of the enamel, the circularly arranged fibers of the dental sac become the periodontal ligament around the tooth root. The periodontal ligament produces the cementum which covers the root dentin. It also produces the lamina dura of the tooth socket. As the cementum and the lamina dura are being produced about the forming root, fibers of the periodontal ligament become entrapped in their substance. The attachment of the periodontal ligament fibers in the lamina dura and in the cementum holds the tooth securely in the socket (Fig. 3–1). As the tooth erupts, the periodontal ligament fibers are reoriented.

As the tooth crown moves occlusally it carries with it the reduced enamel epithelium which covers it. At the cervical border of the reduced enamel epithelium some of its cells seem to pull off in strands which remain stretched like a network in the periodontal ligament around the forming root. This network is called *Hertwig's epithelial root sheath.* The root sheath serves two functions: (1) determines the outline form of the root dentin before cementum formation begins and (2) determines the number of roots a tooth will have. The cells of Hertwig's epithelial root sheath *must* break-up and pull away from the root dentin surface before the cementoblasts can move to the surface and produce the cementum matrix (Figs. 3–1; 3–34; 3–35). Later, when the tooth is fully formed and in function, a few fragments of Hertwig's epithelial sheath may still be found upon microscopic examination of the periodontal ligament. These small groups of cells are called the epithelial *rests of Malassez.* (See Chapter 8).

ANOMALIES

Development of the teeth may vary in a number of ways from the usual standard. Sometimes less than the normal number of tooth germs develop and an individual has too few teeth *(hypodontia),* or perhaps no teeth *(anodontia).* Sometimes more than the usual number of tooth germs develop and the individual has too many teeth. These extra teeth are called *supernumerary teeth* (super = additional; numerary = number) (Fig. 3–36). Sometimes certain teeth have a peculiar shape: the maxillary lateral incisor may be peg-shaped; the maxillary central incisor may be screwdriver-shaped, having a mesiodistal dimensin which is smaller in the incisal third than in the cervical portion.

Again, there may be faulty development of the hard tooth tissues. Enamel development may be so imperfect that the enamel is lost from the surface of the tooth soon after eruption. This condition is hereditary. A more frequent condition is localized enamel hypoplasia (hypo = under; plasia = formation), which is the result of a systemic disturbance during the time the tooth crowns are forming. This is often seen in the form of a pitted line across the facial surfaces of the permanent incisors, the tips of the canines, and the cusps of the first molars in the same mouth. It affects the areas of the teeth that were in the process of formation at the time the systemic cause of the hypoplasia occurred.

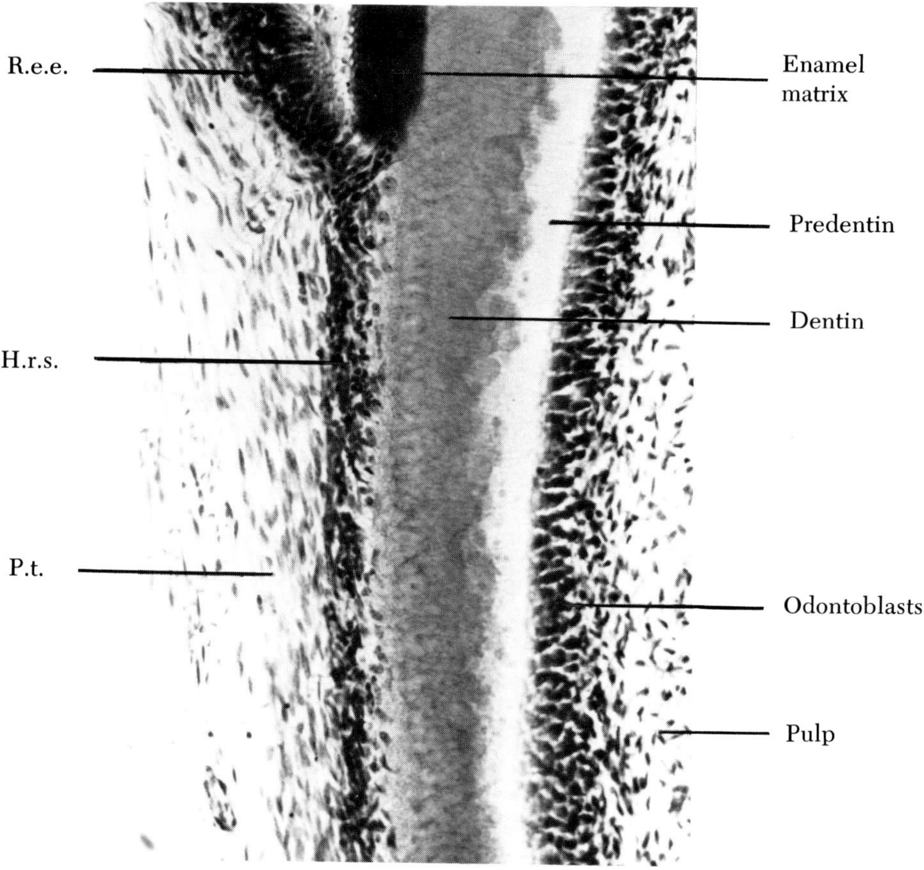

Fig. 3–34. Photomicrograph of the cervical region of a developing kitten tooth. *Hertwig's epithelial root sheath* (H.r.s.) is still intact along the root dentin; it is still continuous with the reduced enamel (dental) epithelium (R.e.e.) over the crown. Cementum is not present at this stage of development. Hertwig's sheath must break up and pull away from the root dentin surface before the cementoblasts can move to the surface and produce the cementum matrix. P.t.—periodontal tissue.

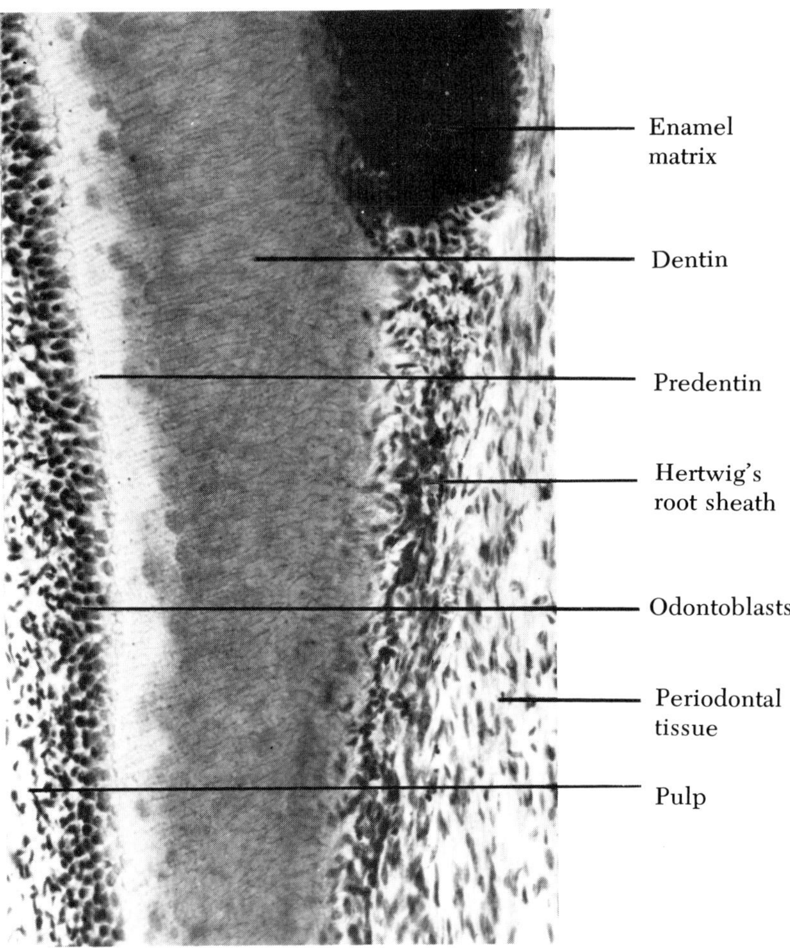

Fig. 3–35. Section similar to that seen in Figure 3–34; it is a more advanced stage. *Hertwig's epithelial root sheath* cells are separated and less concentrated, especially in the most cervical root area just apical to the enamel matrix; the area where the first cementum matrix will form.

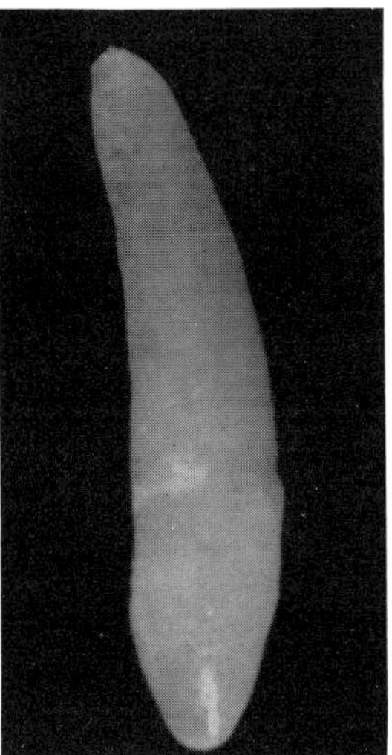

Fig. 3–36. A supernumerary tooth (history unknown). This kind kind of tooth is usually found in the maxilla, lingual to the other teeth.

Still another abnormality is in interference with the calcification of the enamel matrix which produces hypomineralized areas in the enamel. This condition is seen in individuals who have lived during the first eight years of their lives in regions where the drinking water contained over 2 parts per million of fluoride. Fluoride in the drinking water causes enamel hypomineralization only when it is consumed during the period of tooth formation; and such hypomineralization is clinically visible only when the fluoride is in amounts in excess of approximately 2 ppm. The hypomineralized areas of enamel soon become stained brown when exposed to the oral cavity, so that there are unsightly brown spots on the teeth. This condition is called *mottled enamel* or *dental fluorosis.*

Another variation in enamel formation found in molars, chiefly mandibular molars, is an extension of the enamel at its cervical border between the roots of the teeth (Fig. 3–23). Perhaps this pattern of enamel distribution should not be called an anomaly, as it has been reported to occur in 90% of the mandibular first molars in persons of Mongoloid racial stock. It is unusual in teeth of persons of Caucasoid racial stock.

An interesting anomaly which is sometimes seen in the process of examining a collection of extracted teeth is the *enamel pearl.* This is a spot of enamel, usually in the shape of half a sphere, which is found on the roots of teeth. The most frequent location of enamel pearls is said to be on the distal surface of third molars (Figs. 3–37; 3–38; 3–39), although they are sometimes found on the buccal surface of a molar at the root of furcation. Their formation is ordinarily said to be the result of a small group of cells of Hertwig's epithelial root sheath adhering to the surface of the newly formed root dentin instead of becoming separated from the dentin and moving out into the periodontal ligament. These epithelial cells adhering to the root dentin differentiate into ameloblasts just as the cells of the inner enamel epithelium in the crown area differentiate into ameloblasts, and a drop of enamel (enamel pearl) is then produced on the root.

That the production of an enamel pearl is more than merely a simple matter

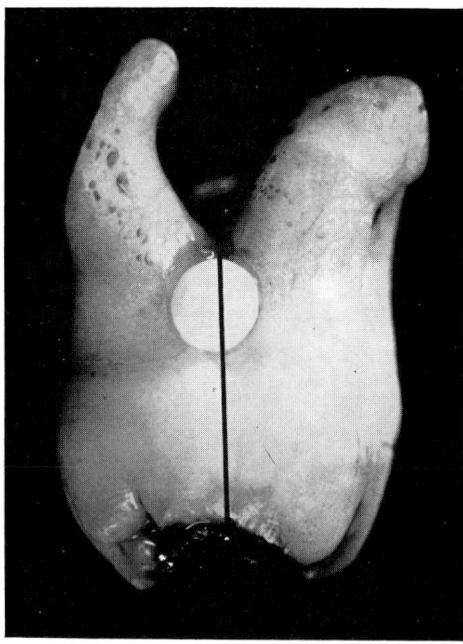

Fig. 3–37. Distal surface of a maxillary right third molar. On the root trunk is an enamel pearl. The tooth was ground to a thin section along the vertical line. (See Figure 3–38.)

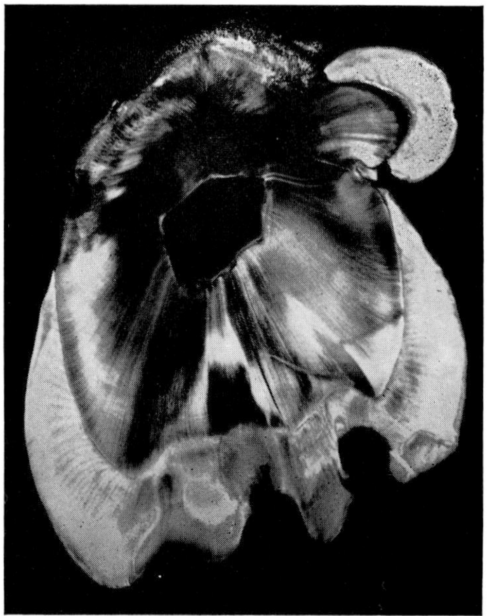

Fig. 3–38. A ground section of the tooth shown Figure 3–37. The enamel pearl is in the upper right. The roots are not present here because the section was made at the root furcation. Notice that besides having a formation of enamel in this unusual location there is a variation in the dentin formation which has resulted in a protrusion of dentin beneath the enamel pearl.

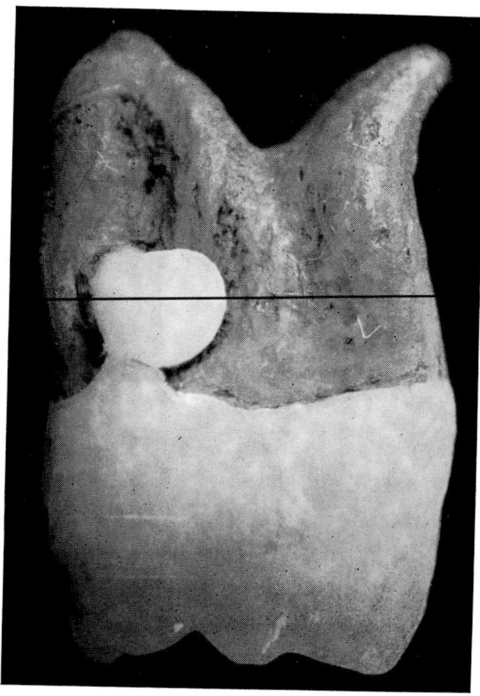

Fig. 3–39. A maxillary right third molar with a very large enamel pearl on the distal surface of the lingual root. The tooth was ground to a thin section along the horizontal line. (See Figure 3–40.)

of the cells of Hertwig's sheath adhering to the root dentin is indicated by the fact that the dentin beneath the enamel pearl in many, if not all, cases protrudes into the pearl. That is, the external dentin surface is not flat, as on the rest of the root: there is a protrusion of dentin which is covered by the enamel pearl (Figs. 3–38; 3–40). In some teeth the configuration of the pulp canal is also altered. In the cross section (Fig. 3–40) of the tooth shown in Figure 3–39, there

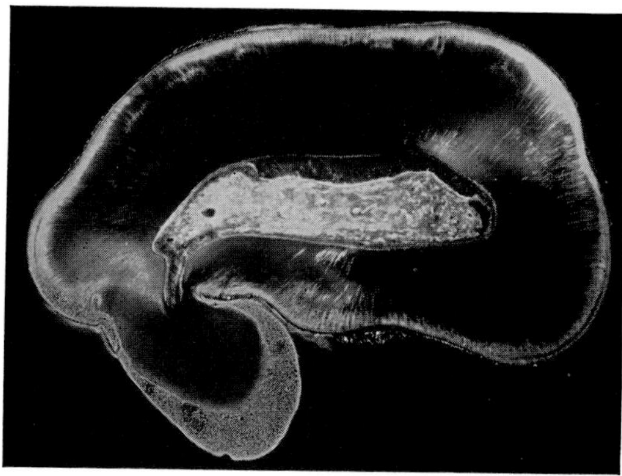

Fig. 3–40. A ground section of the tooth shown in Figure 3–39. The enamel pearl is in the lower left. In this tooth there is not only a protrusion of the dentin beneath the enamel pearl, but there is also an extrusion of the pulp cavity in the location of the pearl.

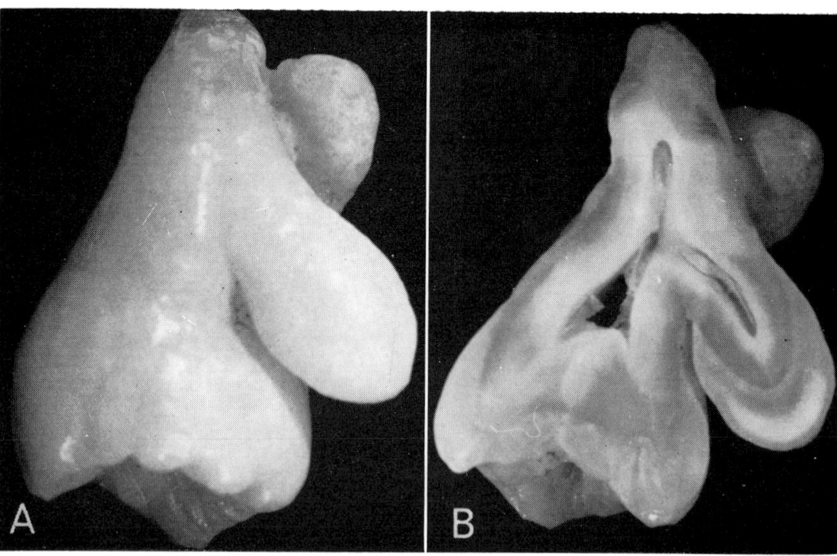

Fig. 3–41. A. Buccal aspect of a left maxillary third molar with a supernumerary tooth growing from its distal side. B. When the buccal surface was ground away, the pulp cavities of the third molar and the supernumerary tooth were found to be joined.

is an extrusion of the wall of the pulp canal beneath the enamel pearl.*

Sometimes on a tooth root there is a projection larger than an enamel pearl: it has an enamel-covered crown and a short cementum-covered root (Fig. 3–41A). It is, in fact, an attached supernumerary tooth, a result of anomalous formation of the tooth germ at an early stage of its development. Usually in such a specimen the pulp cavities of the large tooth and the supernumerary

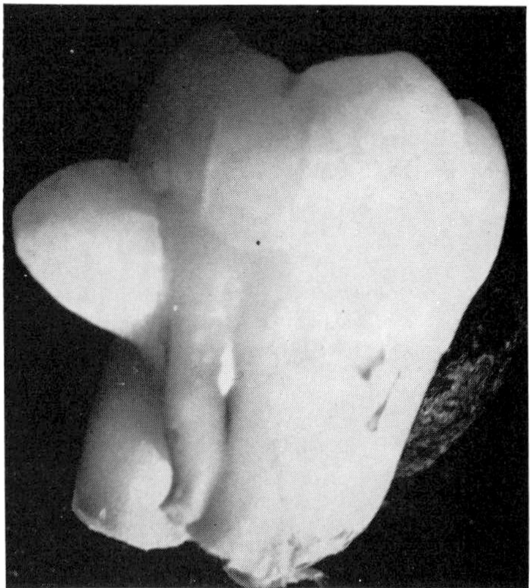

Fig. 3–42. Lingual aspect of a left mandibular third molar with a supernumerary tooth between its roots. The crown of the supernumerary tooth is pointed distolingually. Notice the small extra root on the lingual side of the molar.

*Interesting paper:
Cavanka, A.O.: Enamel Pearls. Oral Surg., *19*:373, 1965.

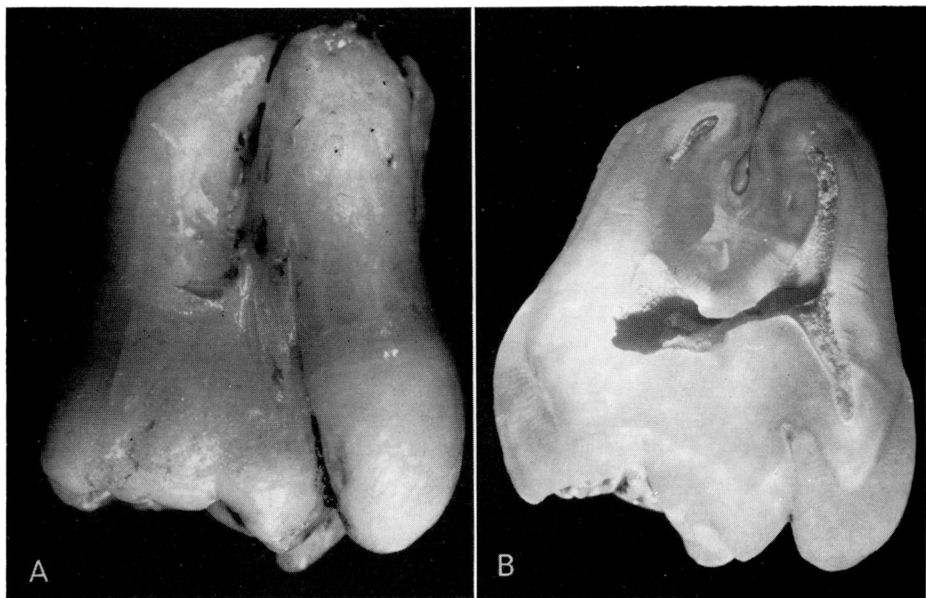

Fig. 3–43. A. Distal aspect of a right maxillary third molar that has a supernumerary tooth attached to the buccal surface of the distobuccal cusp. B. The distal side was ground off, and exposed were the united pulp cavities.

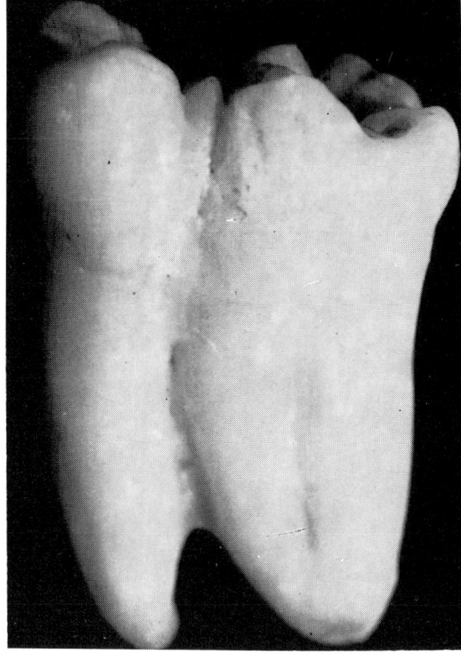

Fig. 3–44. Careful study of this anomaly failed to supply an answer to the question of its probable location in the mouth other than that clearly it came from the mandibular molar area. It was not possible to identify the buccal and lingual aspects with any confidence.

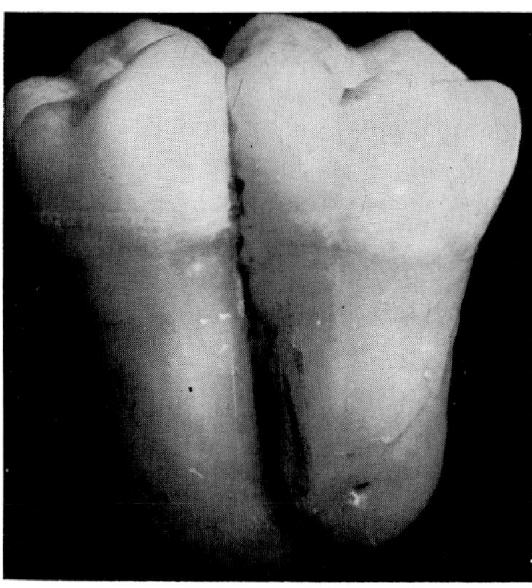

Fig. 3–45. The lingual surface of fused mandibular molars.

tooth are united (Fig. 3–41B). (Compare the pulp cavities of the specimens in Figures 3–40; 3–41B.)

Figure 3–42 is a supernumerary tooth between, or in this case, among the roots of a mandibular third molar: this mandibular molar has a third root beneath the distolingual cusp. When one side of the specimen was ground away the pulp cavities of the molar and the supernumerary tooth were found to be united.

Figure 3–43A is a right maxillary third molar with a supernumerary tooth attached to the buccal surface of the distobuccal cusp and root. When the distal side of the tooth was removed the pulp cavities were seen to be united (Fig. 3–43B).

Figure 3–44 is a picture of fused mandibular molars, the pulp cavities of which formed a common chamber.

The specimen of fused mandibular molars seen in Figure 3–45 had only two roots externally and two root canals internally, but there were two distinct crowns, fused, each with two buccal and two lingual cusps. The pulp chambers in crowns were united.

The shape of these kinds of anomalies are, of course, established in the early stages of the formation of the enamel organ. Before any matrix of hard tissue is produced in a developing tooth the enamel organ takes a shape such that the cells of the inner enamel epithelium, which will, of course, become ameloblasts, have the configuration of the future dentinoenamel junction. The basement membrane located between the ameloblasts and the peripheral cells of the dental papilla is the location of the future dentinoenamel junction. In the developing tooth many of these anomalies would be visible in microscopic examination of sections of tissue obtained at this early stage of tooth formation.

Chapter 4

TOOTH ENAMEL

LOCATION

Tooth enamel makes up the outside layer of the anatomic crown of a tooth (Frontispiece and Fig. 1–11).

COMPOSITION

Enamel is composed of both inorganic (mineral) and organic substances. Mature human enamel is about 96% inorganic. The remaining 4% of its substance is an organic matrix (framework) and water. Enamel is the hardest tissue of the body, its mineral content far exceeding the mineral content of dentin (70%), of cementum (50%), or of bone (50%). See Table 9–1.

MACROSCOPIC STRUCTURE OF ENAMEL

Examine the teeth of several persons who maintain reasonably good oral hygiene. The crown surfaces are composed of hard, shiny enamel. In young individuals who are free from dental caries, no other tooth tissues are exposed in the oral cavity. On some of the teeth of older individuals, due to a normal aging process, the gingiva may have receded to such an extent that cementum is visible. In persons of any age whose teeth have unrepaired caries lesions, dentin will be exposed in the areas where the disease has destroyed the enamel.

On the labial surfaces of the maxillary central incisors of a young person you usually see a number of fine horizontal lines on the enamel. In the cervical part of the crown these lines are close together; incisally on the crown they are farther apart (Fig. 4–1). These lines are called *perikymata.** Their presence is not confined to the maxillary central incisors; they are found on the enamel of all surfaces of all teeth, but they are easier to see on the more accessible surfaces. In older persons perikymata usually are not visible: they have been worn off the less protected surfaces.

Examination of the teeth of persons of different ages will show that generally in older persons the enamel appears darker in color than in younger persons.

Despite its hardness tooth enamel is subject to *attrition*—that is, wearing off under the friction of use (Fig. 1–11). Examine the teeth of several middle-aged persons. Probably you will find the enamel of the molar cusps worn so that the cusp tips are nearly flat. Sometimes the enamel is entirely worn off the cusp tips and the exposed dentin is seen as dark spots (Fig. 4–2). In the anterior teeth the incisal edges of the central and lateral incisors may be sufficiently worn so that dentin is seen as a fine dark line extending mesiodistally on the incisal

*Pronouced *pĕr ĭ kī′ màt àh*. peri (fr. Greek) = around; kymata (fr. Greek) = waves.

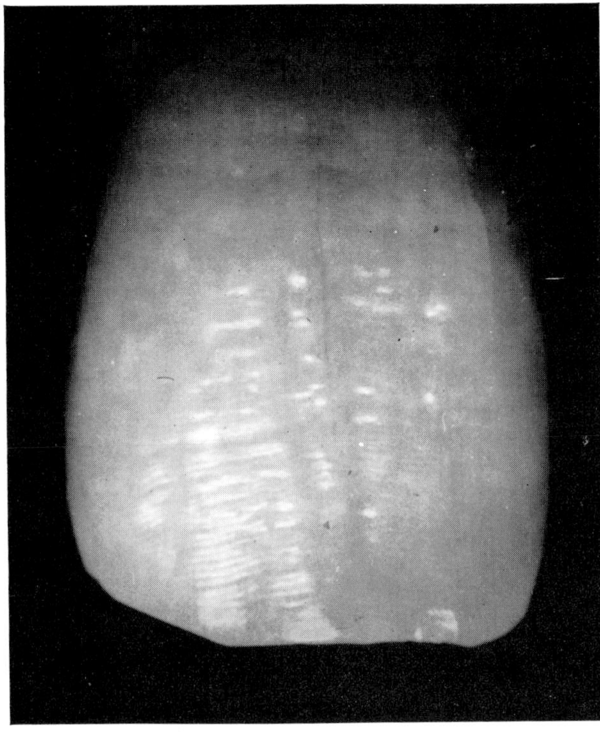

Fig. 4–1. Labial surface of maxillary central incisor. The horizontal lines are perikymata.

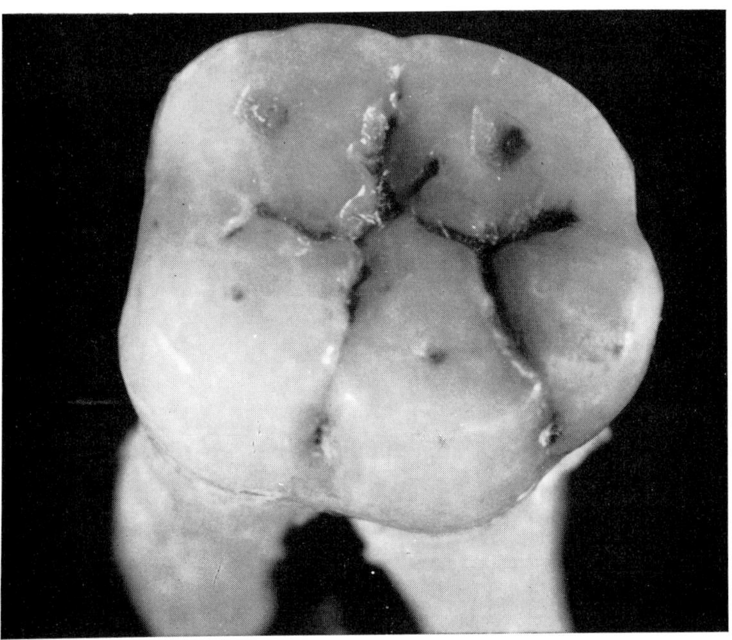

Fig. 4–2. Attrition has almost exposed the dentin on the two buccal and two lingual cusps of this mandibular first molar. There is no apparent attrition on the distal cusp. Notice the pits at the cervical ends of both the mesial and distal buccal grooves.

edge. These conditions of attrition in older individuals are not abnormal but are merely a natural aging process. Accompanying changes in the dentin beneath the worn enamel protect the tooth pulp from damage (Chapter 5, sclerotic and reparative dentin).

Examine the newly emerged incisor teeth of a six- or seven-year-old child. There are probably three prominences, or scallops, along the incisal edge. These prominences are called *mamelons.** They are developmental structures, but are ordinarily of no clinical importance. Usually they are worn off early in the life of the tooth (Fig. 4–3).

In an adult mouth look carefully at the posterior teeth and observe the *grooves* that mark the occlusal surface (Fig. 4–2). Grooves will also be found on the buccal surfaces of maxillary and mandibular molars (Fig. 3–32), on the lingual surfaces of maxillary molars, and sometimes on the lingual surfaces of maxillary and mandibular incisors. The depth of grooves varies: In some teeth they are shallow and smooth, in others they are extended into deep *fissures* (Frontispiece; Fig. 4–7). On occlusal surfaces the grooves and fissures may end in deep *pits* in the mesial and distal triangular fossae or in the central fossa. On the buccal and lingual surfaces the grooves may have a deep pit at their cervical end. It will be impossible to see, in examining the mouth, how deep such fissure are; and usually it will be impossible to insert even the smallest dental instrument or toothbrush bristle into them (Frontispiece; Figs. 4–4; 4–8). The pit or fissure does not extend into the dentin; it always ends in the enamel: there is always a little enamel, however thin, at the bottom of the pit or fissure. Enamel in

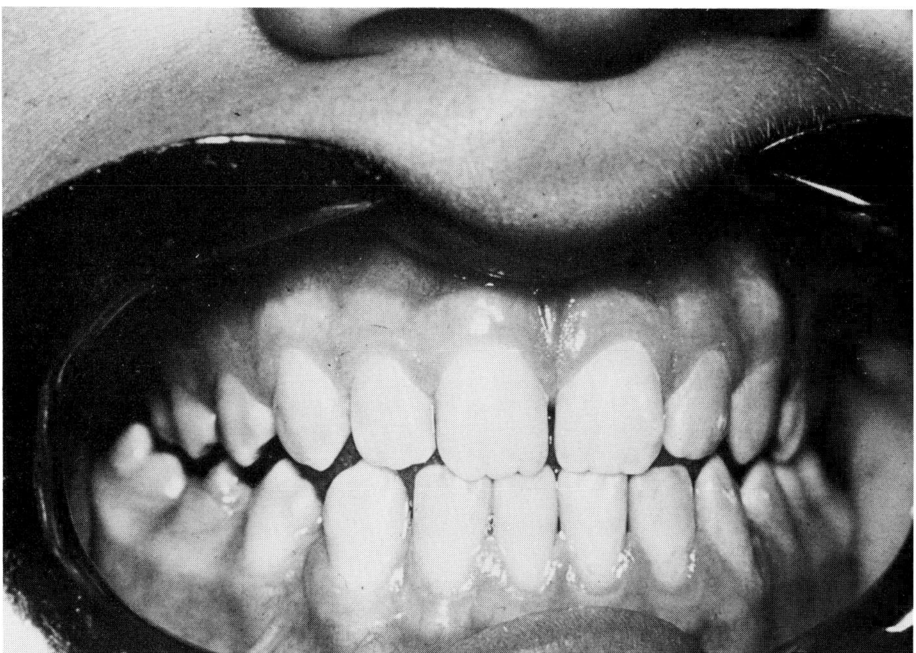

Fig. 4–3. This young subject shows three incisial prominences on the two maxillary central incisors. These are *mamelons.* Note that the mamelons of the left central are less pronounced; wear has taken place.

*Pronounced *măm ĕl ons.*

fissures is studied, of course, not by looking in the mouth, but by examination of ground sections of extracted teeth.*

In thickness the enamel varies in different parts of the tooth crown. At its thickest parts it may be 2 or 2.5 mm thick, while at the cervical line it thins to a knife edge. Examine Figures 1–11, 1–12, and 4–4 for an idea of the relative thickness of the enamel in different locations.

Enveloping the crown of the tooth, and adhering firmly to its surface, is the *enamel cuticle,* a covering which has been the subject of many studies since it was first described by Alexander Nasmyth in 1942. Early histologists called it *Nasmyth's membrane,* and this name is still sometimes used.

Through the years this crown covering has been described in ways so diverse that it seems certain that not one, but several substances were being observed. At different times it has been said to consist of cementum, of denatured hemoglobin, and of substances from saliva. The nature of what Nasmyth saw is not clear, and probably it would be better to refer to the covering, whatever it is, not as Nasmyth's membrane, but as *enamel cuticle.*†

Enamel cuticle is actually two cuticles: *primary enamel cuticle* and *secondary enamel cuticle.* Primary enamel cuticle is the last product of the enamel-forming cells (*ameloblasts,* described in Chapter 3), and it becomes mineralized. Secondary enamel cuticle is a product of the reduced enamel epithelum (Chapter 3), and it does not become mineralized. The secondary enamel cuticle (also called *dental*

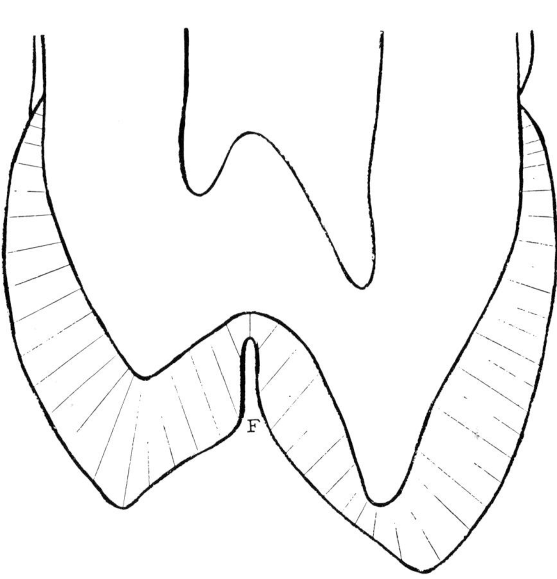

Fig. 4–4. Diagrammatic drawing of a longitudinal faciolingual section of the crown of a maxillary first premolar tooth. The lines in the enamel illustrate the general direction of the enamel rods. Notice the narrowness of the fissure (F) and the thinness of the enamel at the bottom of the fissure. Notice also the radiating pattern of the enamel rods in the fissure.

*Gillings, B., and M. Buonocore: Thickness of Enamel at the Base of Pits and Fissures in Human Molars and Biscuspids. J. Dent. Res., *401*:119, 1961.

†Permar, D.: Our Old Friend, Nasmyth's Membrane. J. Am. Dent. Hyg. Assoc. First Quarter, *44*:31–33, 1970.

cuticle) is the outermost layer and it probably wears away after a period of tooth use.*

The dental cuticle is structurally described as a *basal lamina.* It is similar in appearance to the basal lamina part of basement membranes found at the junction of epithelial and connective tissues (see Chapter 1).

MICROSCOPIC STRUCTURE OF ENAMEL

Enamel can be studied by various methods. With an ordinary microscope you can examine thin ground sections of extracted teeth and see in their natural relationship the organic and inorganic substances that constitute enamel. Or the organic portion, the matrix, which is in the form of a delicate framework, can be examined separately by using special careful techniques to dissolve away the mineral substances. In recent years the electron microscope has enabled the histologist to study enamel and other tissues at magnifications of the order of 5,000× to 160,000×.

Tooth enamel is made up of minute *rods*† which extend from the dentinoenamel junction toward the outer surface of the enamel. They are arranged roughly perpendicular to the dentinoenamel junction (Fig. 4–4). Seldom are the rods perfectly straight; in some parts of the tooth they have multiple curvatures. It has been estimated that a human maxillary central incisor contains 8,586,000 enamel rods, and that a maxillary first molar contains 12,297,000 rods. The average diameter of a rod is about 4 μm (micrometers). Each enamel rod seems to be composed of a series of small units that fit together in a row somewhat like a string of beads (Fig. 4–5). This segmented construction is a result of the manner of formation of the rods.

Each enamel rod appears to be encased in a *rod sheath,* and the sheathed rods seem to be cemented together by an *interrod substance.* Of these three structures, the rods are the most highly mineralized, the cementing substance is slightly less mineralized than the rods, and the rod sheaths are slightly less mineralized than the cementing substance. However, all three are extremely hard. The organic substance which they contain has been shown by the electron microscope to be in the form of a fine fibrillar latticework. This latticework, or framework, of the rods, rod sheaths, and interrod substance is the *organic matrix* of the enamel. In suitable preparations this matrix may be examined with an ordinary microscope, but the fibrils of which it is composed are so minute that its fibrillar character can be seen only by the use of the electron microscope.

The entire organic substance of enamel is only about 4% of its composition. The other 96% of enamel is mineral substance which exists in the form of tightly packed *submicroscopic crystals* (Fig. 4–6). These crystals fill the loose organic matrix. Their size is appreciated when we learn that they are measured in terms of millionths of a millimeter.

Chemically, the organic matrix of enamel has not been fully determined. This is probably due to the small percentage available for analysis and its close chemical bond to the inorganic material. There is some agreement that it is a lacy network of proteins known as *enamelins.*

The chemical nature of the inorganic part has been extensively studied. It is generally agreed to be a crystalline calcium phosphate known as *hydroxyapatite.*

*Carranza F. *Glickman's Clinical Periodontology,* 6th ed. Philadephia, W.B. Saunders Co., 1984.
†Another name for an *enamel rod* is *enamel prism.*

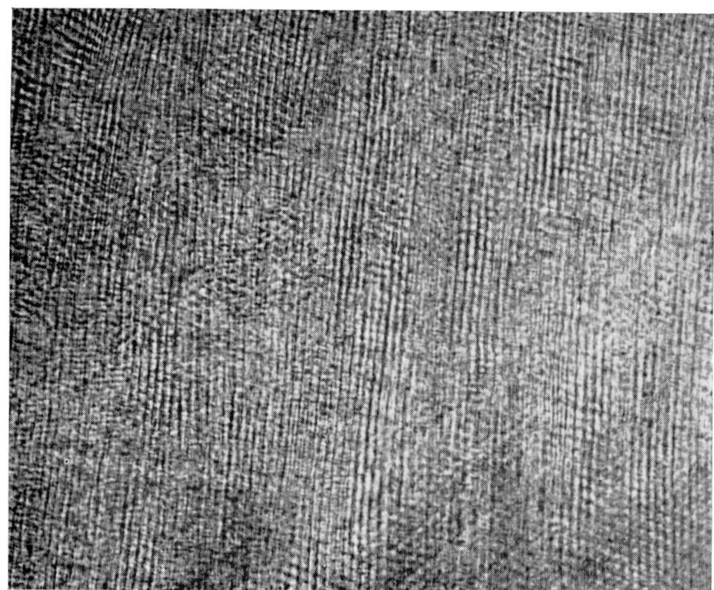

Fig. 4–5. Photomicrograph (high power) of a ground section of human enamel showing the rods extending from the dentinoenamel junction toward the tooth surface. The rods extend from top to bottom of the picture and in this area are nearly straight. The cross striations in the rods are discernible.

In Figure 4–7 the electron micrograph of a replica of human enamel reveals rod outlines. Most of the submicroscopic crystals have been dissolved by the acid-etching which was part of the process of preparation of the specimen. What is seen in the picture is the organic matrix of the enamel.

The student interested in learning more about the ultrastructure of enamel should have the pleasure and satisfaction of starting with a recently published paper and, following its bibliography, tracing the development of the subject back to its beginning.*

Examination with an ordinary microscope of a thin ground tooth section reveals other formations in enamel: *bands of Hunter-Schreger*, *stripes of Retzius*, *enamel lamellae*, *enamel tufts*, and *enamel spindles*. Some of these formations are of little known clinical importance, while others are of great importance.

Bands of Hunter-Schreger are seen when a longitudinal ground section of a tooth crown is examined by reflected light under the low power of the microscope (Fig. 4–8). They are alternating broad light and dark bands which extend per-

*Interesting papers:

Meckel, A.H., W.J., Griebstein, and R.J. Neal: Structure of Mature Human Dental Enamel as Observed by Electron Microscopy. Arch. Oral Biol., *10*:775, 1965.

Poole, D.F.G., and N.W. Johnson: Effects of Different Demineralizing Agents on Human Enamel Surfaces Studied by the Scanning Electron Microscope. Arch. Oral Biol., *12*:1621, 1967.

Hoffman S., W.S. McEwan, and C.M. Drew: Scanning Electron Microscope Studies of Dental Enamel. J. Dent. Res. *48*:242, 1969.

Johnson N.W., D.F. Poole, and J.E. Tyler: Factors Affecting the Differential Dissolution of Human Enamel in Acid and EDTA. Arch. Oral Biol., *16*:385, 1971.

Simmelink, J.W., V.K. Nygaard, and D.B. Scott: Theory for the Sequence of Human and Rat Enamel Dissolution by Acid and by EDTA: A Correlation Scanning and Transmission Electron Miscrope Study. Arch. Oral Biol., *19*:183, 1974.

Hirota, F.: Prism Arrangement in Human Cusp Enamel Deduced by X-Ray Diffraction. Arch. Oral Biol., *27*:931, 1982.

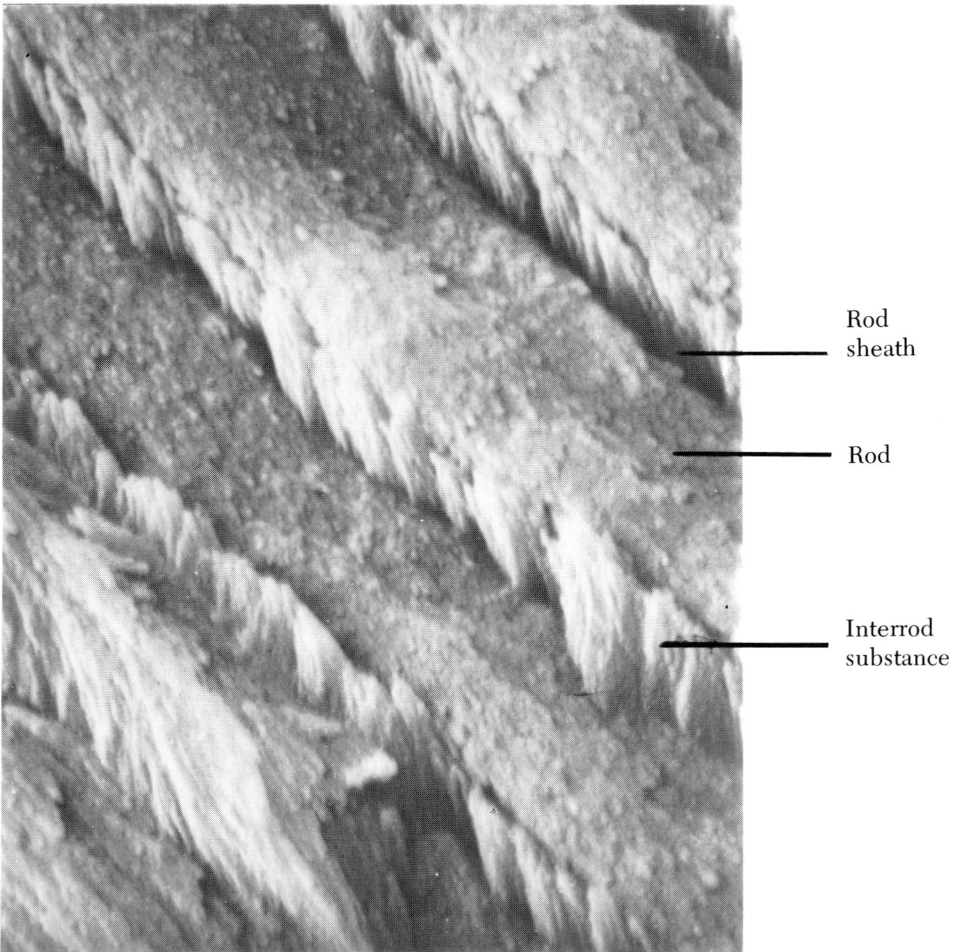

Fig. 4–6. A. Scanning electron micrograph of freeze fractured enamel of a deciduous central incisor. Here, the arrangement and orientation of the apatite crystals can be seen. Note the tight packing of the crystals of the rods and their orientation along the long axis of the rods. Also note in the interrod areas, the slightly less packing of the crystals and their almost perpendicular orientation to the rods. Magnification ×5250. (Courtesy Dr. Ruth Paulson, College of Dentistry, The Ohio State University.)

pendicularly from the dentinoenamel junction toward the tooth surface. Their manifestation is due to the curvature of the enamel rods. In one band the rods are so oriented that they are seen in longitudinal plane; in the adjacent band, as a result of the rod curvatures, they are seen in transverse plane. This pattern can be seen also in a histologic section of a developing tooth which has been processed in such a way that the matrix of the forming enamel has been retained; and it can be seen in specially prepared fully formed enamel examined with the electron microscope (Fig. 4–9). Admittedly, the pattern of curvature of a single rod is difficult to visualize.

The *stripes of Retzius* are a different kind of bands, or lines, in the enamel. In longitudinal ground sections of the tooth crown they are seen under the low power of the microscope as narrow brownish lines extending diagonally outward from the dentinoenamel junction toward the occlusal, or incisal, part of the

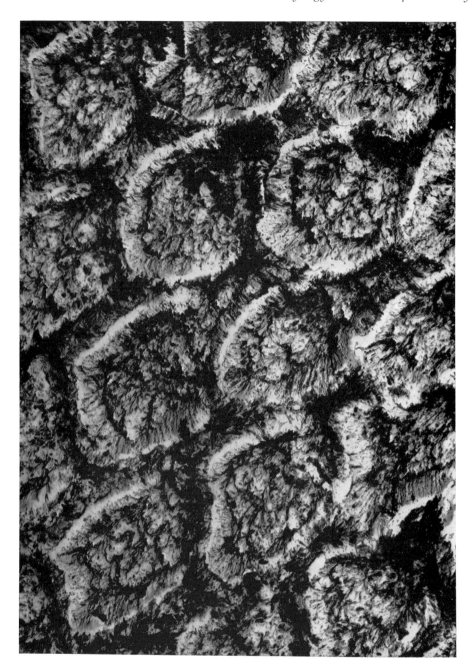

Fig. 4–7. Electron micrograph of a shadowed replica of the end of enamel rods at the buccal surface of a mature human incisor. The clean enamel surface was first lightly acid-etched; then a nitrocellulose film in a softened state was placed over the etched surface. When the dried film was removed, it of course carried the image of the etched surface. This film, called the *replica,* was shadowed at an angle of 40° with a palladium and gold alloy which gave it contrast and a third dimensional character by creating lights and shadows. The original magnification of the electron micrograph of the shadowed replica was ×3,400.

What is seen here is interpreted to be organic matrix of the enamel; most of the mineral substance was removed by the earlier acid-etching. The rods are seen in end view, but there is no way of knowing how near to an exact cross section of the rods we are seeing. The broad white band around each rod conforms to what is considered the rod sheath, and the substance between the rods is interpreted as the interrod substance. (Courtesy Dr. Dennis Foreman, College of Dentistry, The Ohio State University.)

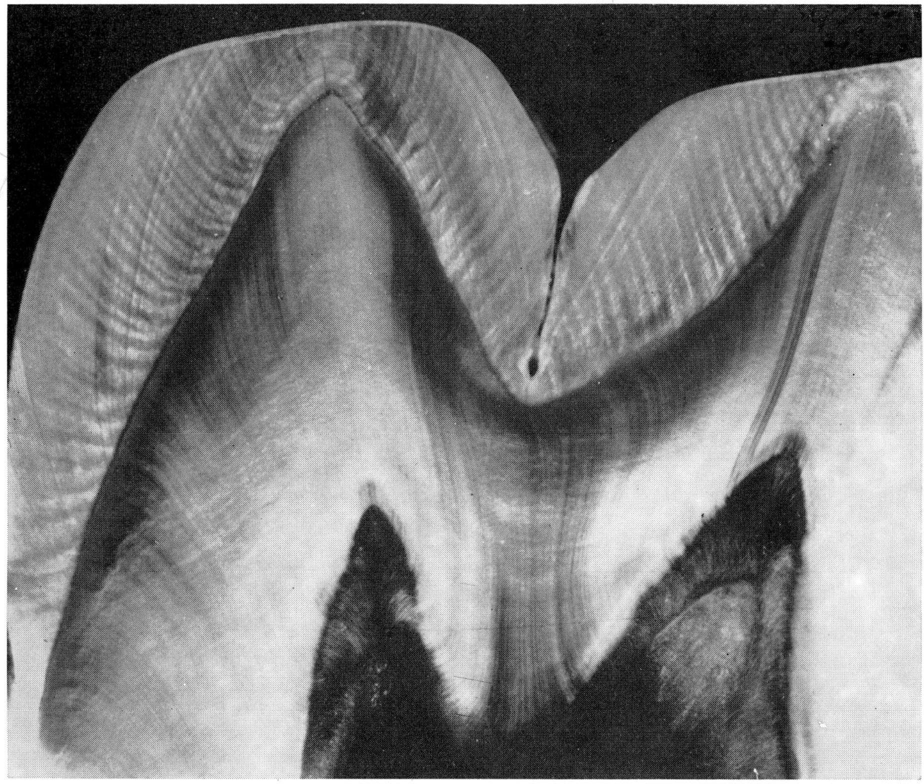

Fig. 4–8. Ground section cut buccolingually through a mandibular molar. In the enamel the dark and light bands of Hunter-Schreger extend from the dentinoenamel junction to the enamel surface nearly perpendicular to the dentinoenamel junction. The stripes of Retzius are faintly visible, starting at the dentinoenamel junction and extending outward and occlusally, reaching the enamel surface excepting near the cusp tip (see Fig. 1–14). In this tooth there is some attrition on the cusp tips. Considering the magnification of this picture, it is clear that the fissure is too narrow to permit the insertion of any dental instrument. The enamel at the bottom of the fissure is thin. It shows no sign of caries. See Figure 4–9.

crown (Figs. 1–13; 4–8; 4–10). These lines are formed during the development of the enamel matrix as a result of the layer-upon-layer pattern of enamel matrix formation. They are due to variations in structure and calcification along the lines corresponding to the formation pattern.* On most of the crown the stripes of Retzius end on the crown surface, and their termination on the surface is marked by a series of shallow depressions. The ridges between the depressions are called the *perikymata* (Fig. 4–1). (It is difficult to see in ground tooth sections this association between perikymata and the stripes of Retzius.) Near the incisal or occlusal part of the crown the stripes of Retzius do not reach the enamel surface and therefore there are no perikymata at the incisal edge or cusp tips. Perikymata often may be seen in clinical examination (Fig. 4–1).

Enamel lamellae (literally the word means *little layers*) have been described by some histologists as faults in enamel matrix formation and by others as cracks in the enamel due to injury. Certainly they are microscopic separations in the

*Osborn, J.W.: A Relationship Between the Striae of Retzius and Prism Direction in the Transverse Plane of the Human Tooth. Arch. Oral Biol., *16*:1061, 1971.

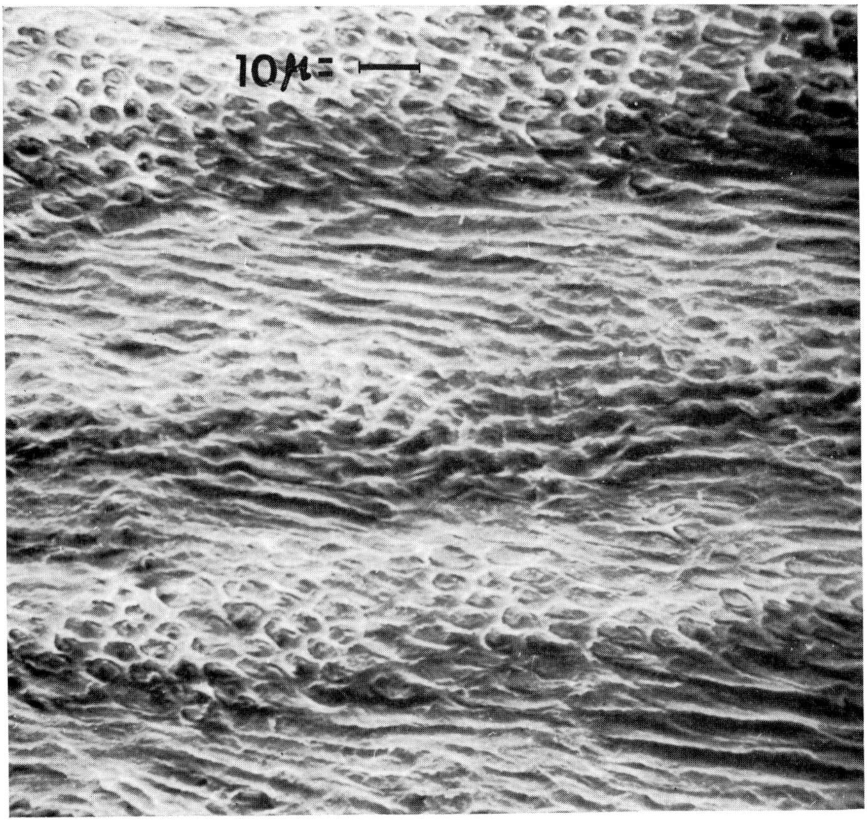

Fig. 4–9. Hunter-Schreger bands in human enamel as seen with a scanning electron microscope. This freeze-fracture specimen from a premolar was taken from an area similar to about the center of the crown on the left side of Figure 4–8. Original magnification ×450. (Courtesy Dr. Ruth Paulson, College of Dentistry, The Ohio State University.)

enamel which extend inward from the enamel surface for varying distances and which are filled with organic material (Figs. 4–11; 4–12).

Enamel tufts also are visible in ground tooth sections. Microscopically they look like small brushes attached to the dentinoenamel junction and extending outward in the enamel to perhaps as much as a fifth of the distance to the surface (Figs. 4–13; 4–14). Histologically they are hypomineralized, or unmineralized, inner ends of some groups of enamel rods, with their rod sheaths and surrounding interrod substance.*

Enamel spindles are peripheral ends of cytoplasmic processes of certain pulp cells (odontoblasts) that extend across the dentinoenamel junction a short distance into the enamel (Figs. 4–16; 4–17; 4–18). Their relationship with the dentin will be understood when you study the structure of dentin.

The *dentinoenamel junction* in many teeth is not a straight line, but rather a scalloped line in which small curved projections of enamel fit into small concavities of the dentin (Fig. 4–15).

*Interesting paper:
Paulson, R.B.: Scanning Electron Microscopy of Enamel Tuft Development in Human Deciduous Teeth. Arch. Oral Biol., *26*:103, 1981.

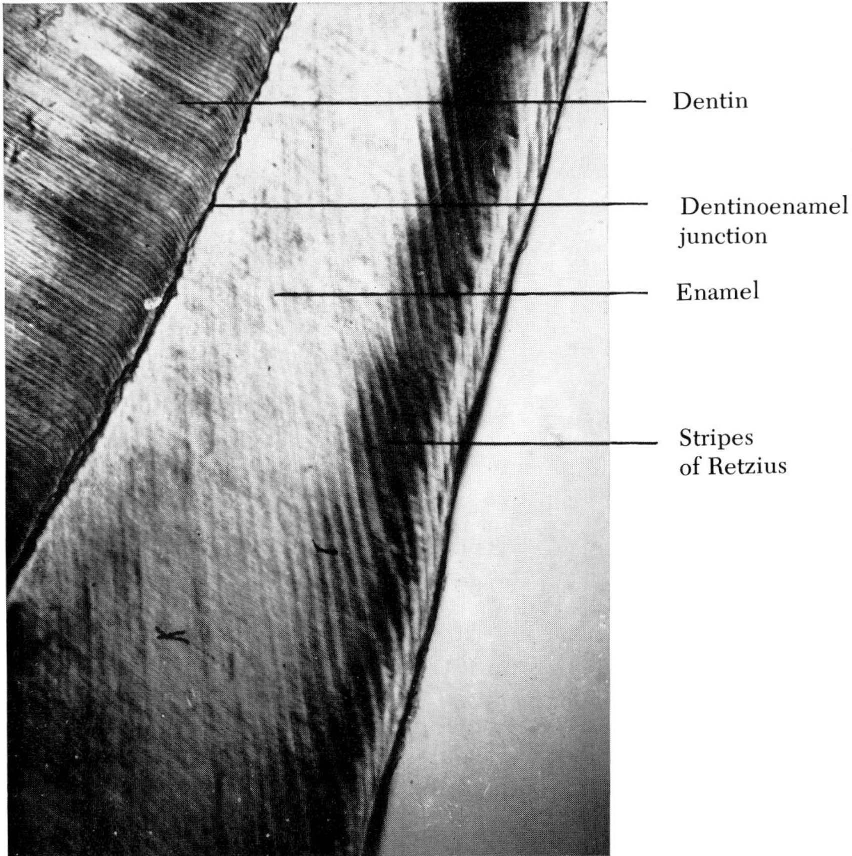

Fig. 4–10. Photomicrograph of a small area of tooth crown cut longitudinally. Stripes of Retzius in the enamel are clearly visible. The direction of the dentinal tubules can also be seen. (Occlusal surface toward bottom of picture; root toward top.)

Enamel contains no cells; it is a product of specialized epithelial cells (ameloblasts). It has no circulation in the form of blood vessels or other structures, but that it is permeable to some substances has been demonstrated in studies using dyes and solutions of radioactive substances.

PERMANENCE OF ENAMEL

Once tooth enamel is formed the mineralization is never decreased by any physiologic process within the tooth. All present evidence indicates that mineral substance is not withdrawn from enamel once it has been deposited there. The notion that pregnancy produces a physiologic withdrawal of calcium from the teeth of the mother is not supported by factual evidence.

Enamel has no possibility of anatomic self-repair following damage by injury or by caries. In the study of tooth eruption it will be seen that the ameloblasts which form the enamel in the developing tooth are lost when the tooth emerges into the mouth, making subsequent enamel formation impossible.

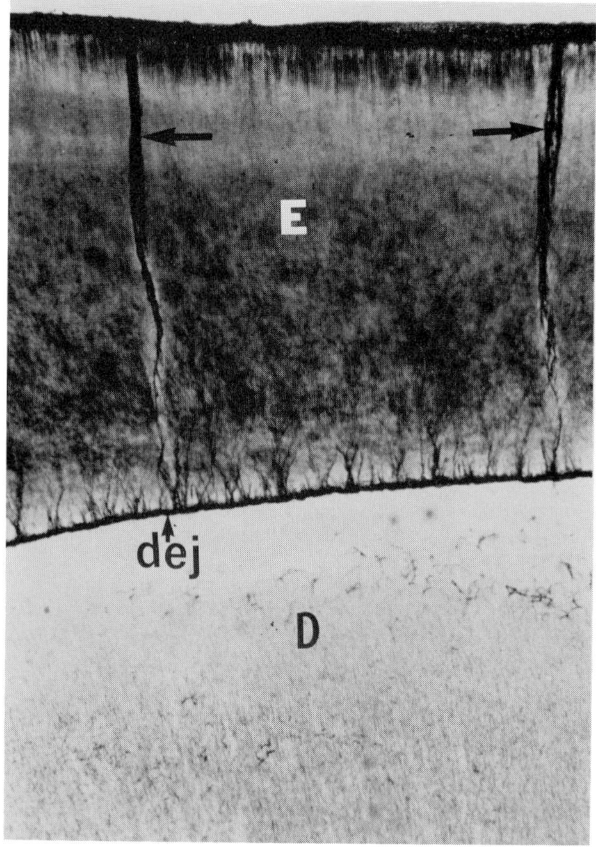

Fig. 4–11. Photomicrograph of a ground section of a portion of a crown showing two enamel lamellae (arrows) extending from the surface into the enamel (E). Dentinoenamel junction (dej). Dentin (D).

CLINICAL IMPORTANCE OF THE STRUCTURE OF ENAMEL

Let us now consider how the character of tooth enamel may affect the clinical condition of the individual.

The high mineral content of enamel makes it a very hard substance which is resistant to, but not proof against, attrition (Figs. 1–11; 4–8). On the incisal edges of anterior teeth and on the cusp tips of posterior teeth, where the teeth of opposing arches meet forcefully in occlusion, attrition may be sufficient to expose the underlying dentin (Fig. 4–3; 4–19).

The microscopic anatomy of enamel in many ways determines the strength and life of a tooth: curvatures of the enamel rods increase its resistance to breakage; areas of low mineralization influence the pattern and speed of progress of caries; and the arrangement of the rods gives direction to the path of pene-

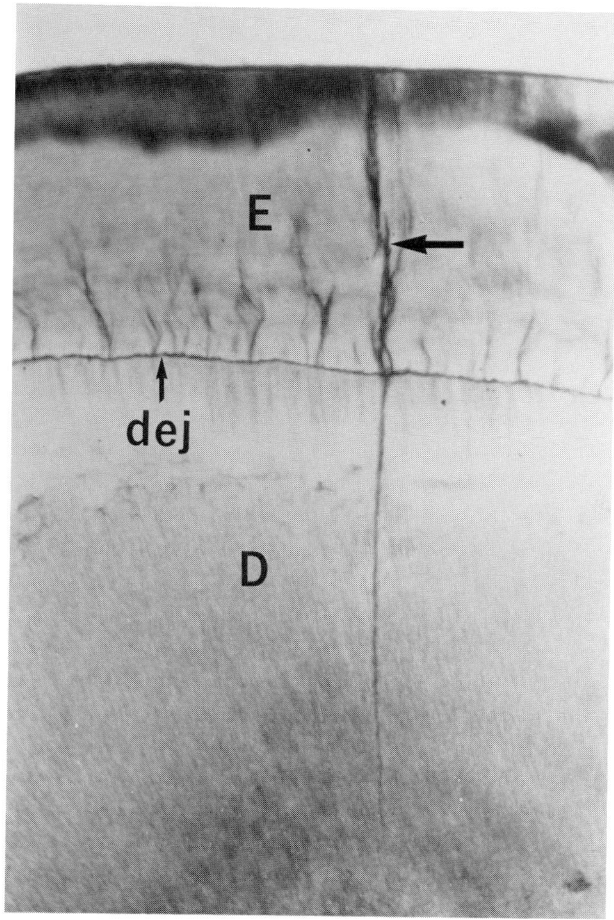

Fig. 4–12. An enamel lamella (arrow) in this ground section, extends from the enamel (E) surface, crosses the dentinoenamel junction (dej) and passes into the dentin (D). Compare to the enamel lamella of Figure 4–11.

tration of caries.* *Perikymata,* which mark the enamel on all surfaces of the crown, are of no known clinical significance.

Bands of Hunter-Schreger, seen in ground sections of a tooth, are an optical phenomenon produced by curvatures in the enamel rods. These curvatures probably reduce the chance of cleavage (splitting) of enamel along the rod length.

Enamel lamellae are believed by some investigators to be areas particularly susceptible to caries.

Stripes of Retzius, areas of slightly less mineralization, facilitate to some degree the lateral spread of caries along the line of each stripe. However, this spread

---

*Interesting papers:

Sognnaes, R.: Reflections on the Reactivity of Dental Enamel. J. Dent. Res. *54*(Special Issue B):B106, 1975.

Kerckaert, G.A.: Electron Microscopy of Human Carious Dental Enamel. Arch. Oral Biol. *18*(6):751, 1973.

Mendis, B.R.R.N. and Darling A.I.: A Scanning Electron Microscope and Microradiographic Study of Closure of Human Coronal Dentinal Tubules Related to Occlusal Attrition and Caries. Arch. Oral Biol. *24*(10–11):725, 1979.

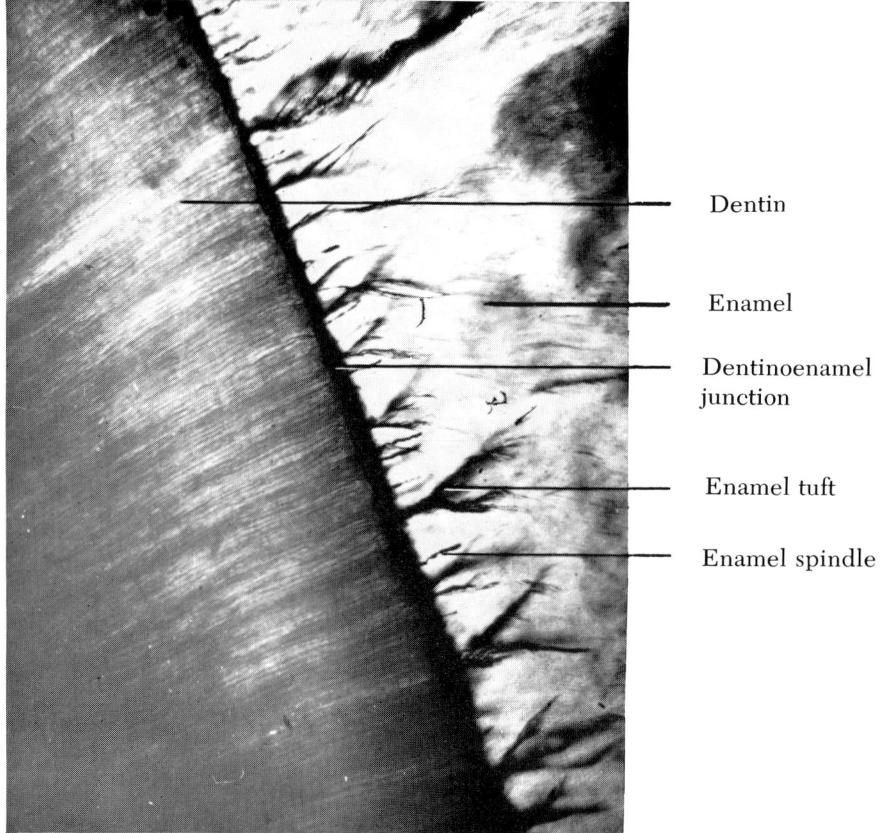

Fig. 4–13. Photomicrograph of a small area of tooth crown cut horizontally. The enamel tufts are clearly visible. Among the tufts, in some places, are seen the much smaller enamel spindles. (As seen under low power magnification.) See Figure 4–14 for a higher magnification.

is considerably less pronounced than the lateral spread of caries that occurs at the dentinoenamel junction in areas of tufts and spindles.

Enamel tufts and enamel spindles, being hypomineralized areas, offer reduced resistance to caries, and a lesion will often spread horizontally in the enamel at the dentinoenamel junction. When the damaging agent enters the dentin, lateral spread of caries is still more extensive.

The arrangement of the enamel rods has an important influence on the pattern of penetration of caries in enamel; and the *configuration of the dentinoenamel junction* determines the pattern of arrangement of the rods—as we shall see later.

DENTAL CARIES PROCESS*

To understand the role of tooth structure in the occurrence and pattern of dental caries, it is necessary to understand the nature of this disease. Dental caries is a disease of the hard tissues of the teeth in which the mineral substance of the tooth is dissolved by acid and the then-exposed organic substance is

*A word about the term *dental caries: Caries* is the correct form of the word. You may say that a person has caries; or that he has a carious tooth; or that he has a cavity in a tooth. Or you may say that caries *is* (singular verb) present in a mouth. But you never say a person has "a carie" —any more than you say a person has a *measle* or a *mump*.

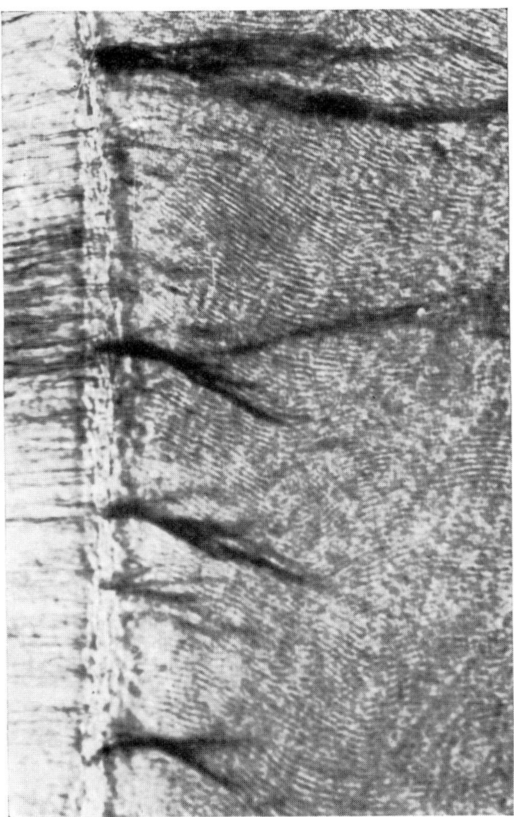

Fig. 4–14. Photomicrograph of a ground section of enamel in an area of enamel tufts. This is a higher magnification of an area similar to that shown in Figure 4–13.

destroyed by proteolysis. The acid is created by the kinds of oral bacteria which, in the process of their metabolism, convert carbohydrates, especially sugars, into acids. Caries-susceptible individuals have in their saliva and in their dental plaques large numbers of these acidogenic (acid-producing) bacteria.

The bacteria which cause the damage are the ones which are located in the dental plaques. A *dental plaque* is a dense accumulation of microorganisms which adheres firmly to the surface of a tooth. In mouths kept ordinarily clean, plaques are found chiefly in protected areas—around contact areas, and in pits and fissures (Fig. 4–20).

A known sequence of events follows the oral intake of sugar by a caries-susceptible person: Food taken into the mouth is retained in the area of the plaque; the acidogenic bacteria of the plaque reduce the sugars to acids; the acids in the plaque are in contact with the tooth surface to which the plaque is attached; and since tooth enamel is soluble in acid, the enamel beneath the plaque is slightly dissolved. This is the beginning of a caries lesion. Repeated eating of sugar results in repeated periods of enamel dissolution.

The manner in which the enamel is destroyed by acid is becoming better understood as studies with electron microscopy progress. The long, narrow submicroscopic crystals that make up the mineral phase of enamel seem to be most readily dissolved when acid attacks them from their ends. The crystals in

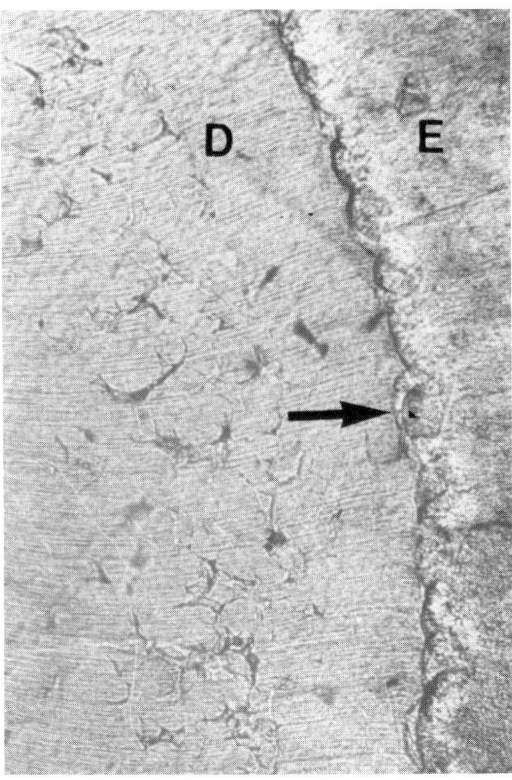

Fig. 4–15. This is a ground section of an area of dentin (D) and enamel (E) along the scalloped appearing dentinoenamel junction (arrow).

the center of each rod are arranged with their long axes parallel to the long axis of the rod. The rods are arranged, generally speaking, perpendicular to the dentinoenamel junction. The relationship of crystal orientation relative to the rod axes, the rod orientation relative to the dentioenamel junction, and the configuration of the dentinoenamel junction determine the pattern of a caries lesion. The whole question of the mechanism of dental caries has been, and is, under study by many people. Answers presently accepted are subject to change as research progresses.*

SMOOTH SURFACE CARIES

Let us first consider a caries attack on the smooth facial, lingual, or proximal surface of a tooth. The dentinoenamel junction in these locations is straight or broadly convex; the rods, although they have curvatures, extend toward the surface in a direction generally perpendicular to the dentinoenamel junction (Fig. 4–4). Therefore, a lesion occurring around a contact area, for instance, penetrates more or less in a straight line toward the dentinoenamel junction.

---

*Interesting papers:

Scott, D.B., J.W. Simmelink, and V. Nygaard: Structural Aspects of Dental Caries. J. Dent. Res., *53*:165, 1974.

Gustafson, G., and B. Sundstrom: Enamel: Morphological Considerations. J. Dent. Res., *54*:B114, 1975.

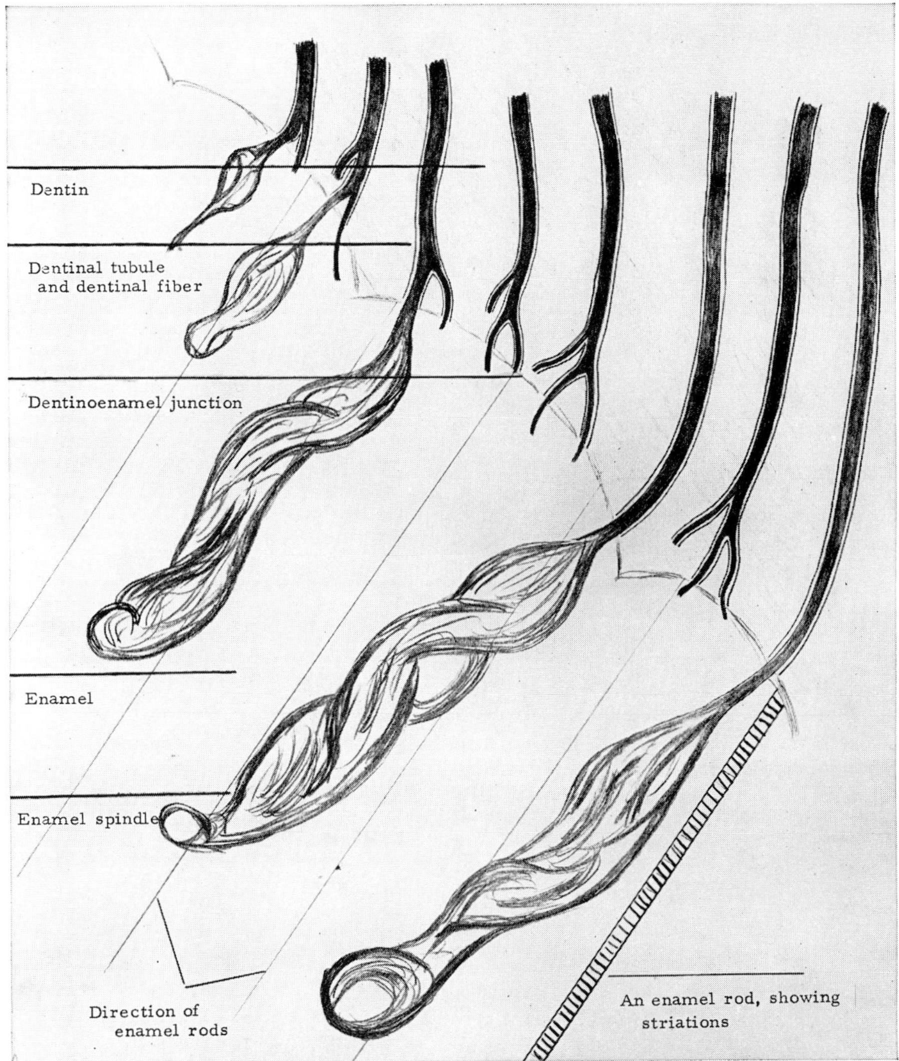

Fig. 4–16. Diagrammatic drawing of details of area A in Figure 1–12 showing enamel spindles.

PIT AND FISSURE CARIES

Particularly prone to caries are the grooves, fissures, and pits of the posterior teeth. While teeth without fissures and pits (Figs. 4–20 and 4–21) often—not always—remain intact in their shallow grooves, teeth with fissures and pits have in the depths of these narrow depressions an ideal environment for the growth of microorganisms. Although the fissure or pit may be so narrow and so deep that even the smallest dental instrument cannot be inserted to the bottom (Figs. 4–8; 4–22; 4–23; 4–24), it still permits the entrance of microorganisms and food into this sheltered, warm, moist, richly provided incubator, and a dental plaque can be expected to form here (Figs. 4–23; 4–24). In a caries-susceptible person, when sugar is eaten and comes in contact with the plaque, acid is created by

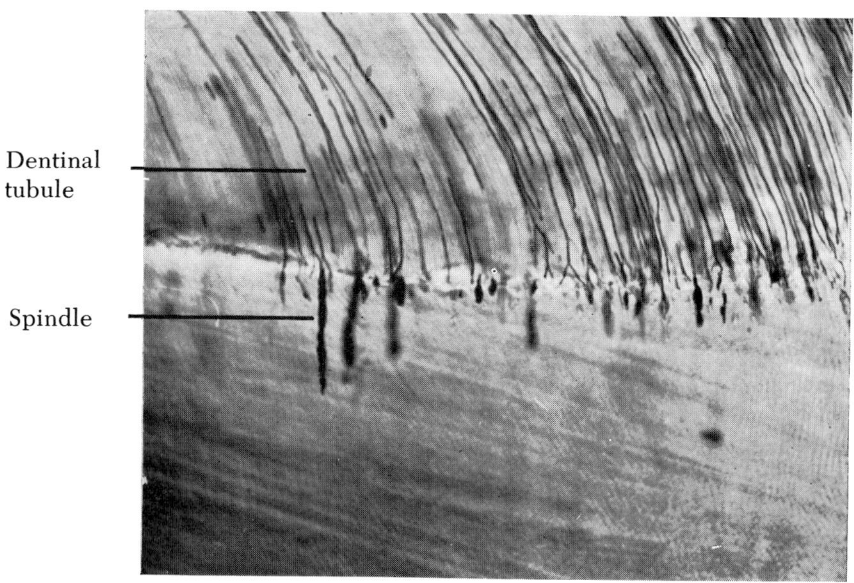

Fig. 4–17. Photomicrograph of a ground section of a tooth crown near the cusp tip. Dentin is at the top of the picture, enamel is below. Many enamel spindles are seen in the enamel. Branching of the dentinal tubules is clear. Compare with Figure 4–18.

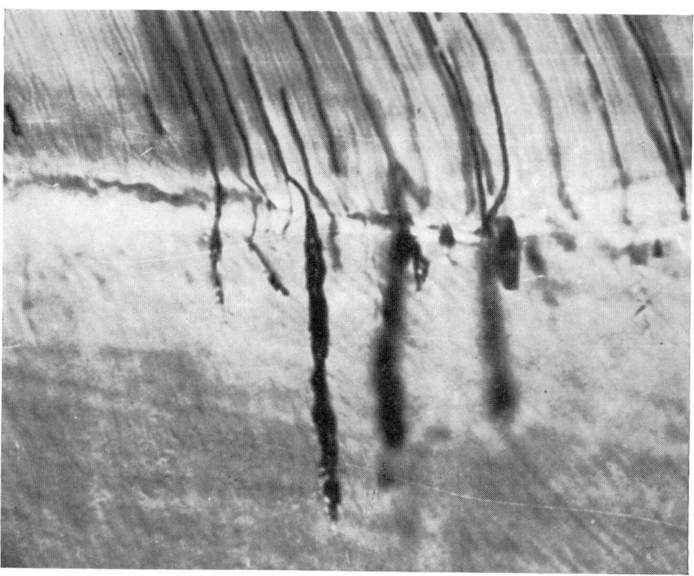

Fig. 4–18. An enlargement of the spindles seen in Figure 4–17. It is possible to see that the spindle is a continuation of the odontoblastic process.

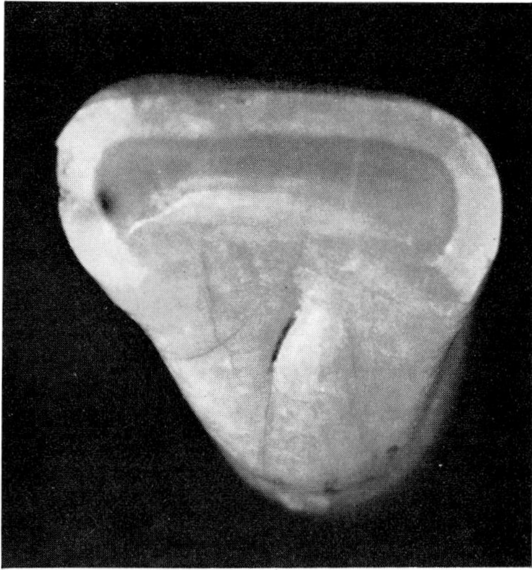

Fig. 4–19. An extracted maxillary left central incisor photographed from the incisal aspect. The facial surface is toward the top. Attrition on the incisal edge has exposed the dentin. This edge was not ground off; this is the result of wear from the friction of use. Notice the thickness of the enamel. The caries lesion showing in the dentin on the mesial side (to the left) started on the enamel surface around the mesial contact area. A diagonally placed groove can be seen on the cingulum.

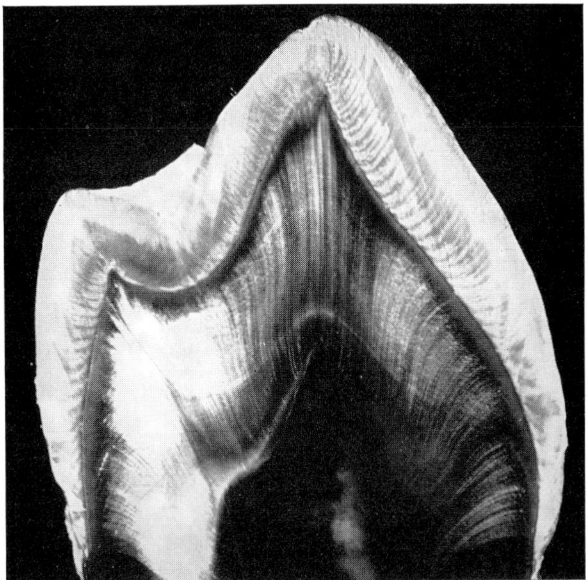

Fig. 4–20. Ground section cut buccolingually through a mandibular first premolar. The groove on the occlusal surface of the tooth is not deep, and there is no fissure at the bottom of it. No caries is present in this groove. A plaque is retained in the groove. If the plaque is mineralized, it is called calculus. Notice the direction of the dentinal tubules which extend from the dentinoenamel junction to the pulp chamber (Chapter 5).

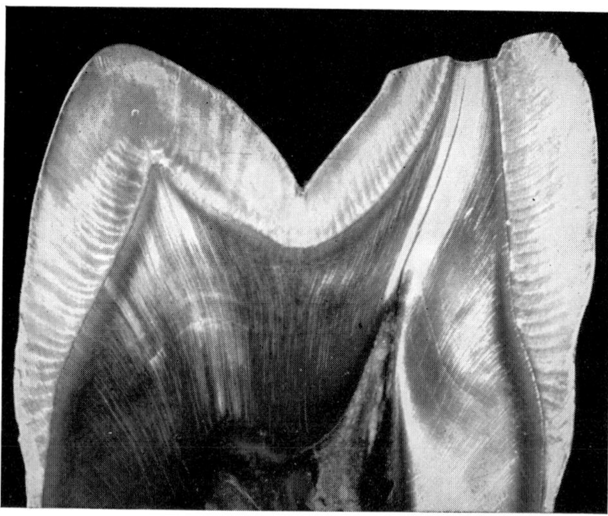

Fig. 4–21. Ground section of a molar. The groove on the occlusal surface does not have a fissure at the bottom of it. No dental caries is present in the groove. Notice the direction of the dentinal tubules. The pulp horn extends far into the cusp (Chapter 6).

acidogenic bacteria in the plaque and this acid damages the enamel walls of the pit or fissure. Caries result.

In occlusal fissures or pits the form of a caries lesion is different from that of a smooth surface lesion. Here the enamel rods still lie nearly perpendicular to the dentinoenamel junction, but the sharp concavity of the junction in this location results in a radial pattern, a fanning out, of rods (Figs. 4–4; 4–23). Seldom does one see, in microscopic examination of a tooth section, a caries

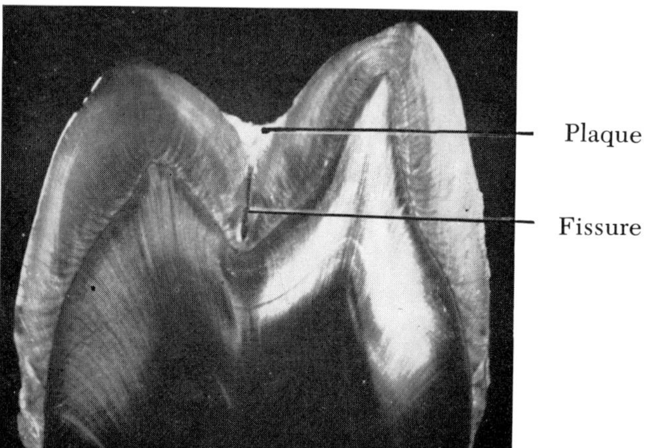

Fig. 4–22. Ground section through a maxillary first premolar cut buccolingually. The central groove has a deep fissure at its base. The thin enamel at the bottom of the fissure seems to be intact, but the appearance of the dentin immediately beneath it suggests that caries was present in the fissure at one side or the other of the section here seen, and that the lesion had spread near the dentinoenamel junction, undermining the sound surface enamel. A dense plaque is present in the groove, but in this particular area it seems not to be dense enough within the *fissure* to be visible in the photomicrograph.

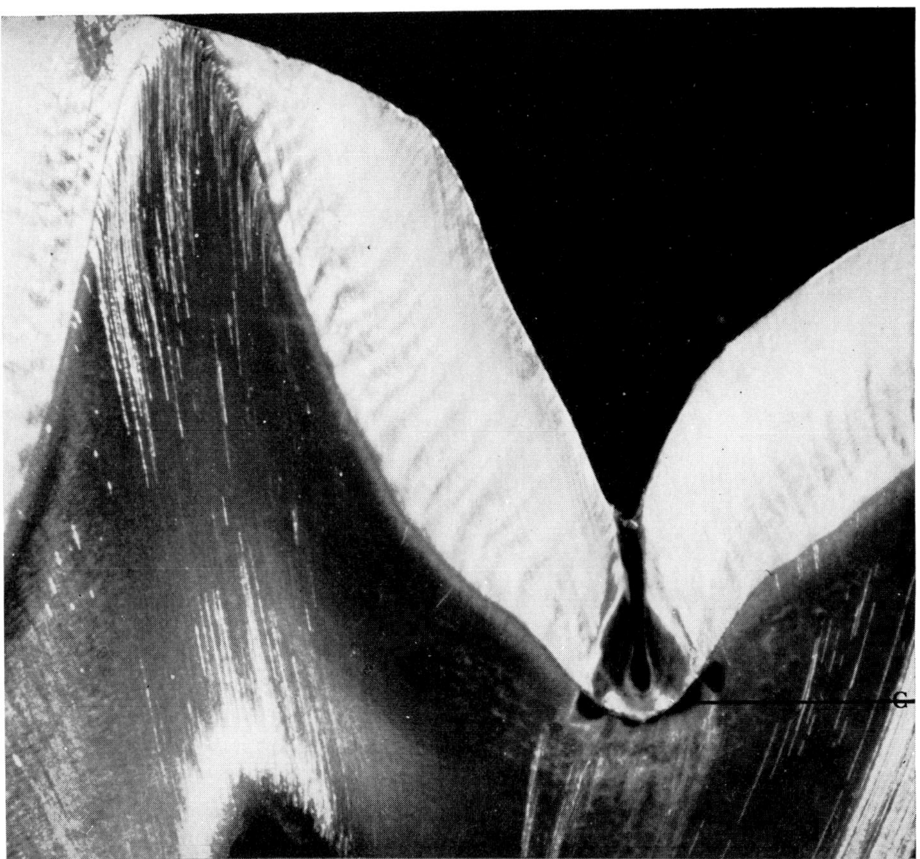

Fig. 4–23. Ground section of a molar. The fissure in the occlusal groove clearly is affected by dental caries. Notice the radiating pattern of the lesion in the enamel near the bottom of the fissure. This is due to the fanning out of the enamel rods. (See Figure 4–4.) The dentin beneath the bottom of the fissure is destroyed near the dentinoenamel junction (C), leaving the enamel unsupported. There is little evidence of sclerosis of the dentin beneath this lesion. The bacteria here have probably penetrated well into the dentinal tubules (Chapter 5). The plaque is indistinctly seen in this ground section. Often plaques are destroyed in the process of grinding a specimen. Notice attrition on the cusp tip.

lesion at the bottom of a fissure that has not an acute angle at the occlusal surface and a broad curved base at the dentinoenemal junction, (Fig. 4–23). The result is a deceptive clinical picture. Clinical examination may reveal only a small carious area visible in a groove; but at the dentinoenamel junction, invisible without x-ray pictures, the broadening of the lesion has left the surface enamel unsupported (Figs. 4–24; 4–25; 4–26).

While fissures and pits are commonly thought of as occurring on occlusal surfaces of molar and premolar teeth, they are found also in other places. In some molar teeth pits are found at the cervical end of buccal grooves (Figs. 3–32; 4–3). Examine Figure 4–26A, B. The pit at the end of the buccal groove (Fig. 4–26A) has a caries lesion, not obvious from the outside, that penetrates some distance into the dentin (Fig. 4–26B).

Again, at the junction of the cusp of Carabelli and the mesiolingual cusp of

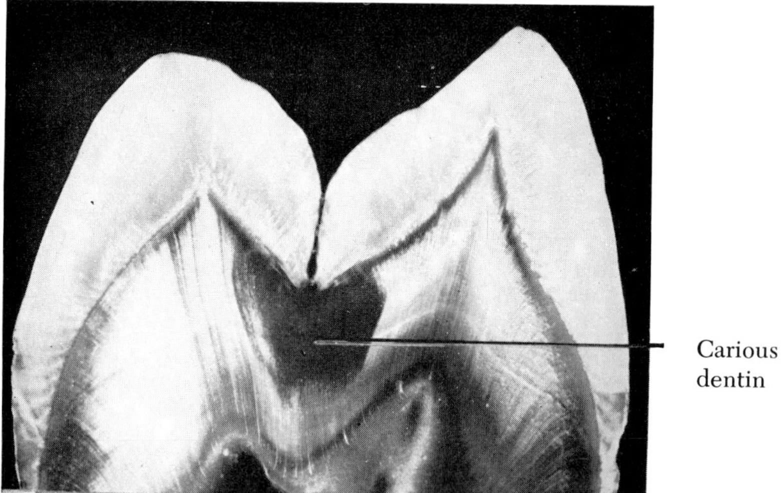

Fig. 4–24. Ground section of a molar tooth. In this tooth the caries started in the enamel at the bottom of the fissure spread along the dentinoenamel junction. In this area the lesion has visibly penetrated the dentin, and the effect of caries is seen in the dentin over a broad area of the dentinoenamel junction and pulpward. The dark region in the dentin beneath the fissure, broad near the dentinoenamel junction and more narrow nearer the pulp, is carious dentin (see Chapter 5). Caries will spread downward, destroying the unaffected dentin beneath it and around it. Destruction of dentin will leave the superficial enamel unsupported.

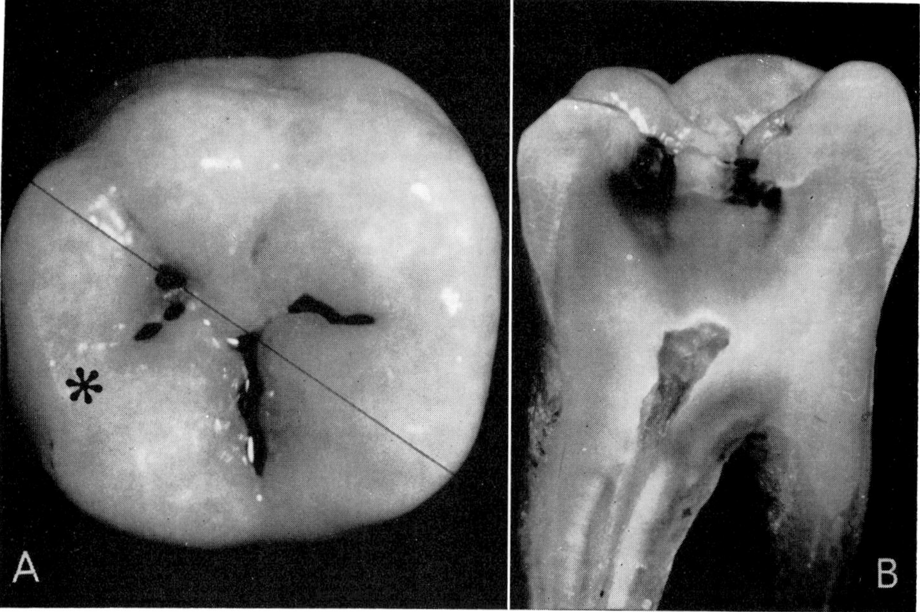

Fig. 4–25. *A.* Even the casual observer can see that this mandibular first molar is carious in the occlusal fissures. The extent of the lesion is partly seen when the distolingual portion of the tooth (asterisk) is ground off. *B.* Caries had probably penetrated farther into the dentin in an area beyond the cut surface here seen. Under the triangular ridge of the distal cusp caries in the dentin has noticeably undermined the enamel.

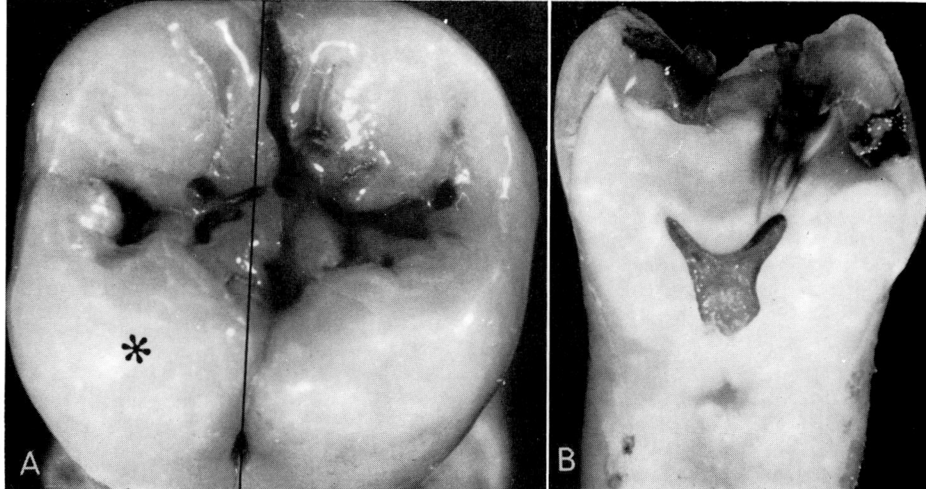

Fig. 4–26. *A.* Clearly there is caries in the occlusal grooves of this mandibular second molar. The buccal pit at the end of the buccal groove (bottom of picture) appears to be deep but undamaged. *B.* Removal of the mesial side of the tooth (asterisk in A) reveals considerable caries damage in the buccal pit and a deep penetration into the occlusal dentin beneath the bucco-occlusal groove.

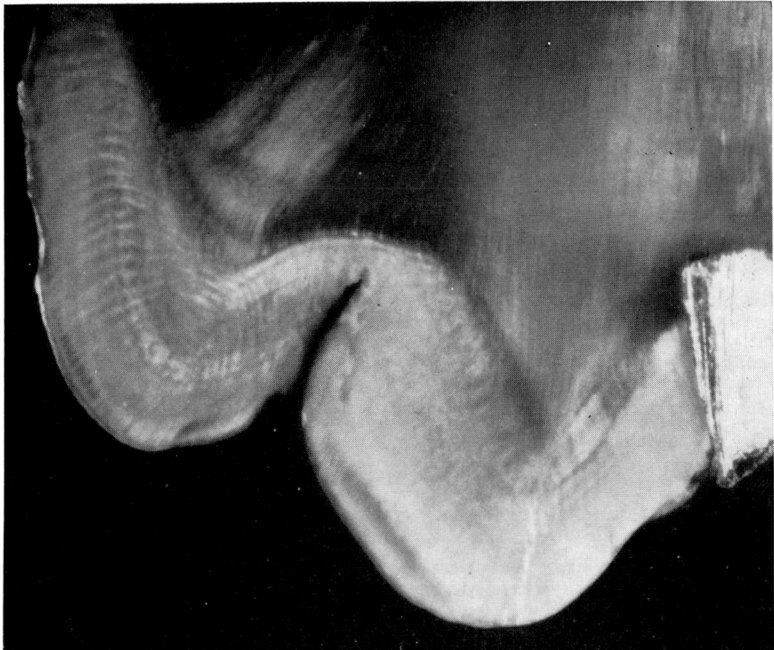

Fig. 4–27. A maxillary first molar with a prominent cusp of Carabelli was ground to reveal the deep fissure at the line of attachment of this fifth cusp to the mesiolingual cusp. In this tooth the enamel of the fissure appears to be intact. In some similar fissures, caries is present. (The cusp of Carabelli is at the left of the picture. The oblong object at the right is part of an amalgam filling in the occlusal surface.)

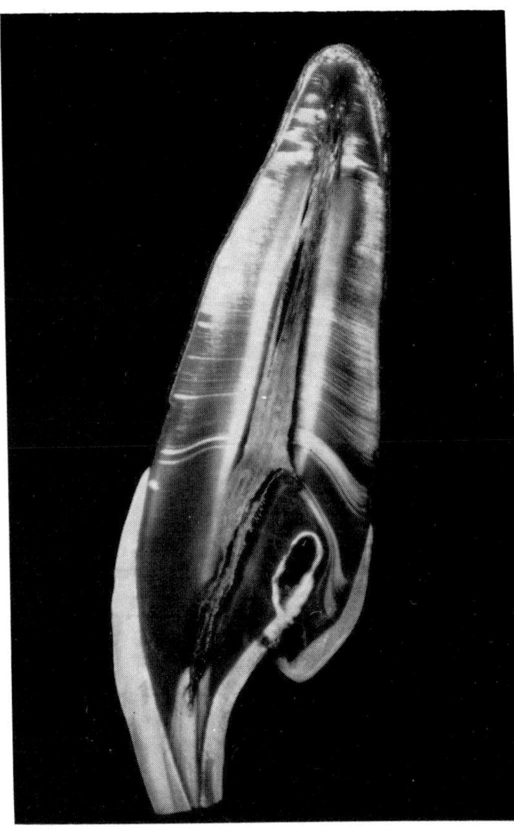

Fig. 4–28. This maxillary central incisor had a deep lingual fossa, pronounced marginal ridges, and what appeared to be a pit at the incisal border of the cingulum. It was ground to a thin center section. In this photomicrograph what appeared to be a small lingual pit is seen to extend into the tooth and to be lined with a thin layer of enamel. No caries was evident in this tooth even when the section was examined under high magnification. However, caries frequently is found in such invaginations. In some teeth this kind of developmental invagination is much deeper, and is called *dens in dente* (tooth within a tooth).

the maxillary molar to which it is attached there is a groove, often deep enough to be called a fissure, which is susceptible to caries (Fig. 4–27).

Unexpectedly, a pit may be present at the incisal border of the cingulum of a maxillary incisor tooth that has a deep lingual fossa and heavy marginal ridges. This was the external appearance of the maxillary central incisor pictured in Figure 4–28. A ground section of this tooth reveals a deep developmental depression. Such an invagination is at times so deep that it protrudes into the pulp cavity. It is called a *dens in dente* (a tooth in a tooth). Notice that enamel lines the surface of this invagination.

In some mongoloid peoples deep grooves, oriented apicoincisally, occur characteristically on the cingulum of mandibular incisors. In such places caries often develops.

Surprisingly, pits often are on the incisal edges of mandibular incisor teeth when there are prominent mamelons. The pits seen in Figure 4–29 are not carious, but sometimes in such pits early caries can be detected in the study of a ground section.

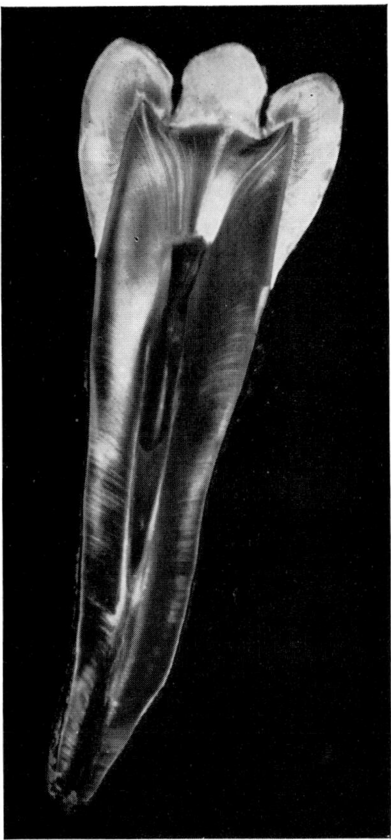

Fig. 4–29. Ground section of mandibular incisor cut mesiodistally. The intact tooth had mamelons that appeared unusually pronounced. The ground section shows deep pits in the depressions between the mamelons, with a very thin layer of enamel at the bottom of the pits. In ground sections of a number of teeth that had unusually pronounced mamelons, it was found that such pits were generally present. Notice the curvature of the dentinal tubules in the tooth crown. In the root the tubules are nearly straight and are directed slightly apically from the cementodentinal junction.

With these several structural characteristics of enamel tending to facilitate the spread of caries beneath the enamel surface, it is easy to see how one day an individual may bite on something firm and part of the surface of a seemingly (to the patient) good tooth will cave in. An understanding of the subsurface spread of dental caries motivates the dentist and the dental hygienist to instruct patients on the importance of regular dental examinations and on the necessity for prompt attention to even seemingly small cavities.*

AGE CHANGES

Enamel undergoes changes with age. Some of the changes are clinical observations, others are supported by scientific data.

The most common age change of enamel is *attrition*—the wearing away of tooth substances due to mastication. Cusp tips and incisal edges may wear away

*Important references:
Menaker, Lewis: *The Biologic Basis of Dental Caries*. Hagerstown, MD, Harper & Row, 1980.
Newbrun, Ernest: *Cariology*, 2nd ed., Baltimore, William & Wilkins, 1983.

completely, exposing the dentin. Excessive wear may also lead to the elimination of pits and fissures.

Other age changes of enamel are: less permeablility, darker color, reduction of caries, and an increase of fluoride content at the surface. Many of these changes are associated with the eating habits and the environment of the individual.

Chapter 5

DENTIN

LOCATION

Dentin is located in both the crown and the root of a tooth, making up the bulk of the tooth. In an intact tooth the dentin is not visible because in the crown it is covered by enamel and in the root it is covered by cementum (Figs. 5–1; 5–2).

COMPOSITION

Dentin is a mineralized tissue, and like all mineralized tissues of the body it is composed of both *organic* (protein) and *inorganic* (mineral) substances. Although not nearly so hard as tooth enamel, dentin is harder than cementum and bone. Mature dentin is about 70% inorganic substance and about 30% organic material and water. (Compare these figures with those given for enamel in Chapter 4.)

STRUCTURE OF DENTIN

The organic part of dentin known as the *organic matrix,* is composed of small *fibrils,* and a surrounding structureless *ground substance.* In dentin development the organic matrix is formed first; then minerals in solution, similar to the minerals of enamel, cementum, and bone, are deposited in the cementing substance (see Table 9–1). Dentin becomes a hard tissue when the minerals crystallize out of solution, the crystals forming on and around the fibrils.

The organic matrix of dentin consists of *collagen* fibrils and a ground substance of mucopolysaccharides. The inorganic material consists of hydroxyapatite crystals, as in enamel, cementum, and bone.

Dentin is perforated by innumerable holes called *dentinal tubules* which contain cell processes. The tubules lie close together and extend from the tooth pulp to the dentinoenamel junction in the crown of the tooth and to the dentinocemental junction in the root (Figs. 5–2; 5–3). At their outer ends the dentinal tubules are divided into a number of branches (Figs. 4–7; 4–18). Much smaller branches connecting adjacent dentinal tubules are often found along the length of the tubules. In diameter (Figs. 5–4; 5–5; 5–6) the dentinal tubules measure about 3 μm at the pulpal ends and somewhat less at the other ends. In the cusp area in the tooth crown (Fig. 5–7) and in the apical half of the root (Figs. 4–29; 5–1) the dentinal tubules are nearly straight and are arranged nearly perpendicular to the dentinoenamel or dentinocemental junction. In the facial, lingual, mesial, and distal areas of the crown (Figs. 4–20; 4–29) and in the cervical portion of the roots (Fig. 5–2) the dentinal tubules are S-shaped. The outer ends of the S-

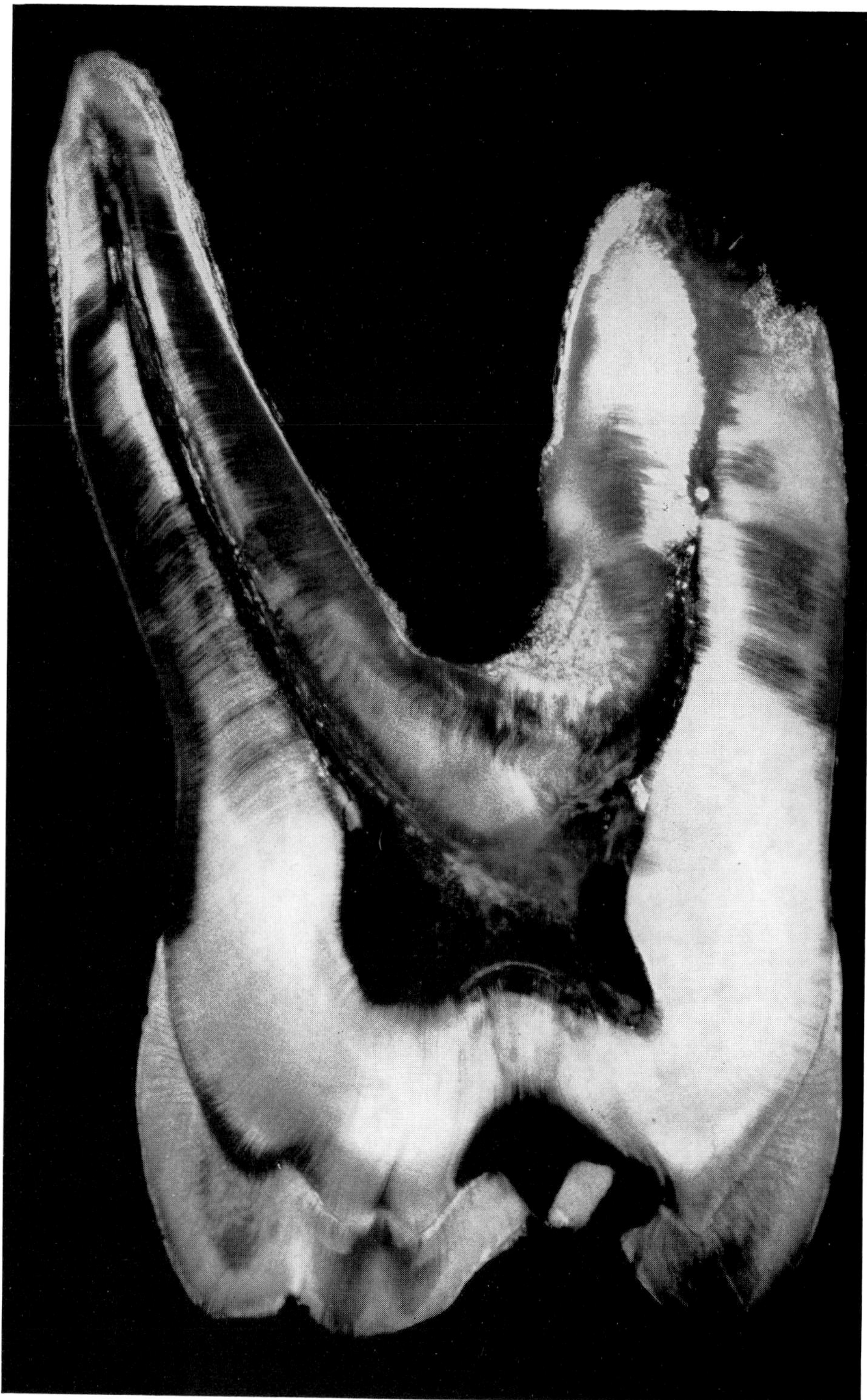

Fig. 5–1. Photomicrograph of a ground section cut faciolingually through a maxillary first molar. This tooth is shown diagrammatically in Figure 5–2.

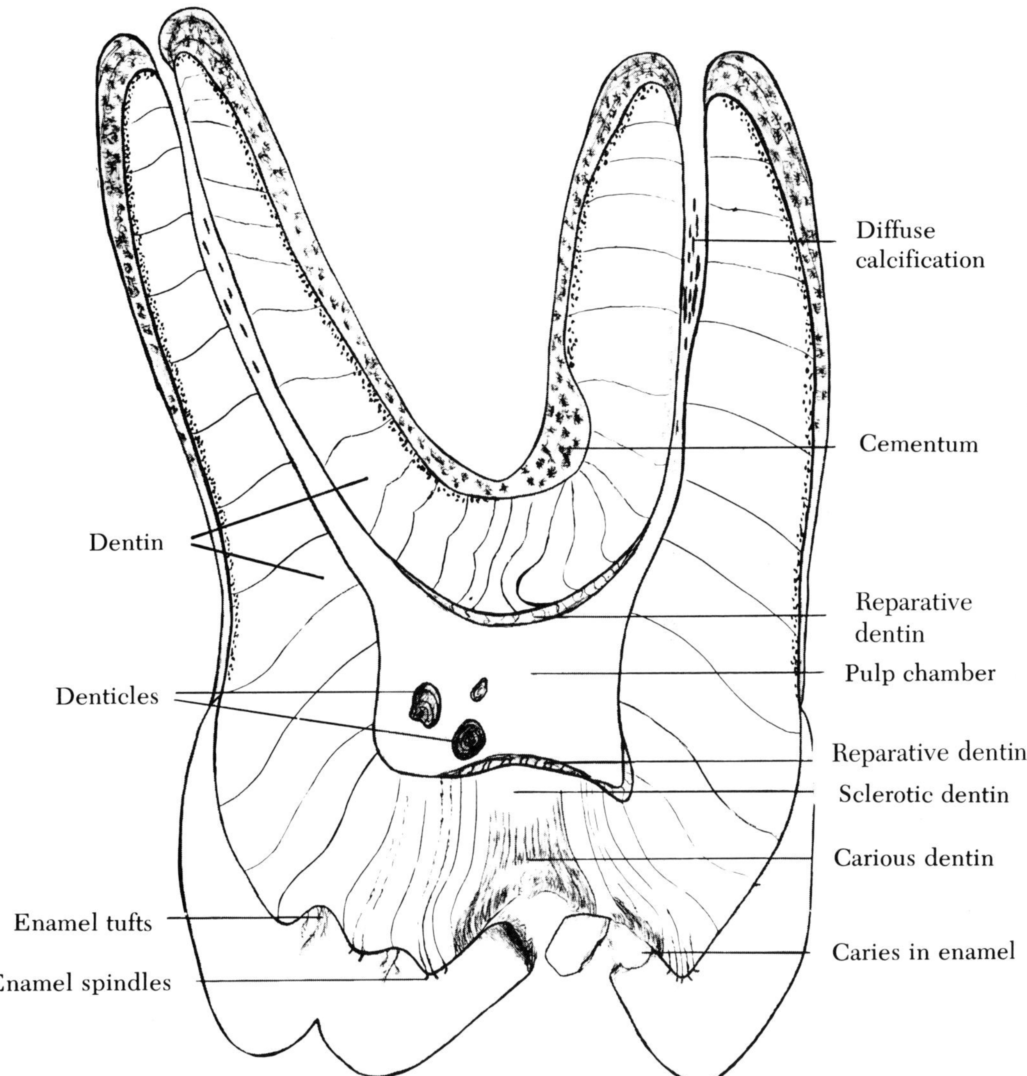

Fig. 5–2. Diagrammatic drawing of a longitudinal faciolingual section of a maxillary first molar. Dental caries has destroyed the enamel in the area around a groove on the occlusal surface. The caries has spread horizontally at the dentinoenamel junction, with a resultant undermining of enamel. Caries has spread pulpward in the dentinal tubules to about two thirds the thickness of the dentin. The dentin close to the pulp is sclerotic dentin: the tubules are filled with mineral salts. On the pulpal wall beneath the caries lesion a small amount of reparative dentin has formed. The reparative dentin on the floor of the pulp chamber (next to the root) was not caused by caries; reparative dentin in this location is not unusual. (See Figure 5–1).

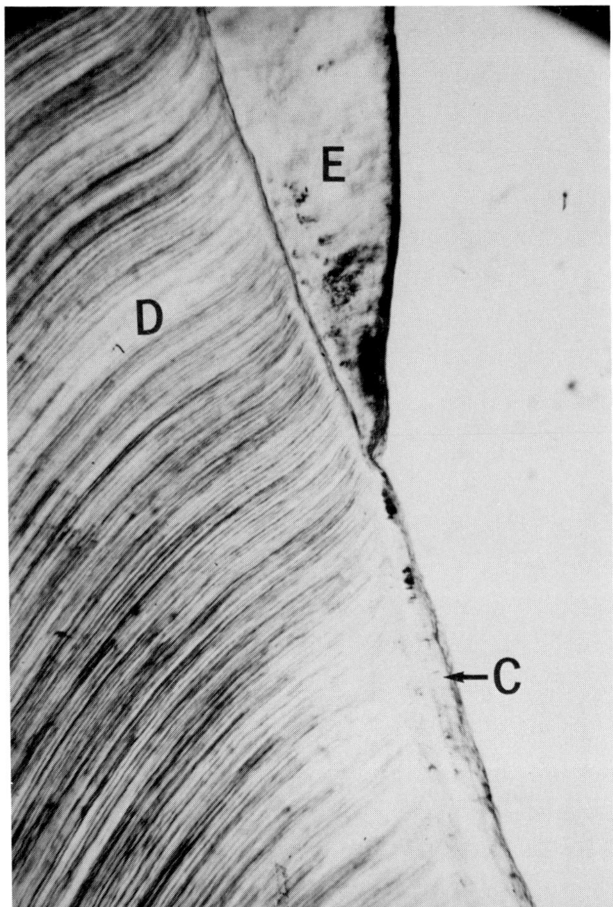

Fig. 5–3. Ground section of the cervical part of a tooth showing relation of the dentinal tubules of dentin (D) to the enamel (E) and to the cementum (C). The tubules appear dark here. Due to processing, the tubules are filled with air.

shaped tubules are always occlusal to the pulpal ends of the tubules (Figs. 5–2; 5–3).

A cell process occupies each dentinal tubule (Fig. 4–15). It is the cytoplasm of a pulp cell. Those cells of the pulp which lie next to the dentin have the somewhat surprising distinction of being cells of the dentin also. They are named *odontoblasts*. These cells form the *organic matrix* of dentin. They also serve to provide nutrition to dentin and possibly play a role in the pain sensation of a tooth. The nucleus of the odontoblast cell remains in the pulp surrounded by part of the cell's cytoplasm. The remainder of the cytoplasm of the odontoblast cell is stretched out like a long, thin tail and extends into a dentinal tubule (Fig. 5–8). This cytoplasmic extension of the odontoblast is the *odontoblastic process*. In young teeth each process extends through the tubule to the dentinoenamel or dentinocemental junction. At their peripheral ends the processes are branched just as the tubules are branched (Figs. 4–15; 5–8). In older teeth the processes apparently, in some manner, have been withdrawn so that they are found only in the pulpal ends of the tubules.

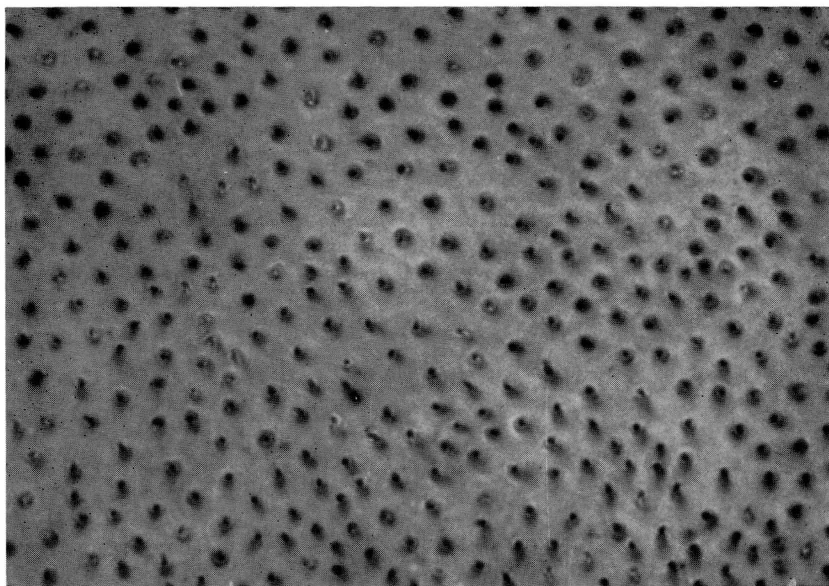

Fig. 5–4. Photomicrograph of a ground section of dentin cut in such a direction that the dentinal tubules are seen in cross section. The specimen was dipped in a histologic stain which remained in the tubules, making them appear dark in the picture. The tubules in this section, taken from near the pulp of the tooth (rather than close to the enamel), are probably about 3 micrometers in diameter.

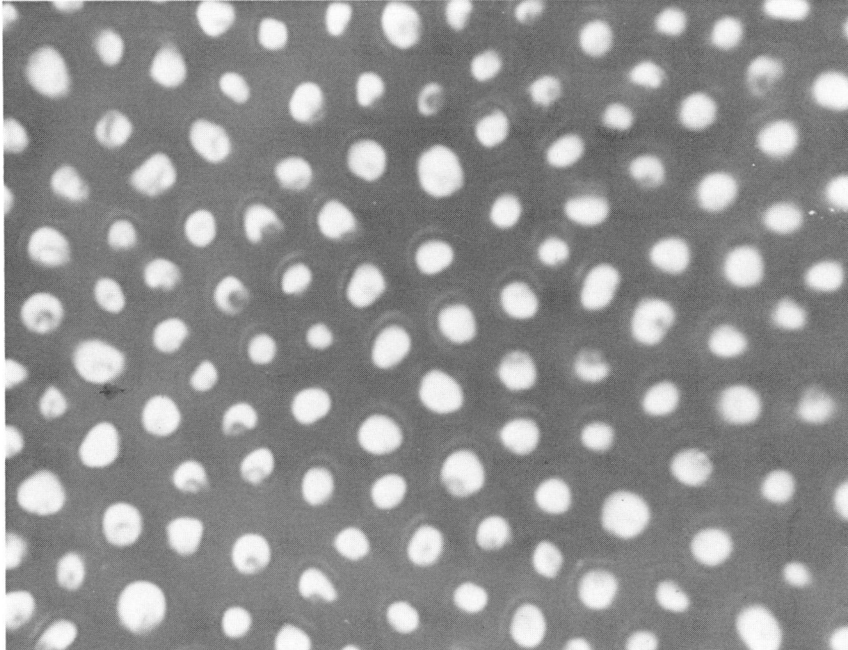

Fig. 5–5. Cross-section of the dentinal tubules. This demineralized specimen is more coronal than that seen in Figure 5–4. Most of the tubules are empty; some contain shrunken odontoblastic processes.

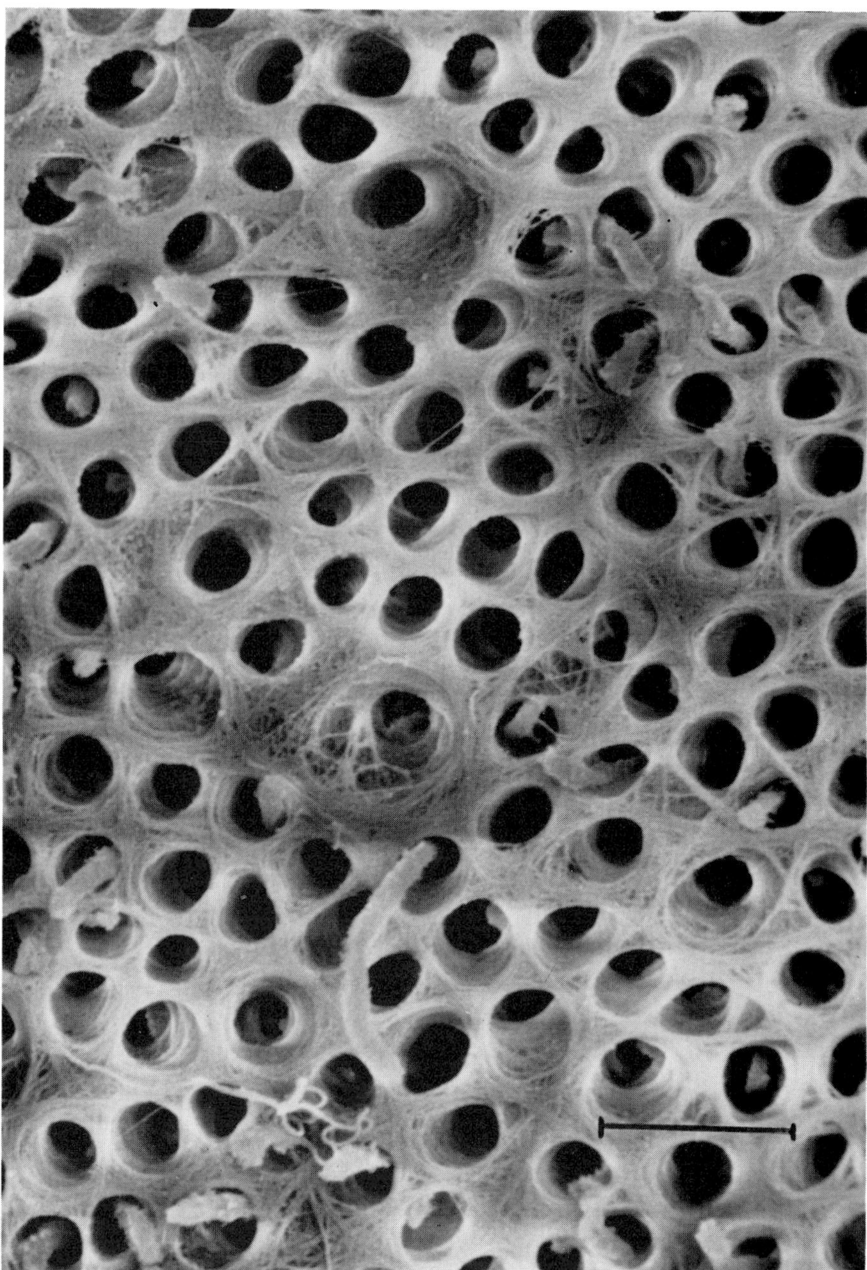

Fig. 5–6. Scanning electron micrograph of the cross section of dentinal tubules adjacent to the pulp chamber of a human tooth. A rinse with NaOCl solution produced the strikingly clear dentinal tubule orifices enclosed in some of which are odontoblastic processes not removed by treatment. The black line engraved in the lower right is 10 μm long. (Courtesy of Dr. Dennis Foreman, College of Dentistry, The Ohio State University.)

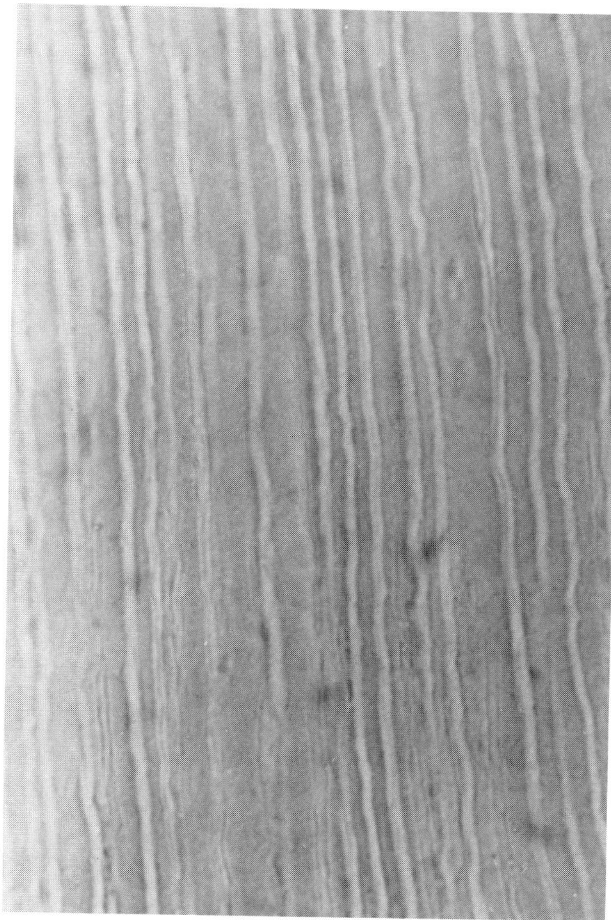

Fig. 5–7. Photomicrograph of a demineralized section of dentin cut in such a direction that the dentinal tubules are seen in longitudinal section. Some of the tubules in this section (cusp area, near the enamel) contain shrunken odontoblastic processes, while others are empty; this is caused by section preparation.

In some places in the crown of a tooth the peripheral ends of some odontoblastic processes cross the dentinoenamel junction and protrude into the enamel. Here they appear as short, slightly thickened objects. These ends of processes in the enamel, or the empty spaces once occupied by ends of the processes are *enamel spindles* (Figs. 4–15; 4–16; 5–8).*

Young teeth always have a layer of dentin adjacent to the pulp that is less mineralized than the rest of the dentin. This layer is called *predentin* or *dentoid.*

*Interesting papers:

Brannstrom, M., and R. Garberolio: The Dentinal Tubules and the Odontoblast Processes. A Scanning Electron Microscopic Study. Acta Odont. Scand., *30*:291, 1972.

Scott D.B., J.W. Simmelink, and V. Nygaard: Structural Aspects of Dental Caries. J. Dent. Res., *53*(2):165, 1974.

Thomas, H.F.: The Effect of Various Fixatives on the Extent of the Odontoblast Process in Human Dentin. Arch. Oral Biol., *28*:465, 1983.

Thomas, H.F. and Payne, R.C.: The Ultrastructure of Dentinal Tubules from Erupted Human Premolar teeth. J. Dent. Res., *65*:532, 1983.

Proceedings: International Workshop on the Biology of Dentin and Pulp. J. Dent. Res., *64*:Special Issue, 1984.

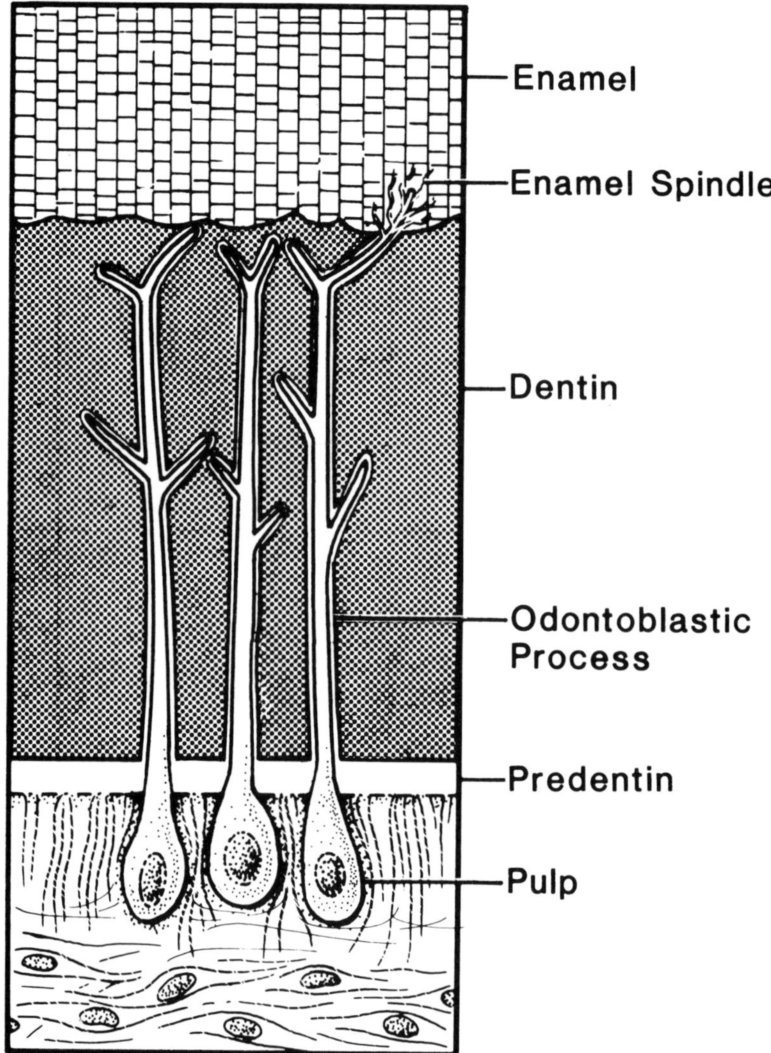

Fig. 5–8. Diagrammatic illustration of a small portion of the crown area showing three odontoblasts. The cell body (nuclear part) of the odontoblast lies in the pulp and its process extends into the dentinal tubule. Notice the branching of the processes, and the entrapped end of a process within the enamel—an enamel spindle

It is actually the organic matrix of dentin that has not yet mineralized. Figure 5–9 is a photomicrograph of a section cut through the root of a young tooth that was demineralized and prepared for histologic viewing. Predentin is clearly visible in this section because of the way it stains. Since predentin is less mineralized, it stains lighter than the mineralized dentin.

In the crowns of some teeth the dentin has in it spots which are unmineralized or are hypomineralized (hypo = under, less than ordinary). These unmineralized spots, irregular in shape, usually occur in a layer a short distance inside the dentinoenamel junction (Figs. 1–12; 1–13; 5–10). In this location such an area of unmineralized dentin is called *interglobular* dentin. The reason for failure

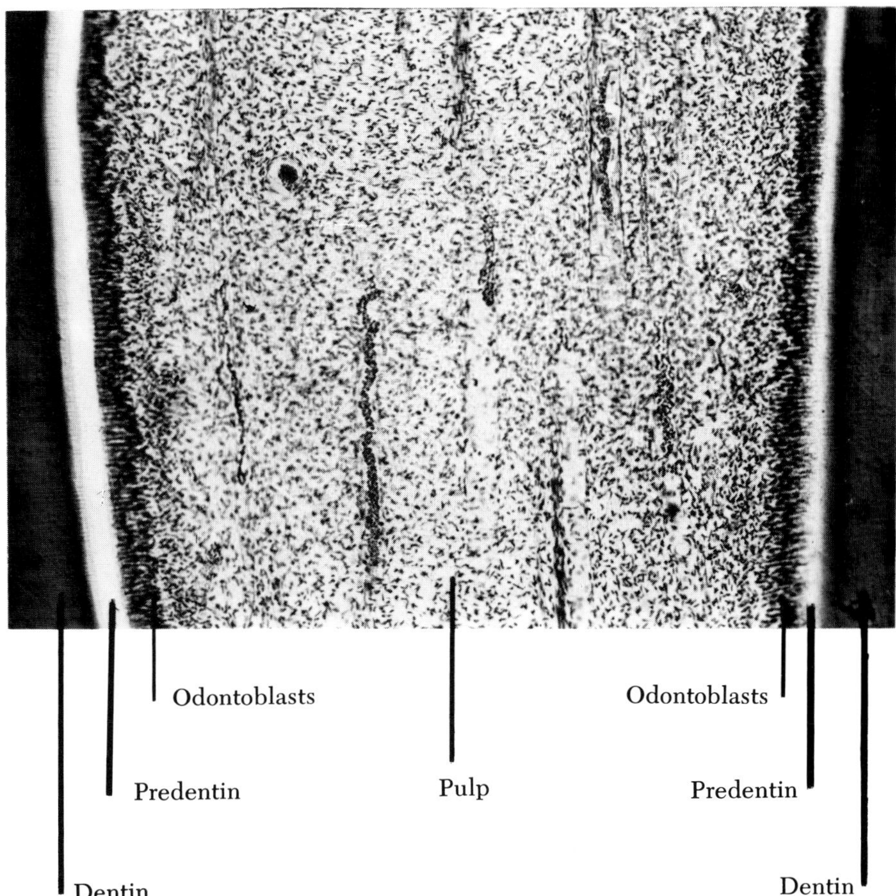

Fig. 5–9. Section cut through the root of a young tooth showing the unmineralized *predentin* layer. Note the striking contrast between the predentin and the mineralized dentin. Chemically, predentin and dentin differ, therefore, when they are stained for histologic viewing, they stain differently.

of proper mineralization here is believed to be some metabolic disturbance which occurred at the time this part of the tooth was forming.

Root dentin invariably contains a band of minute unmineralized spots almost immediately beneath the cementum. This is called *Tomes granular layer* (Figs. 1–13; 1–14; 5–11; 5–12). It was first described by the dental histologist Sir John Tomes (1815–1895) who thought that this region of the dentin had a granular appearance. Later is was found that this area is not really granular, but is made up of very small unmineralized spots in the dentin. There is good evidence that these spots, these seeming granules, are produced by looping of the terminal portions of dentinal tubules.* Tomes' granular layer has considerable clinical importance which will be discussed later.

In the root dentin of some teeth a short distance beneath Tomes' granular layer there may be also a layer of interglobular dentin similar in size and configuration to the interglobular dentin found in the crown of the tooth (Fig. 5–11).

A modified type of dentin known as *reparative dentin* is usually found in older

*Ten Cate, A.R.: An Analysis of Tomes' Granular Layer. Anat. Rec., *172*(2):137, 1972.

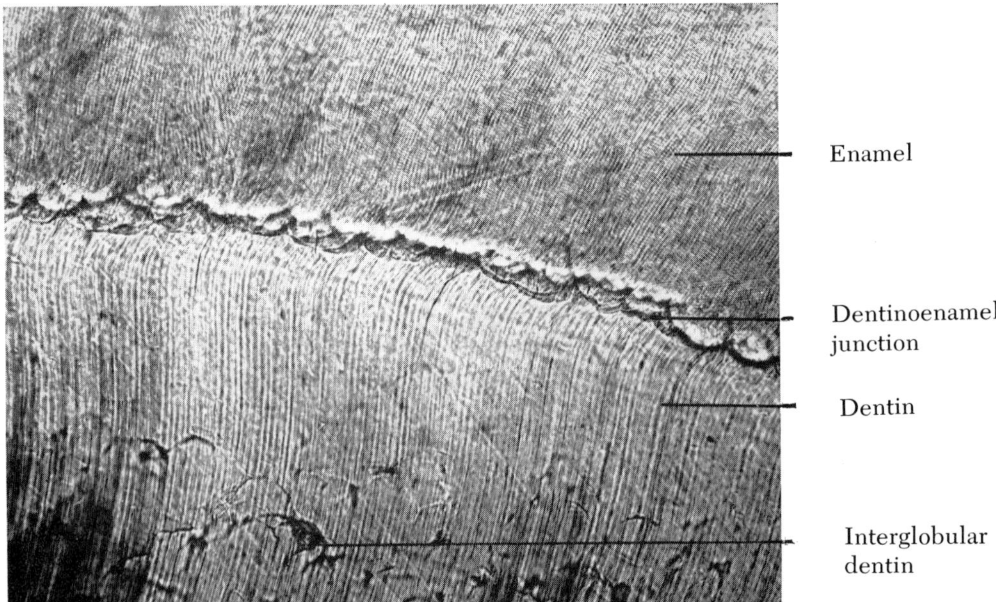

Fig. 5–10. Photomicrograph of part of a ground section of a tooth crown. The enamel is attached to the dentin at the scalloped dentinoenamel junction. Curvatures in the enamel rods are evident and in some areas cross-striations of the rods can be seen. In the dentin at the bottom of the picture are irregular areas (dark) of interglobular dentin.

teeth along the pulpal wall. Aside from the fact that in varying degrees it has fewer and less regular dentinal tubules than the first dentin produced, reparative dentin is similar to the earlier dentin. Reparative dentin may be formed throughout the life of the tooth as long as the pulp is healthy.

In certain areas on the pulpal wall reparative dentin is formed in larger amounts. In posterior teeth it is formed in larger amounts in the pulp horn—that is, in the part of the pulp that extends toward the cusp tips—and on the floor of the pulp chamber (Figs. 5–1; 5–2; 5–13; 5–14; 5–15). In anterior teeth it is formed in larger amounts beneath the incisal edge when there has been considerable attrition (wearing off) (Figs. 1–12, 5–14). It may occur in larger amounts also on the pulpal wall in areas where dental caries has penetrated to the dentinoenamel junction (Figs. 5–1; 5–2; 5–13). Its greater formation in these areas is often a result of the reaction of the tooth pulp to the irritation of attrition or caries.

Reparative dentin produced in response to attrition, caries, operative procedures, or other damaging stimuli usually has fewer and more irregular dentinal tubules than dentin produced merely as a result of aging. Dental clinicians, at times, use the term *secondary dentin* when referring to reparative dentin.

Sclerotic dentin is a modified dentin found in some areas of most old teeth and sometimes in young teeth. Dentin is said to be sclerotic when the odontoblastic processes have degenerated and the dentinal tubules have become filled with calcium salts. Sclerotic dentin is often found beneath worn enamel such as occurs in the incisal area of anterior teeth, and beneath slowly progressing dental caries in locations where reparative dentin is being produced on the pulpal wall (Fig.

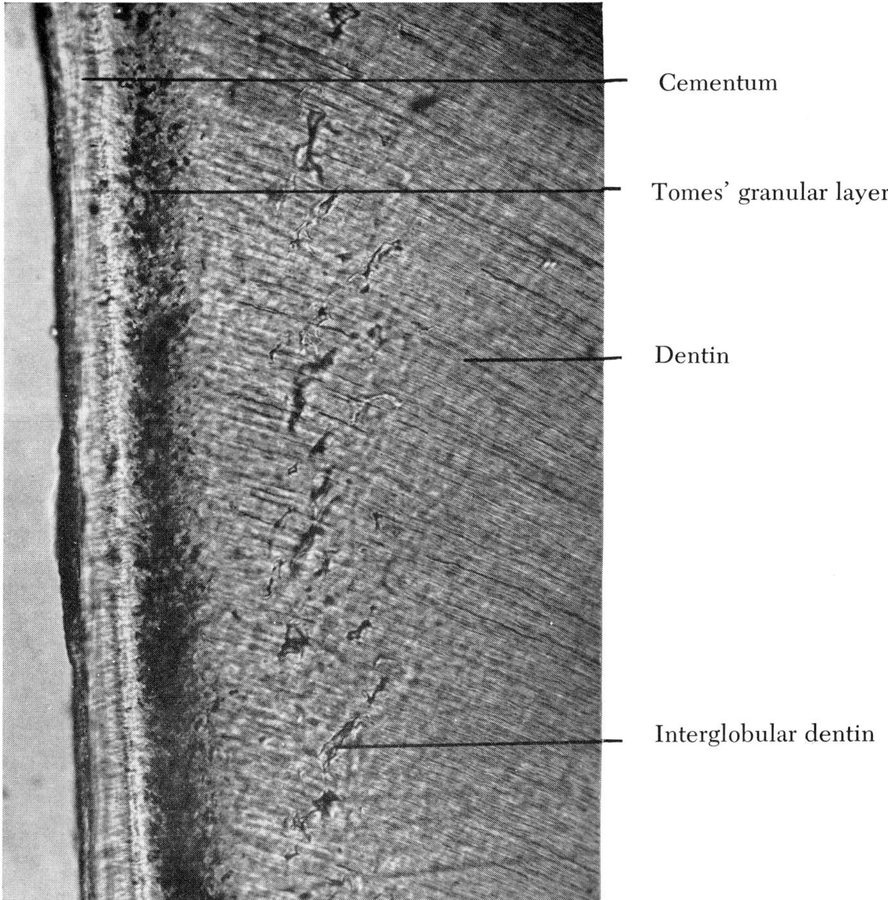

Fig. 5–11. Photomicrograph of part of a ground section of tooth root. The cementum is the relatively narrow light band at the left of the picture; the dentin is the wide area at the right of the picture. In the dentin close to the cementum is the band of closely packed small areas of uncalcified dentin called Tomes' granular layer. Deeper in the dentin are larger, irregular areas of interglobular dentin (dark areas). Notice that the dentinal tubules are straight, and are now quite at right angles to the cementodentinal junction. In the cementum are small lines, perpendicular to the cementum surface, which are spaces once occupied by Sharpey's fibers (Chapter 7). (High power magnification.) Was the crown of this tooth located beyond the top or beyond the bottom of this picture?

5–2). Sclerotic dentin is also found beneath Tomes' granular layer in the cervical area of older teeth where the cervical cementum has become exposed to the oral cavity as a result of recession of the gingiva (Chapter 11).

In the mandibular incisor tooth shown in Figure 5–16 the odontoblastic processes have degenerated beneath the worn incisal edge, but the dentinal tubules have not become filled with calcium salts. Such an area has been referred to as a *dead tract*. The pulp beneath the dead tract in this tooth is protected by the presence of reparative dentin. At the cervix on the facial side of this tooth there is a change in the dentin beneath the cervical abrasion. The white area, indicated by the pointer, is probably a dead tract. Outside of the dead tract, nearer the surface of the tooth, the dentin appears to be sclerotic—*i.e.*, the tubules are filled, or are becoming filled, with calcium salts.

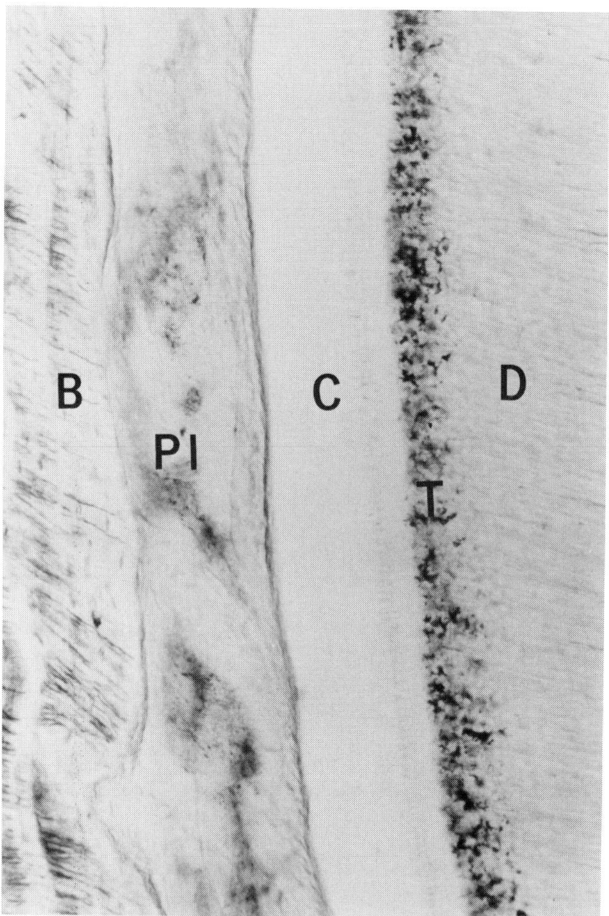

Fig. 5–12. This is a ground section of a tooth and a portion of its surrounding tissues. The hypomineralized Tomes' granular layer (T) is seen within the dentin (D) near the cementum (C) (acellular here). Bone (B). Periodontal ligament (PI). Since this is a ground section, cellular detail of the bone and the periodontal ligament is lacking.

CLINICAL IMPORTANCE OF STRUCTURE OF DENTIN

The structure of dentin influences both the pattern of a caries lesion and the speed with which dental caries destroys a tooth; and it accounts for the sensitivity frequently experienced by patients during the performance of an oral prophylaxis or during the eating of hot or cold foods.

In the preceding chapter it is explained that dental caries is a disease of the hard tissue of the tooth: acidogenic bacteria convert sugars into acids which dissolve the minerals out of the hard tooth tissues; and proteolytic (protein-destroying) bacteria destroy the organic component of the hard tooth tissue in the same area.

When at any point the caries process has penetrated the enamel as far as the dentinoenamel junction, the caries-producing bacteria will also reach this depth and will come in contact with the peripheral ends of the dentinal tubules. Since the bacteria are smaller than the diameter of the dentinal tubules, they enter the tubules. The odontoblastic processes which occupy the tubules are de-

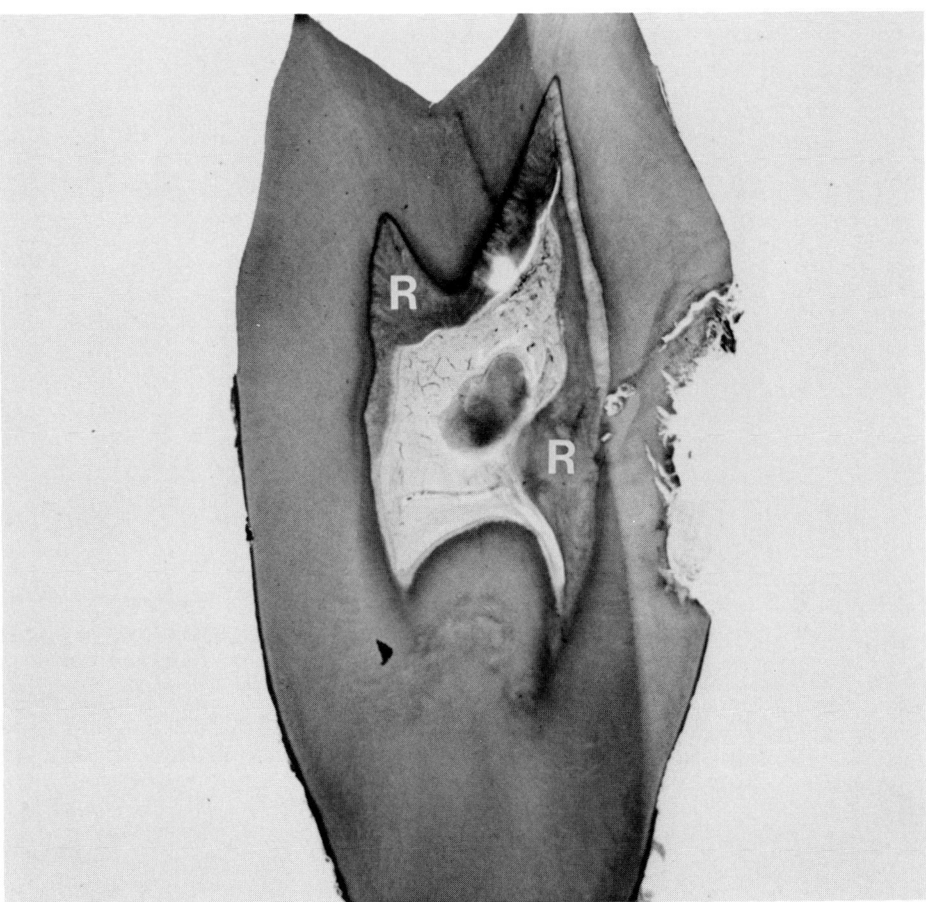

Fig. 5–13. Section of a demineralized tooth with reparative dentin (R) in the pulp horn regions and under caries (right side). The structure surrounded by pulp tissue is a pulp stone. Enamel was lost during histologic processing.

stroyed. The bacteria travel pulpward in the opened tubules and the dentin is slowly destroyed. Because the bacteria follow the course of the dentinal tubules, a caries lesion originating around a contact area or in the cervical area of a tooth extends in an apical direction as it approaches the pulp. Notice the direction of the dentinal tubules in Figures 5–1, 5–2, and 5–16.

The horizontal spread of caries is considerably more rapid in dentin than in enamel. A tooth with only a small area of caries visible on the surface may be so extensively carious in the dentin that clinical restoration is impossible. It is not difficult to understand why the teeth shown in Figures 5–17 and 5–18 were lost. The occlusal surfaces of these teeth, particularly in Figure 5–17, showed too little damage to impress even an observing patient with the probably serious condition inside the tooth.

The teeth shown in Figures 5–19, 5–20 and 5–21 had a larger surface area of visible caries, and the enamel around the point of entry was so seriously undermined that a large part of it was unsupported. With this kind of condition,

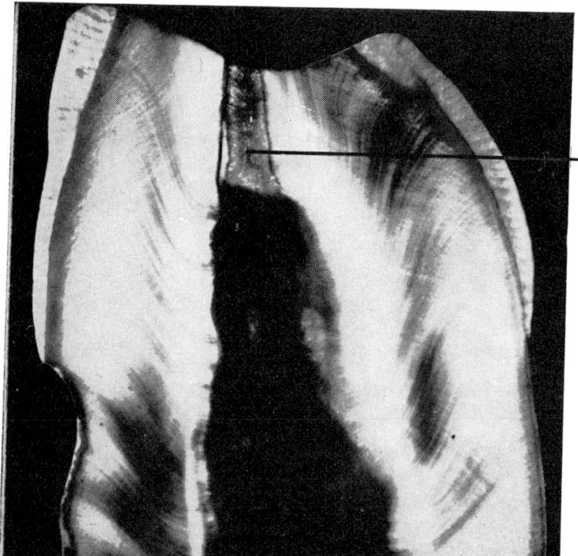

Fig. 5–14. Photomicrograph of a ground section (cut faciolingually) of a canine tooth. Extensive attrition has resulted in the loss of the enamel and part of the dentin of the cusp. The formation of reparative dentin in the incisal part of the pulp cavity has protected the pulp from exposure.

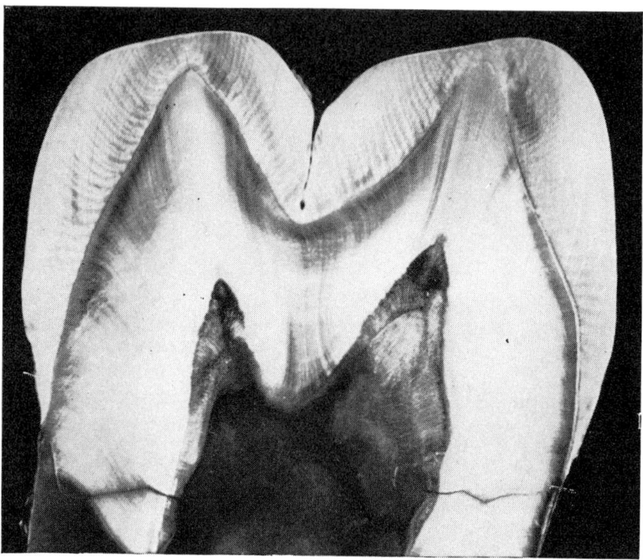

Fig. 5–15. Photomicrograph of a ground section of a mandibular molar. A large amount of reparative dentin has formed in the pulp horns of both the buccal and lingual cusps. Notice the attrition of the enamel on the cusp tips.

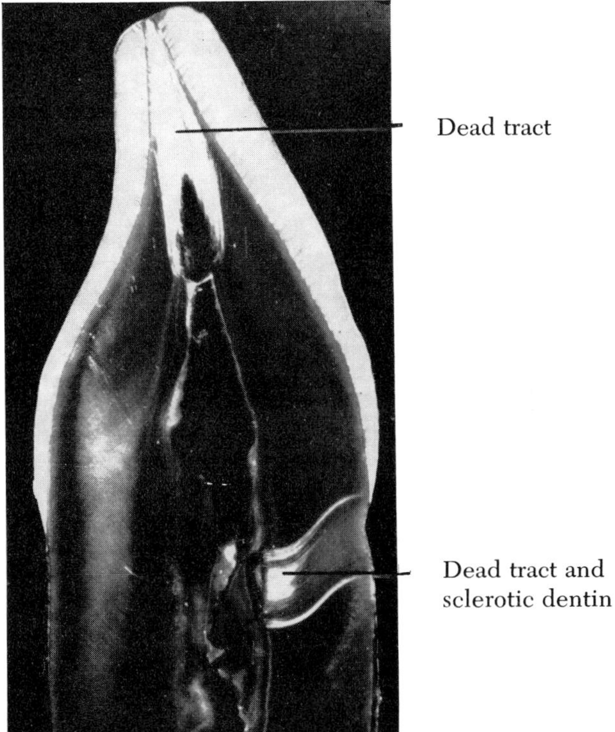

Fig. 5–16. Photomicrograph of a ground section of a mandibular incisor cut faciolingually. Beneath the worn incisal edge is a dead tract in the dentin. Deposition of reparative dentin beneath the dead tract has protected the pulp from damage. On the facial side of the tooth in the cervical area there is abrasion: the cementum is gone and some of the dentin has been worn away. (See Figure 11–12.) Beneath this abraded surface there is an alteration in the dentin. Near the pulp is an area of dead tract, which appears white. Superficial (nearer the surface) to this tract the dentin seems to be sclerotic. On the pulp wall in this region reparative dentin has been produced; it protrudes into the pulp cavity inside the dead tract. Notice the curvature of the dentinal tubules in the cervical area.

the occlusal enamel often collapses completely when the patient bites on some relatively soft food.

The progress of dental caries through the dentin is often retarded, but not stopped, by defense reactions that take place in the pulp. One such reaction is the production of *sclerotic dentin*. From the pulp tissue calcium salts are deposited in the dentinal tubules causing them to become filled with mineral substances, and so the progress of bacterial invasion is slowed down. Another defense reaction against caries is the formation of reparative dentin, at the location where the bacteria-filled tubules reach the pulp. This increases the thickness of the dentin wall and helps to protect the tooth pulp, for a time at least, against the invasion of the disease. In a tooth from which the pulp has been removed these defense changes which are dependent upon the pulp cannot occur.

Another characteristic of dentin of particular interest to dentist and dental hygienist is the location of Tomes' granular layer and its effect on the comfort of the patient. As we have seen, Tomes' granular layer consists of a narrow band of unmineralized areas in the root dentin immediately beneath the cementum. A natural aging process which occurs in nearly all mouths is the gradual recession of the gingiva and a resulting exposure of the cementum at the necks

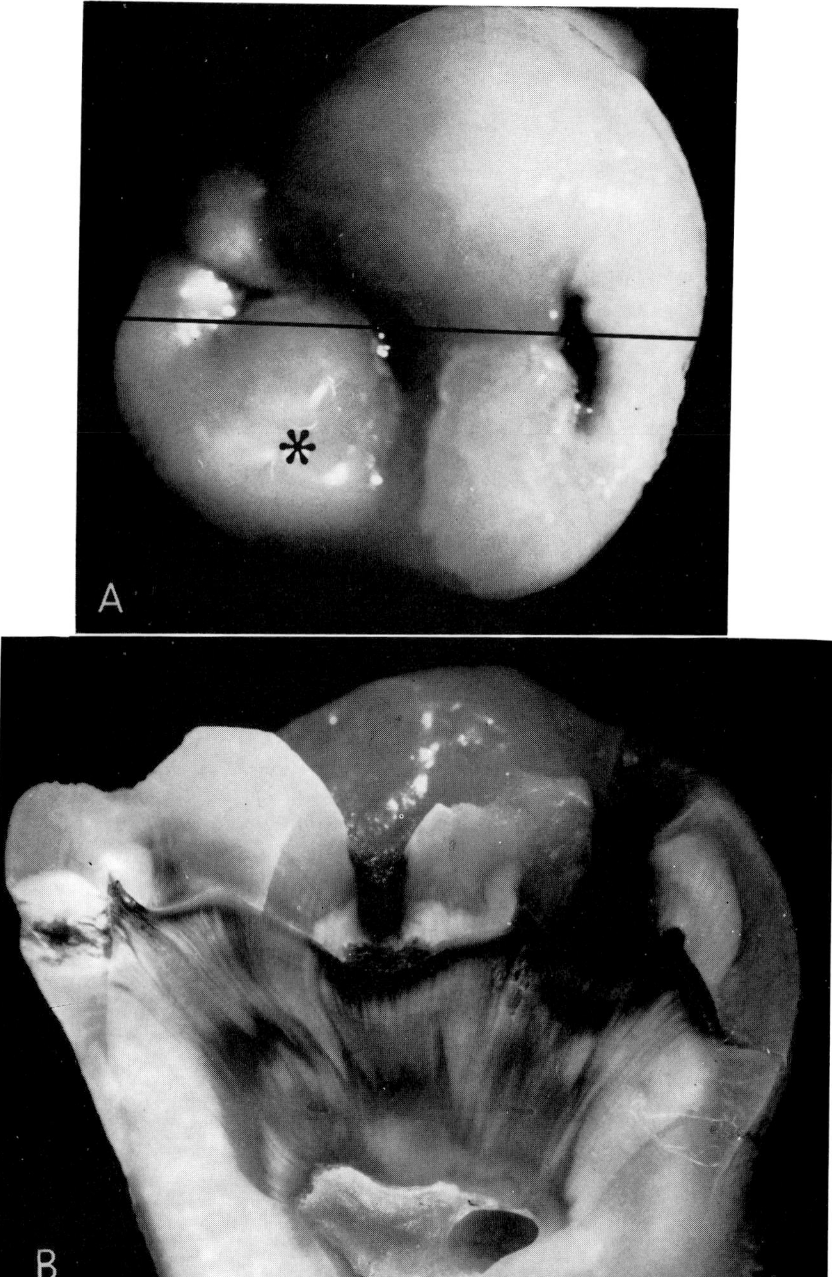

Fig. 5–17. *A.* This maxillary molar shows evidence of caries in the central fossa and in the mesial triangular fossa, but the casual observer scarcely expects what is revealed when the buccal side of the tooth (asterisk) is ground away. *B.* Caries has penetrated to the pulp cavity and has spread laterally, undermining the enamel of the entire occlusal surface. (Notice the curvatures of the dentinal tubules.)

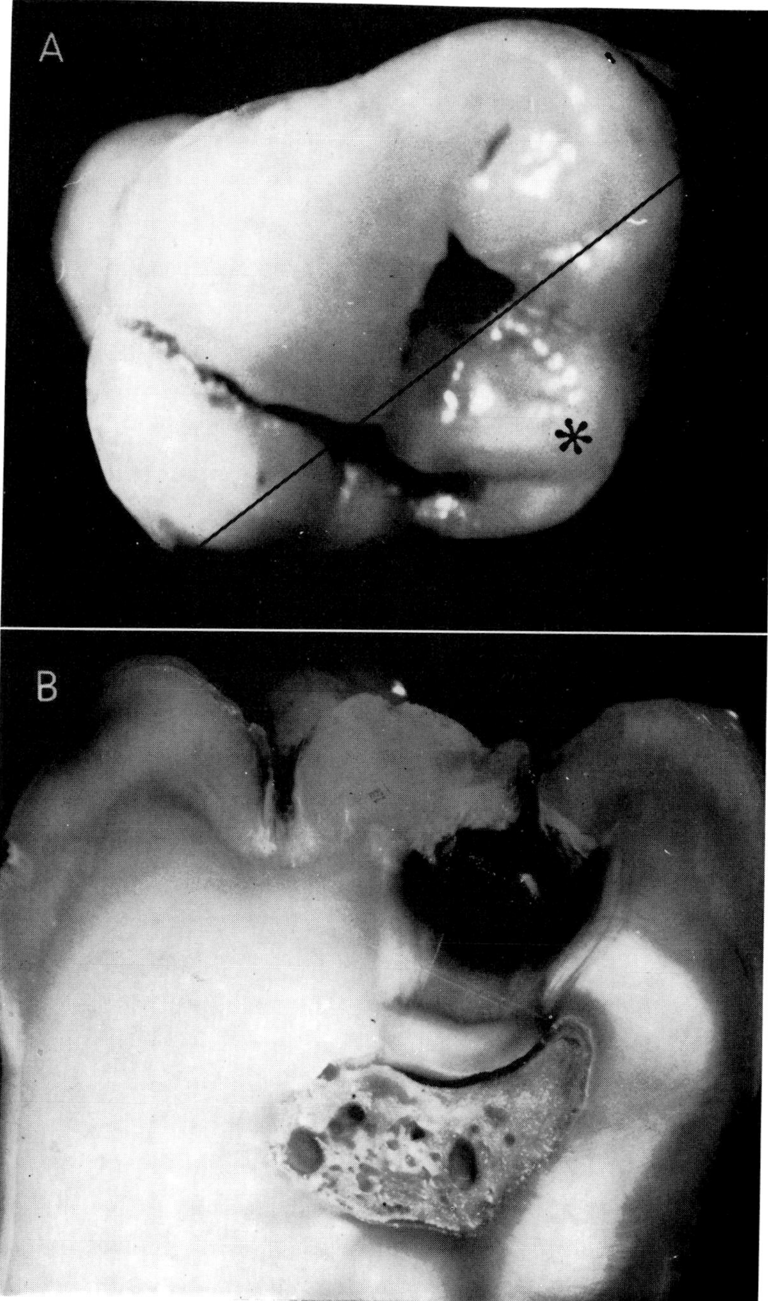

Fig. 5–18. *A.* This maxillary molar was clearly carious in the central fossa, and probably also in the groove between the lingual cusps. *B.* Removal of the distobuccal side of the tooth (asterisk in A) exposed a deep lesion in the central fossa, but little evidence of caries in the distolingual groove at this particular point. The groove may have been carious either buccal to or lingual to the area we see here.

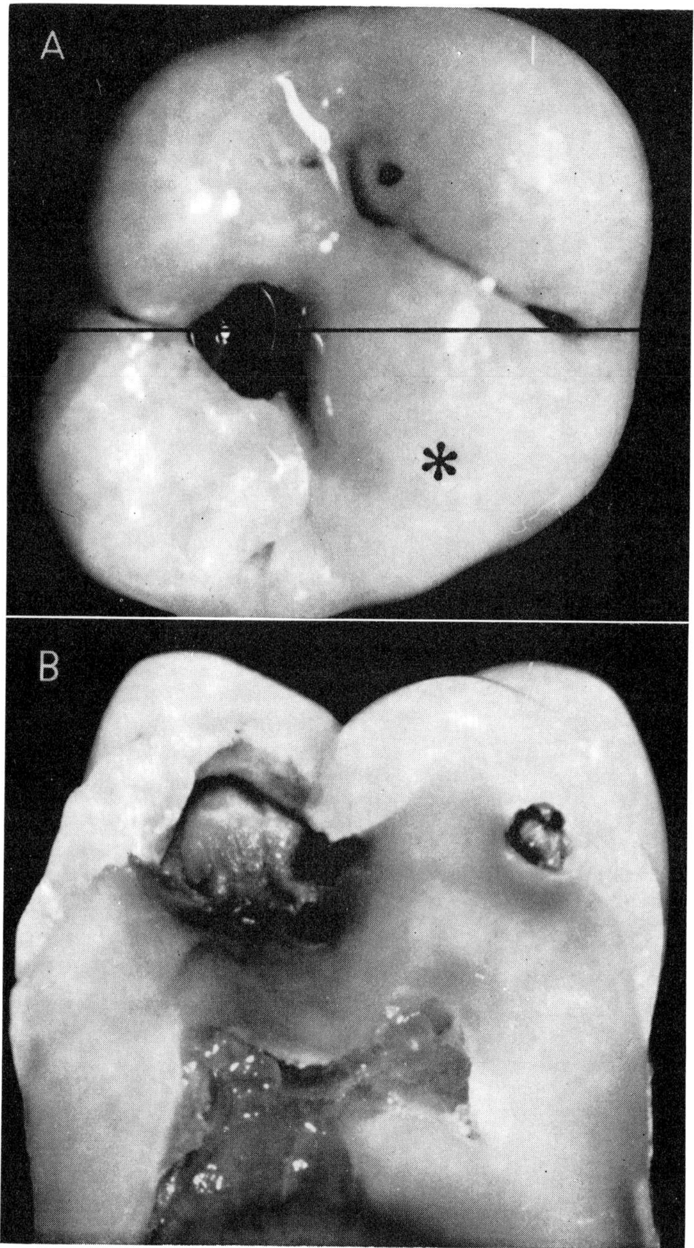

Fig. 5–19. *A*. Caries is obvious in the central fossa of this maxillary molar, and an area of possible caries is seen in the lingual developmental groove. When the mesial surface of the tooth was removed (asterisk in *A*) completely unsupported enamel was exposed around the central fossa and around the suspicious area in the groove. *B*. Notice the extent of caries in the dentin.

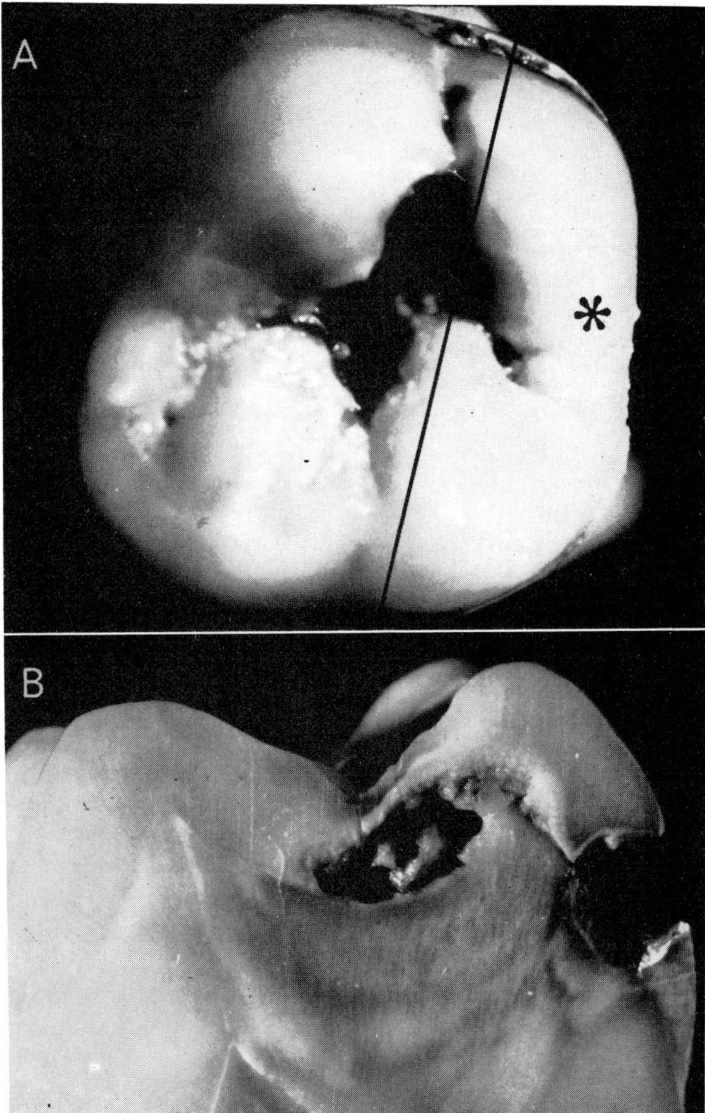

Fig. 5–20. *A.* The extent of destruction beneath the occlusal surface of this maxillary molar is seen when the distal side of the tooth (asterisk) has been removed. *B.* The occlusal enamel is undermined around the occlusal opening of the lesion. Caries has penetrated also from the lingual groove.

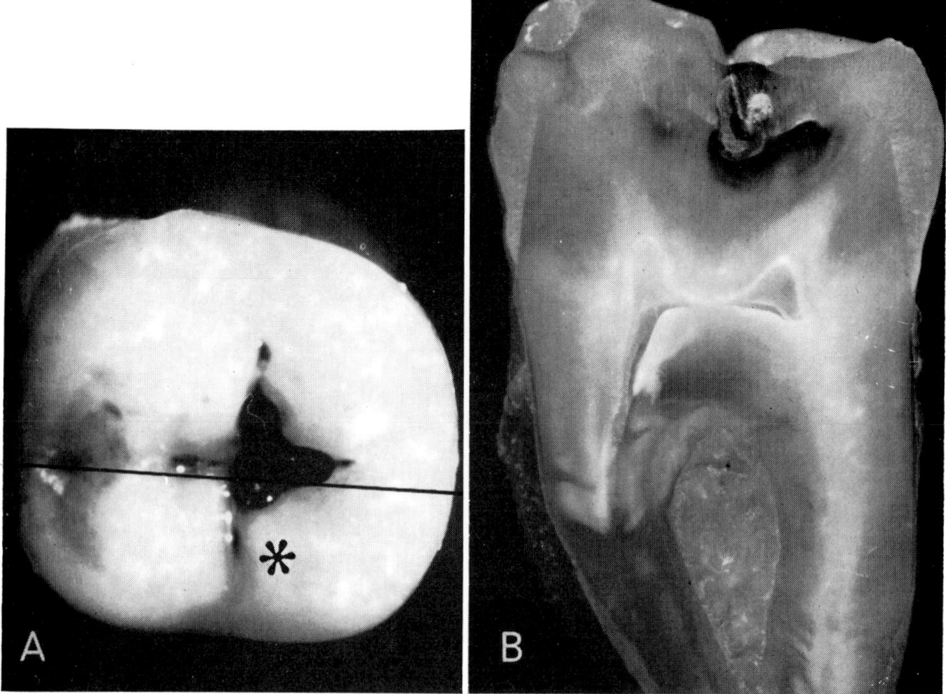

Fig. 5–21. *A*. This mandibular second molar has caries in the central fossa. *B*. Removal of the lingual side of the tooth (asterisk in *A*) exposed a lesion in the dentin that extended horizontally beneath enamel that on the surface appeared undamaged.

of the teeth. (This will be discussed in Chapter 11.) In the performance of an oral prophylaxis it is necessary to clean this exposed cervical cementum. This means working very close to Tomes' granular layer which, being unmineralized and in close contact with the odontoblastic processes, causes this area to be very sensitive. Therefore the patient may experience pain. The patient may also find this area of exposed cementum sensitive to hot or cold foods. A patient with exposed cervical cementum may believe that he has caries in this area because of the pain he experiences during eating or while brushing his teeth. These discomforts are more noticeable when the cervical cementum first becomes exposed. After the cervical cementum has been exposed to the oral environment for a few weeks or months the dentin beneath the exposed surface usually becomes sclerotic (Fig. 5–16), and the patient ceases to notice discomfort.

Chapter 6

TOOTH PULP

LOCATION

The pulp of a tooth is located in the interior of the tooth. It occupies the pulp chamber in the crown and the root canal in the root and connects with the periodontal ligament at the apical foramen (Figs. 1–12; 6–1).

ORIGIN

The *dental papilla* (mesenchyme) of the *tooth germ* undergoes growth and development and becomes the tooth pulp.

COMPOSITION

Tooth pulp is the only nonmineralized tissue of a tooth. It is a soft connective tissue, and like other connective tissues it is made up of *cells, intercellular substance* and *tissue fluid* (Fig. 6–2). The pulp tissue of older teeth has relatively fewer cells and more intercellular substance than that of young teeth.

While the *cells* of young pulp tissue are chiefly *fibroblasts,* specialized types of cells also are present: *histiocytes, undifferentiated mesenchymal cells, odontoblasts.*

The *intercellular substance* of the pulp consists of two kinds of material, the *ground substance* and the *fibrous substance* The ground substance is a jelly-like material in which are suspended all of the cellular and fibrous elements of the pulp tissue. The fibrous substance is a meshwork of minute collagen fibrils.

Tooth pulp contains *blood vessels* and *nerves.* In many teeth there are also mineralized structures called *denticles* (pulp stones) and *diffuse mineralizations.*

COMPONENTS OF THE PULP

Fibroblast cells are more numerous than any other kind of cell in the pulp (Figs. 6–2; 6–3). Often they are described as star-shaped because of the irregular pointed outlines of their cytoplasm. Fibroblasts are responsible for the formation of the intercellular substance of pulp tissue.

Histiocytes and *undifferentiated mesenchymal cells** are located throughout the pulp near the capillaries. They are part of the pulp's defense mechanism and they respond to pulp injury by changing into the defense cells of the sorts seen in any inflammatory reaction.

The *odontoblasts* are specialized connective tissue cells located next to the dentin (Figs. 6–4; 6–5; 6–6). They are roughly cylindrical in shape, being somewhat longer than they are wide, and they contain an oval-shaped nucleus. They are peculiar cells in that their cytoplasm does not remain entirely in the pulp. While

*Pronounced *mĕs ĕn′ kĭ màl.*

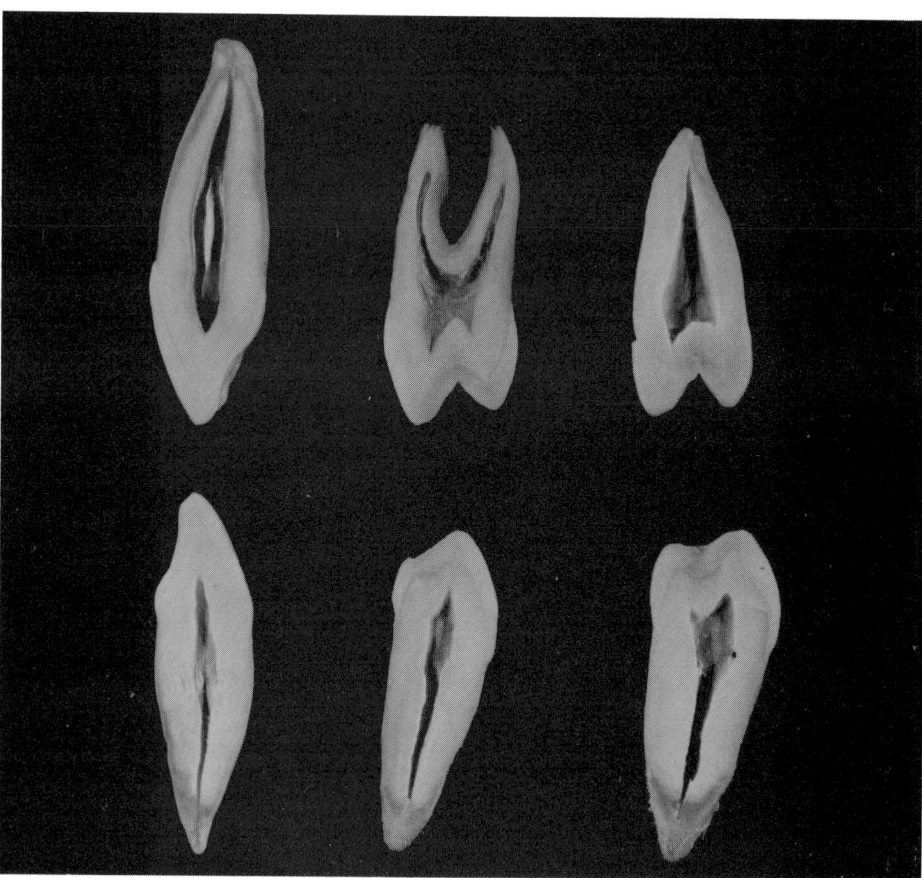

Fig. 6–1. These human teeth were ground down in a faciolingual direction to illustrate the anatomic features of the pulp cavity. Notice that the outline of the pulp cavity somewhat mirrors the outer surface of the tooth. The maxillary (above) and mandibular teeth shown here are, from the left: canine, first premolar, and second premolar.

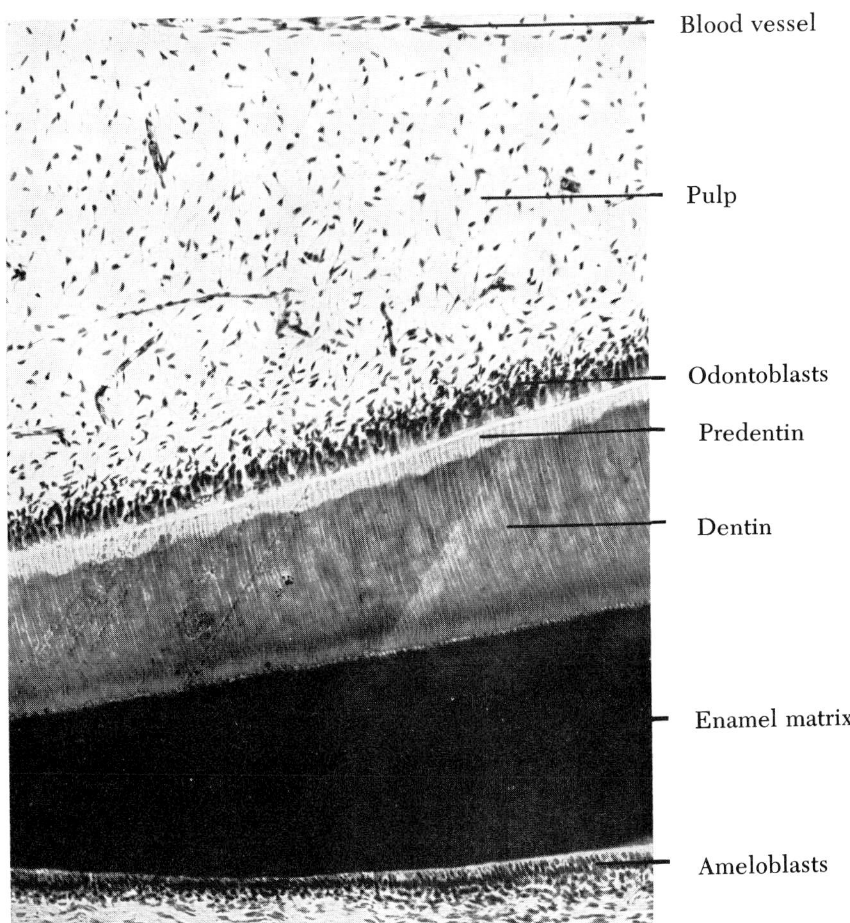

Fig. 6–2. A section through a developing tooth of a pig. The tissues are similar to those of a human tooth. The dark-stained, as yet unmineralized, enamel matrix is covered on its outer surface by the layer of ameloblasts which are beginning to lose their columnar shape. (See Chapter 3). The dentin contains dentinal tubules which extend from the dentinoenamel junction to the pulp. The layer of dentin next to the pulp is unmineralized, and is called predentin, or dentinoid. In this section it is stained a lighter color than the earlier formed, mineralized dentin. The pulp cells next to the predentin are the odontoblasts. Most of the other cells seen in the pulp are fibroblasts. Collagen fibers are not seen in this preparation. They require a special stain. Nerves are not seen in this preparation. Small blood vessels are scattered throughout the pulp tissue, and a larger blood vessel is seen at the top of the picture.

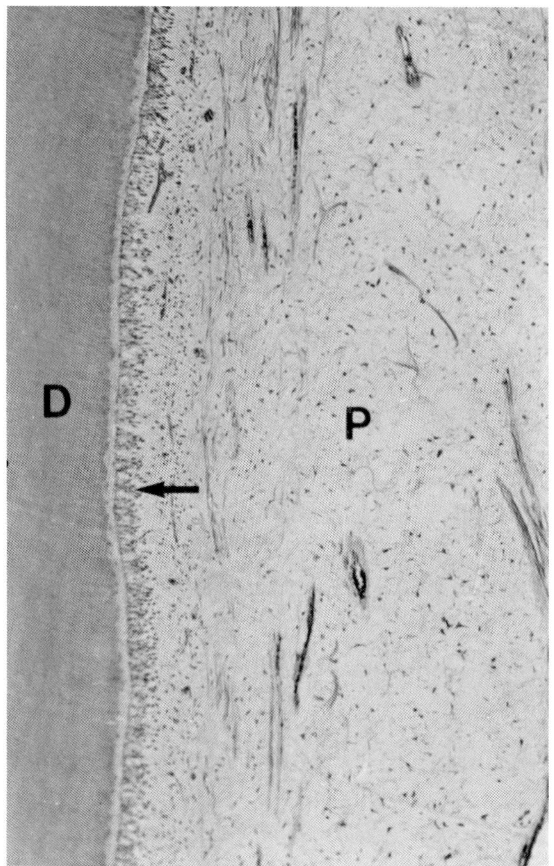

Fig. 6–3. Histologic section through a young human tooth showing the relation of the pulp (P) tissue to the dentin (D). Most of the cells scattered throughout the pulp tissue are fibroblasts. Here, they appear as dots. The clear area around the cells is intercellular substance. At this magnification, the processes of the odontoblast (arrow) are not seen passing into the dentinal tubules.

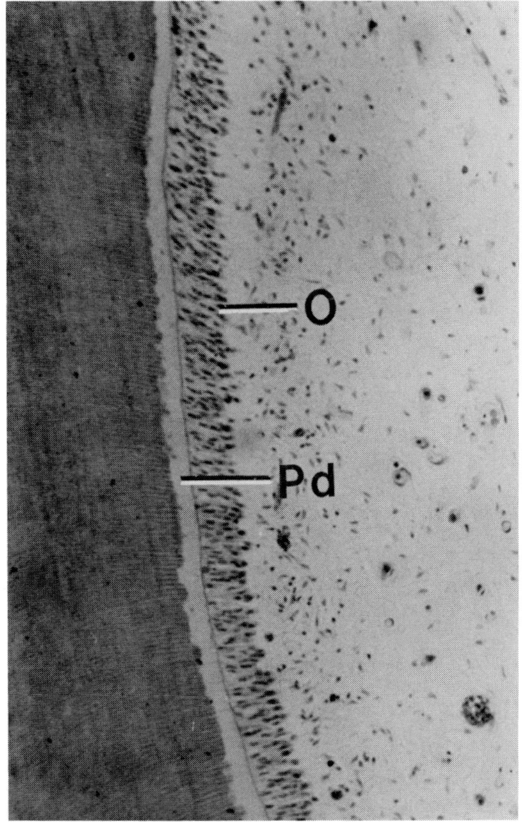

Fig. 6–4. Section of young, healthy human tooth pulp showing normal arrangement of the odontoblastic cell bodies (O) next to the predentin (Pd) layer of the dentin.

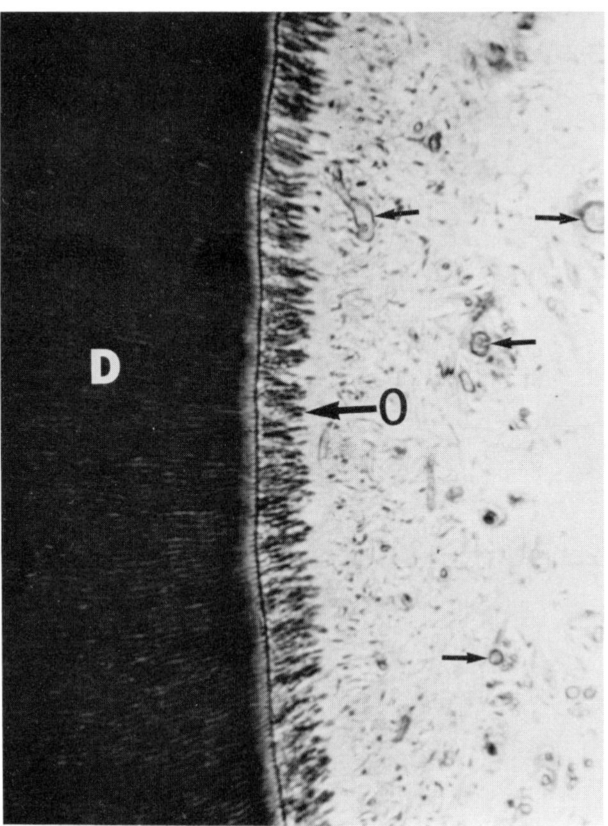

Fig. 6–5. Higher magnification of the odontoblast cell bodies (O). The cell bodies are roughly cylindrical in shape. At this magnification, the cell processes of the ododontoblasts are not visible (see Figure 6–7). Notice the blood vessels scattered throughout the pulp (arrows). Dentin (D).

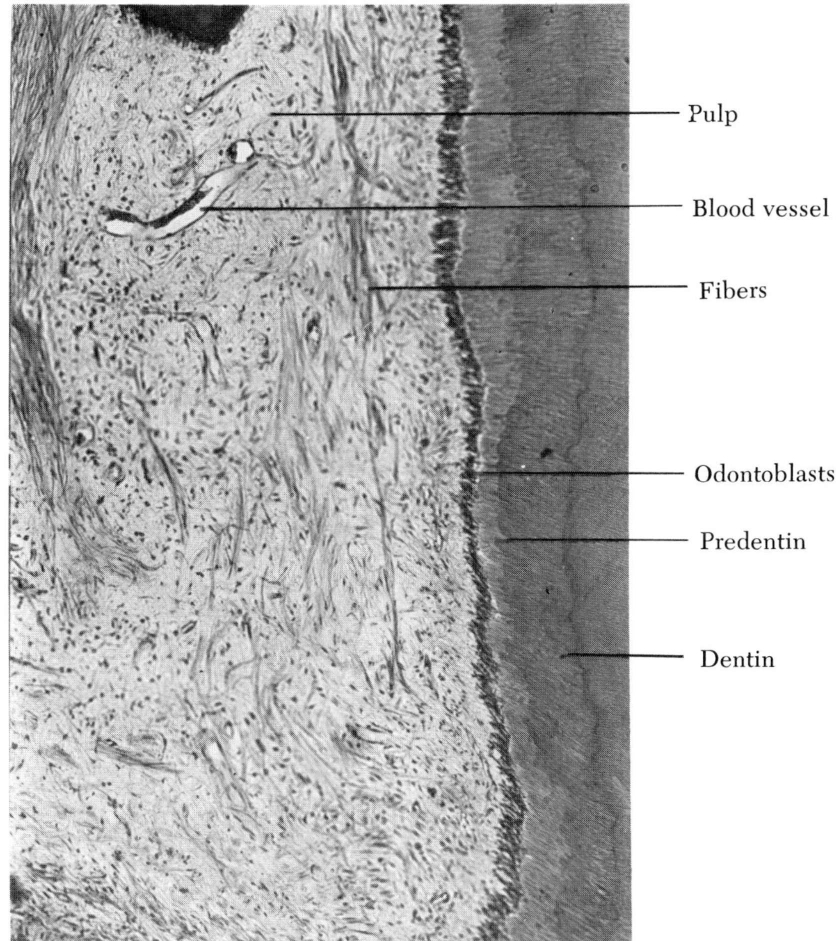

Fig. 6–6. Section through the pulp and dentin of an older human tooth showing an increase of fibers within the pulp. Compare this section to that of the younger tooth seen in Figure 6–3.

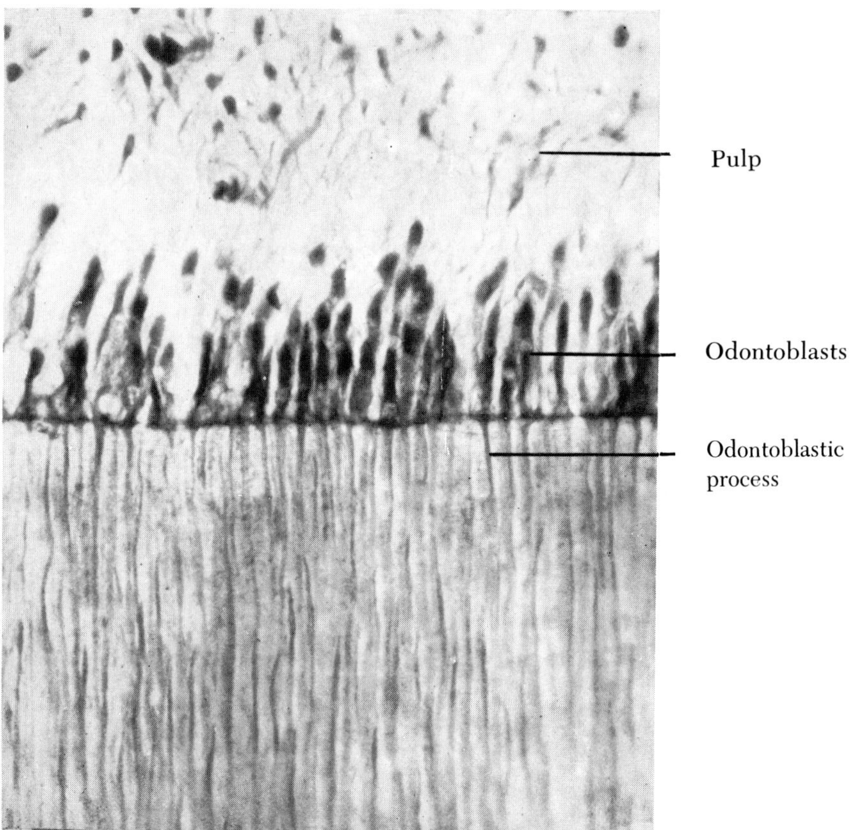

Fig. 6–7. A section through the pulp and predentin of a young human tooth. The ododontblasts are dark-stained columnar cells. The nuclei and part of the cytoplasm of the odontoblasts are in the pulp. Long cell processes extend into the dentinal tubules. These are the *odontoblastic processes.*

part of the cytoplasm of the odontoblast remains surrounding the nucleus in the usual manner of cells, the remainder of it is stretched out in a long, thin tail which enters a dentinal tubule and extends in the tubule to the dentinoenamel or the dentiocemental junction (Figs. 5–8; 6–7). This cytoplasmic tail of the odontoblast is called an *odontoblastic process.* When a process crosses the dentino-enamel junction into the enamel, the portion of it that is in the enamel is called an *enamel spindle* (Figs. 4–16; 4–17).

Korff's fibers are minute rope-like, corkscrew-shaped structures that lie among the odontoblasts during early dentin formation. They have been believed to be the result of the merging of the fibrils of the fibrous intercellular substance of the pulp.* Korff's fibers may be made visible for microscopic examination by special staining techniques applied to thin sections of young pulp tissue.

Blood vessels are plentiful in young pulp (Figs. 6–6; 6–8). Small branches from the superior or the inferior alveolar artery enter the tooth through the apical foramen. As they pass through the root canal to the pulp chamber, they divide into capillaries. The circulating blood is collected into veins which pass out from the pulp through the apical foramen. *Lymphatic vessels* also have been demonstrated in the pulp.

Along the blood vessels, *nerves* enter the tooth through the apical foramen, giving the pulp a rich nerve supply (Fig. 6–9). The maxillary teeth are supplied by branches from the second division, and the mandibular teeth by branches from the third division of the trigeminal nerve. At the inner ends of the odontoblast cells the nerves in the pulp form a network, with some nerve fibers having endings on the odontoblasts. This arrangement helps to account for the sensitivity of the dentin, since the odontoblasts have part of their cytoplasm in the dentinal tubules. Some investigators have seen structures in the dentinal tubules which they have identified as nerves.

Denticles (pulp stones) are mineralized bodies of an irregularly rounded shape frequently found in the pulp (Figs. 5–2; 6–10). They may lie free in the soft tissue or they may be attached to the dentin wall. They vary in shape and size, the size increasing with the age of the tooth (Fig. 6–11). Generally they are regarded as of little clinical importance excepting when they interfere with endodontic treatment. They are never a source of infection.

Diffuse mineralizations are small, thin scatterings of calcified material frequently found in the pulps of older teeth, usually in the root canals (Figs. 1–13; 5–2; 6–12). Clinically they are usually unimportant.

FUNCTIONS OF THE PULP

Tooth pulp has several functions. For purposes of description these functions may be listed as follows: (1) formative, (2) sensory, (3) nutritive, (4) defensive.

The *formative function.* The odontoblasts, whose *cell bodies* (nuclear part) lie at the periphery of the pulp, are responsible for the formative function. They produce the collagen fibrils and the ground substance (organic matrix) of dentin. The odontoblasts will continue to form the organic matrix while the pulp is young and healthy. Naturally, the formative function ceases if the odontoblasts degenerate, or if the entire pulp is removed during endodontic therapy.

---

*Ten Cate, A.R., A.H. Melcher, G. Pudy, and D. Wagner: The Non-fibrous Nature of Von Korff Fibers in Developing Dentine. A Light and Electron Microscope Study. Anat. Rec., *168*(4):491, 1970.

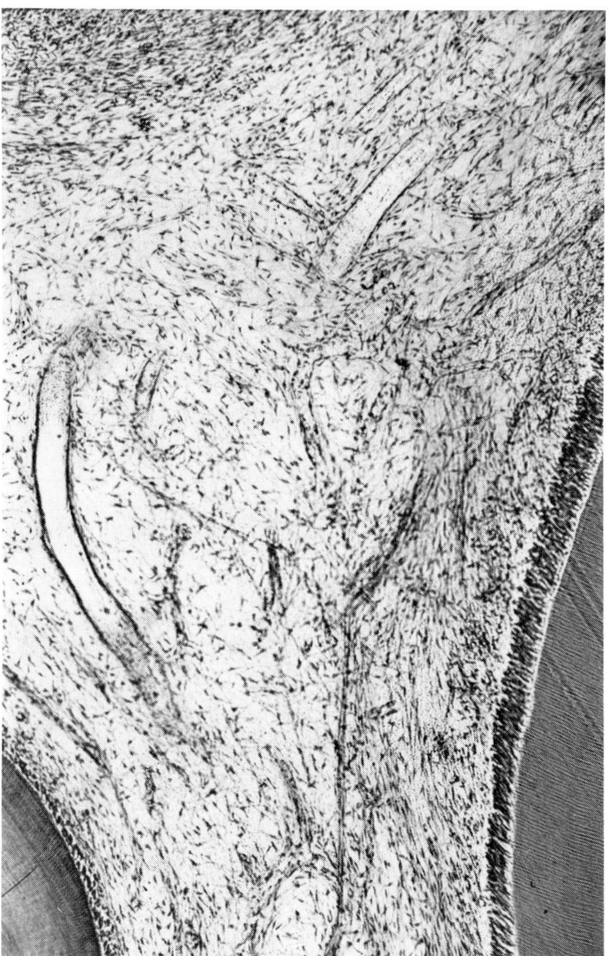

Fig. 6–8. Section cut through a young tooth showing the abundant blood supply of its pulp. Odontoblasts and dentin are seen at the lower left and lower right corners of the picture. Pulp of the crown is above and pulp of the root is below.

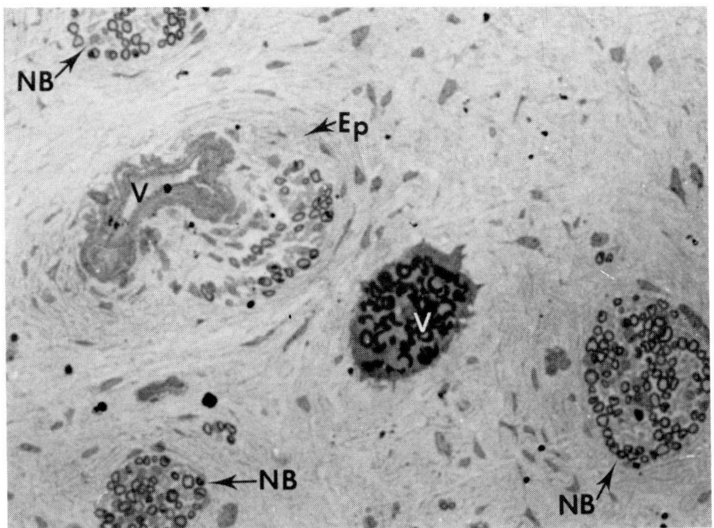

Fig. 6–9. Photomicrograph of center of apical human pulp tissue, cut in cross section. Nerves are grouped in bundles (NB). Note thickness of nerve sheath (Ep) (epineurium) when nerves are associated with blood vessels (V). (Courtesy Dr. Al Reader, College of Dentistry, The Ohio State University.)

The *sensory function*. Tooth pulp is sensitive to external stimuli. The nerves in the pulp are responsible for some of the sensation experienced by an individual when a stimulus is applied to the tooth. It is an interesting fact that the sensation educed by stimuli received by a tooth pulp is a sensation of pain. A person cannot differentiate between extremes of heat (hot coffee) and of cold (ice cream) applied to the tooth. If sensation is experienced it is merely pain in either case. Slight pressures on a tooth will produce a sensation of pressure or touch. Most of this sensation is due to pressure on the periodontal ligament.

The *nutritive function*. Since tooth pulp is a living tissue with a blood supply, it receives nutrients from the blood stream. It may be supposed that nutrients enter the dentinal tubules either by way of the odontoblastic processes or around the outside of the odontoblastic process. Such nutrients may be carried in this way as far as the dentinoenamel and dentinocemental junctions.

Since unwarranted deductions are sometimes made from a set of briefly presented facts such as those given above, it should be made clear that whatever the manner of nutrition of the dentin this is a matter entirely apart from the question of dental caries. We cannot associate the nutritive function of the pulp and the general nutrition of the individual with the presence or absence of dental caries activity. Such association should not be attempted from the above discussion. Dental caries is a disease which starts on the outside surface of the tooth and is a process of an entirely different nature.

The *defensive function*. Defense reactions of the pulp are expressed in several ways: pulp may show an inflammatory reaction; pulp may change the character of existing dentin (sclerosis); pulp may produce additional dentin (reparative dentin).

In case of pulp damage the pulp shows an inflammatory reaction. Cells appear which are commonly found at any site of inflammation. Some of these defense

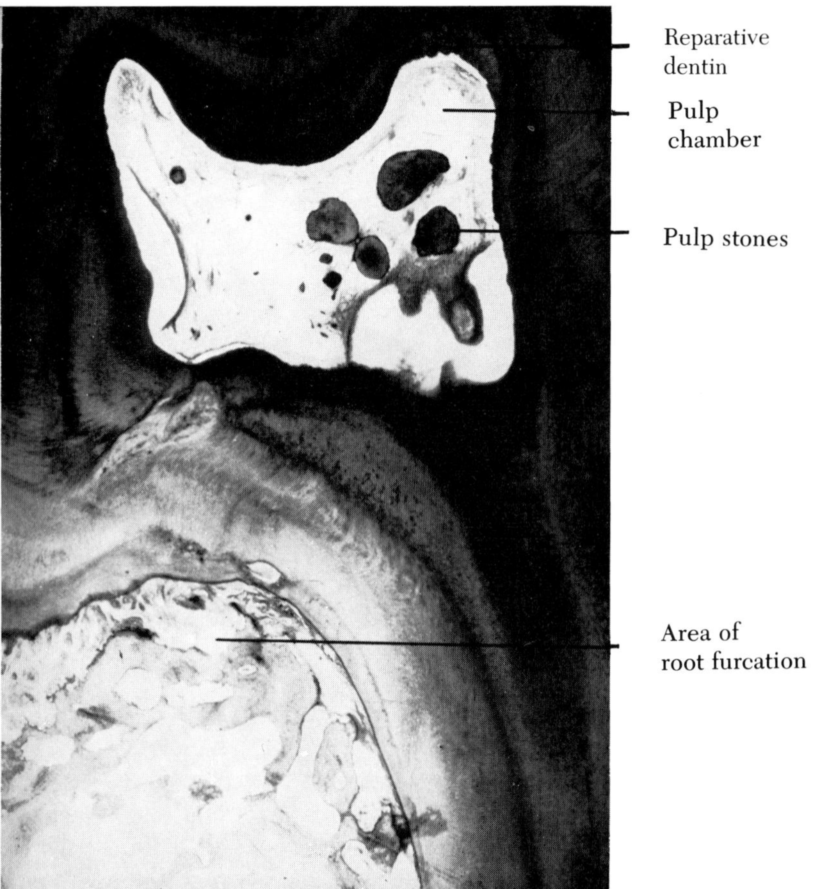

Fig. 6–10. A longitudinal section of a human molar. This was an old tooth. The soft tissue has been shrunken and damaged in the preparation of the specimen but the denticles (pulp stones) are clearly seen. Reparative dentin is seen in the pulp horns. This section was cut at such an angle that it does not pass through the narrow root canal, but of course a root canal was present. The lower left corner of the picture is the area of the root furcation.

cells are derived from histiocytes and undifferentiated mesenchymal cells of the pulp; some are carried into the pulp by the blood stream from their points of origin in the bone marrow and lymph nodes. As the defense cells become effective in controlling the damaging process, the pulp may produce sclerosis of the existing dentin and may also lay down reparative dentin along the pulpal wall (Fig. 5–13).

Sclerosis (sclero = hard) of the dentin involves the filling in of the dentinal tubules, usually in a restricted area, with calcium salts so that the dentin in this area is a solid mineralized tissue instead of a tissue perforated with tubules which contain odontoblastic processes (Fig. 5–2). Sclerotic dentin usually occurs beneath a caries lesion and its presence tends to retard the progress of the destruction of the tooth tissue. The stimulus to the pulp which causes dentin sclerosis is received through the dentinal tubules.

On the inner or pulpal surface of the sclerotic dentin, odontoblasts of the pulp

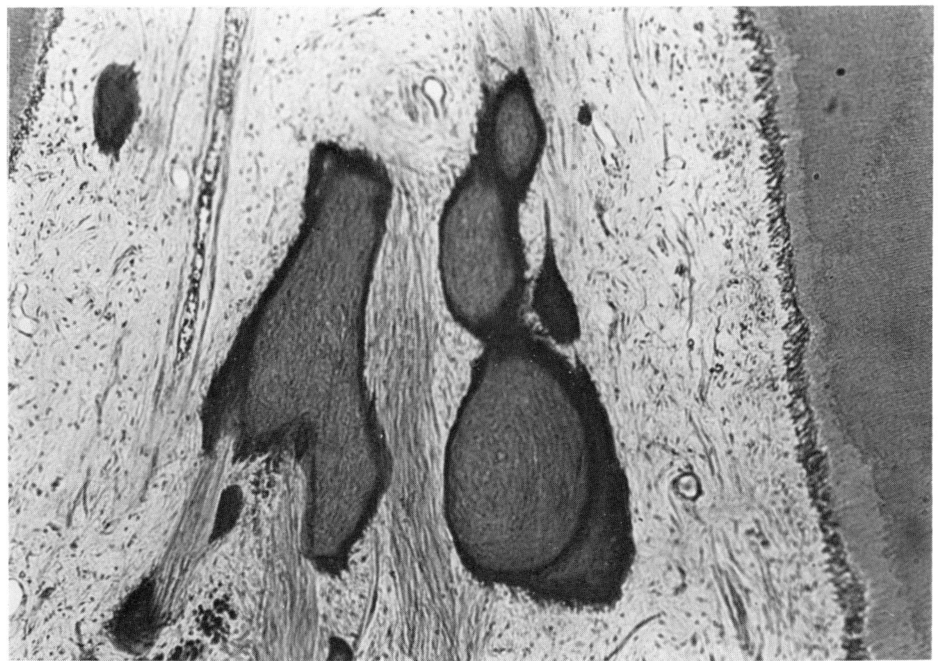

Fig. 6–11. Section through pulp of a human molar showing pulp denticles surrounded by a normal appearing pulp tissue.

may produce, as a defense reaction, varying amounts of *reparative dentin* which gives the pulp additional protection against external irritation. The formation of reparative dentin and sclerotic dentin occurs in aging teeth, where infection is not a factor, as a result of the stimulation produced by attrition (Fig. 5–16).

The saying "A chain is as strong as its weakest link" may be applied to the functions of the pulp. Consider each function as an interlocking link in a chain. If any link is altered, the others will be weakened and a break in the chain of function will occur. If an individual receives a severe blow to a tooth from an outside source and the tooth is displaced, it is possible that the blood vessels entering the apical foramen will be severed. Such damage to the blood supply to the pulp will result in the loss of the nutritive function and a weakening of the other functions. There will follow the complete degeneration of the pulp tissue.*

AGE CHANGES IN THE PULP

Just as age brings about changes in other parts of the body, it brings about changes in the pulps of teeth. These changes are universal and normal and are not to be regarded as pathologic. The continued formation of reparative dentin with increasing age causes the pulp chamber to become smaller and the root canals to become narrower. In some old teeth which show heavy attrition or dental caries of long standing, the pulp chamber may be entirely filled by the deposition of reparative dentin. The cells of the pulp, numerous in young teeth, decrease in number with age, and the fibrous intercellular substance is relatively

*Important references:
Seltzer, S., Bender, I.B., *The Dental Pulp*, 3rd ed., Philadelphia, J.B. Lippincott Co., 1984.

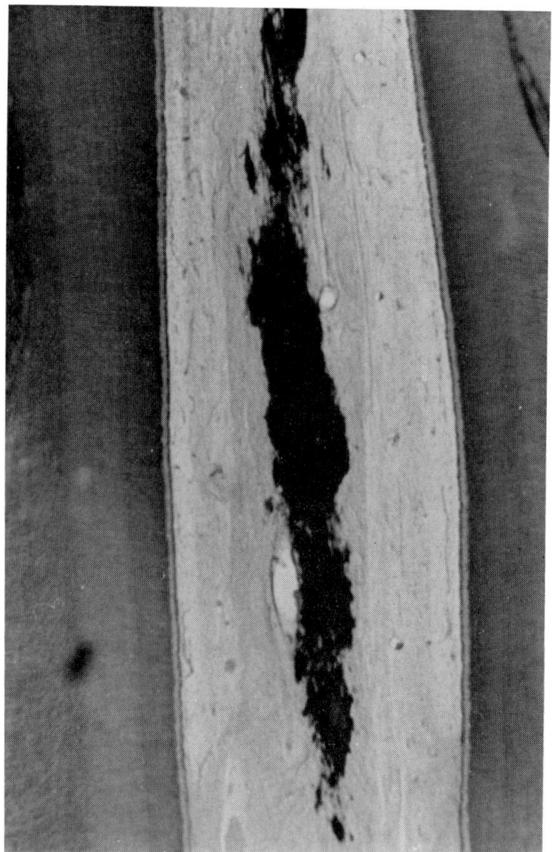

Fig. 6–12. Photomicrograph of a portion of a root canal showing diffuse mineralization within the pulp tissue.

increased (Fig. 6–6). Old tooth pulps are composed mostly of fibrous intercellular substance. The blood and nerve supplies of the pulp decrease with age. Denticles are larger and more numerous in old teeth and diffuse mineralizations are increased. These changes of the pulp do not alter the function of the tooth.

CLINICAL IMPORTANCE OF THE PULP

A fully developed tooth may function for many years after its pulp has been removed and the pulp canal filled. Although the enamel of the tooth becomes more brittle its function is not affected by the loss of the pulp. The cementum is not affected, nor is the process of continued cementum formation. A tooth without a pulp cannot, however, produce reparative dentin or sclerotic dentin. Loss of a tooth pulp usually comes about as a result of caries or of tooth fracture, with accompanying pulp infection. Careful treatment by the dentist is essential in either case to prevent the infection from traveling through the root canal and apical foramen into the tissues surrounding the tooth, with possibly a consequent loss of the tooth.

Chapter 7

CEMENTUM

LOCATION

Cementum is the layer of mineralized tissue that makes up the surface of the root of a tooth (Figs. 1–12; 7–1). It overlies and is attached to the root dentin. Around the cervical part of the root, cementum is about 0.05 mm thick; on the apical part of the root of a functioning tooth it is usually considerably thicker. In the area of the cementoenamel junction the cementum may have any one of three relationships with the enamel of the tooth crown: it may exactly meet the enamel; it may not quite meet the enamel, leaving a little dentin exposed; or it may slightly overlap the enamel (Figs. 7–1; 7–2; 7–3; 7–4). This last arrangement is the most common.

Cementogenesis is the name given to the origin and formation of the cementum.

COMPOSITION

Like enamel, dentin, and bone, cementum is made up of *organic matrix* which contains crystallized mineral substances. Cementum may have cells, called *cementocytes,* irregularly scattered through it. It does not contain blood vessels or nerves. Cementum is not quite so hard as dentin, being about 50% inorganic (mineral) material and about 50% organic substance and water. It has about the same hardness as bone.

STRUCTURE OF CEMENTUM

Compared to dentin, cementum has some similarities and some differences in structure (see Table 9–1). As in dentin, the organic matrix is composed of a framework of fine collagen fibrils held together by a ground substance which becomes mineralized. Unlike dentin, cementum may contain whole cells. You will recall that dentin contains processes of pulp cells, but it does not contain entire cells.

Histologically, two types of cementum may be seen around a tooth. One type is without cells and is called *acellular* cementum, (Fig. 7–1; 7–5); the other type contains cells and is called *cellular* cementum (Figs. 7–1; 7–6).

The organic matrix of both types of cementum is produced by *cementoblasts.* These cells are located in the periodontal ligament next to the cementum; more specifically, they lie next to the *cementoid* layer (Fig. 7–5). The cementoid layer is the most recent organic matrix formed by the cementoblasts.

The cementoblasts may become surrounded by the organic matrix and thus are converted into the cells of the cementum *(cementocytes).*

Cementocytes are connected with one another by numerous thread-like pro-

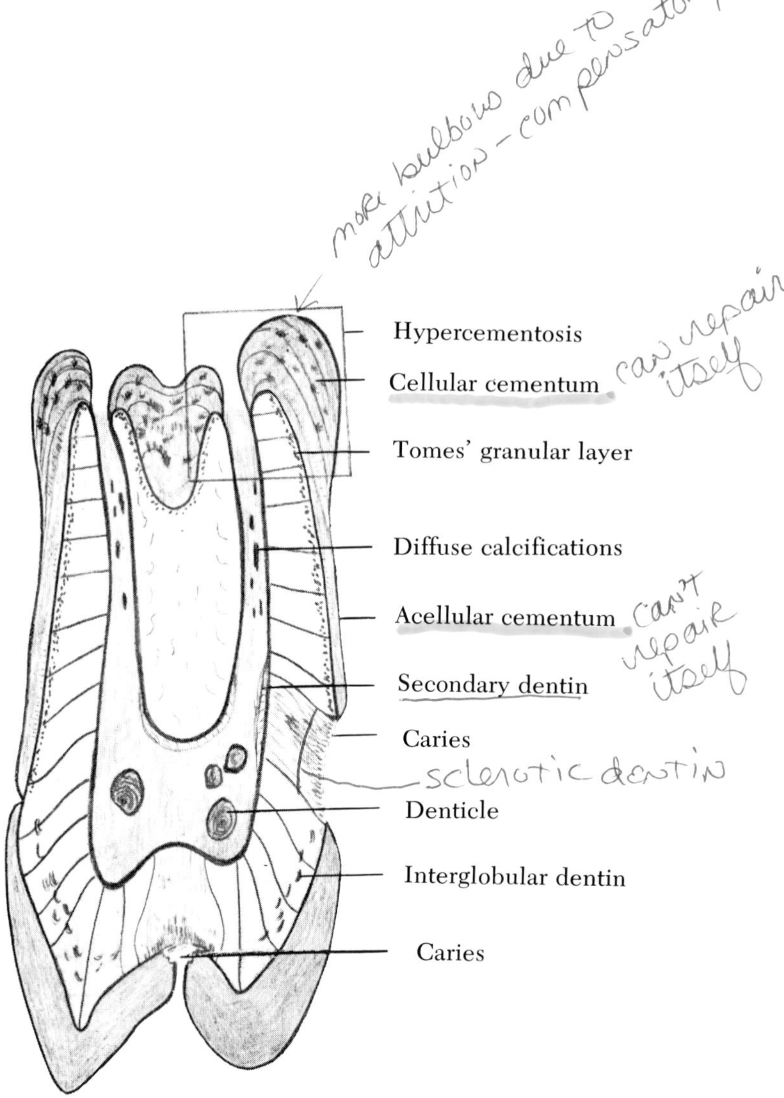

Fig. 7–1. Diagrammatic drawing of a longitudinal faciolingual section of a maxillary first premolar. The tip of the lingual root shows a large amount of cementum which is sometimes referred to as hypercementosis. For a photomicrograph of such thick cementum see Figure 7–12.

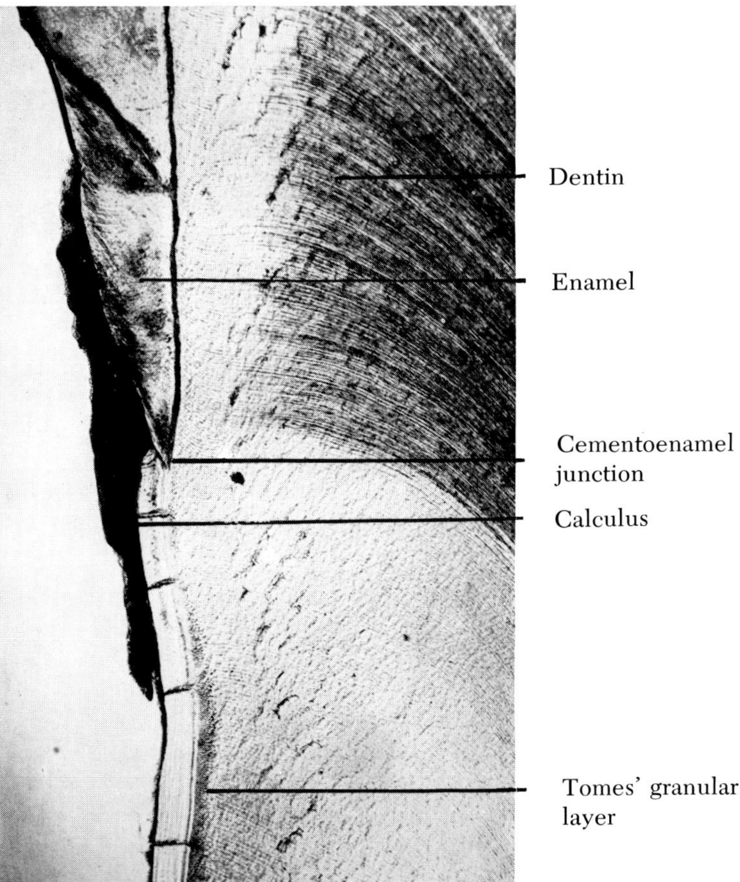

Fig. 7–2. Photomicrograph (low power) of a ground section of a tooth in the area of the cementoenamel junction. The cementum overlaps the enamel slightly. Calculus adheres to both the enamel and the cementum. The four conspicuous lines in the cementum are cracks produced by the grinding of the section. Tomes' granular layer lies beneath the cementum in the dentin. Deeper in the dentin in both the root and the crown are irregular dark areas of interglobular dentin. The dentinal tubules are distinct. The darkness of the tubules in the upper right is caused by air that got into the tubules during the preparation of the section; it is not evidence of any structural change.

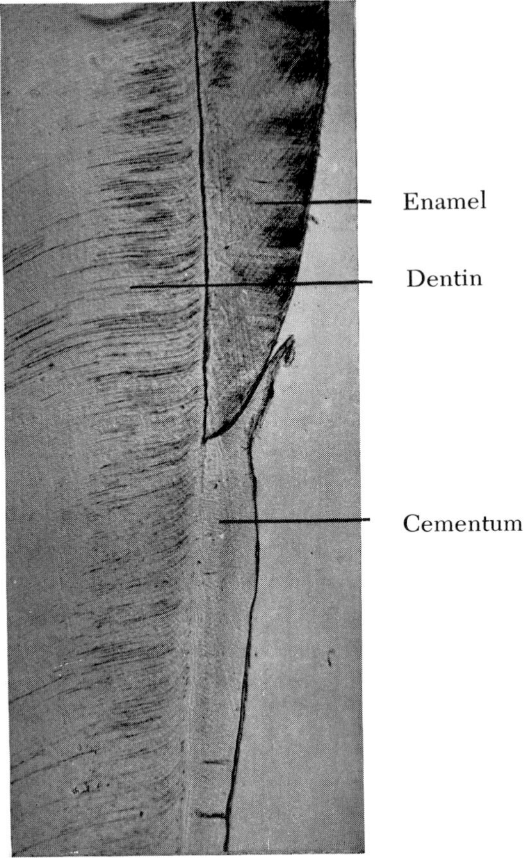

Fig. 7–3. Photomicrograph of a ground section of a tooth in the area of the cementoenamel junction. The cementum overlaps the enamel considerably. The separation of the cementum from the enamel at the border of the cementum is an artifact probably caused by the drying of the specimen during preparation of the section; in life the cementum was probably fixed firmly against the enamel surface.

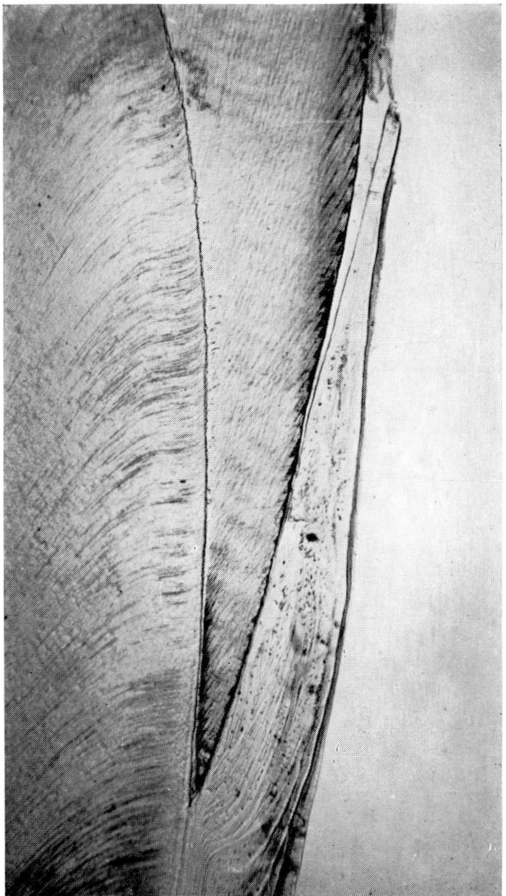

Fig. 7–4. Photomicrograph of a ground section of a tooth in the area of the cementoenamel junction. The cementum on this tooth overlaps the enamel to an unusual extent. Not many teeth show this amount of overlapping. The separation of the cementum from the enamel is probably due to the drying of the specimen during the preparation. In life the cementum undoubtedly was firm against the enamel. This is the mesial side of a mandibular molar.

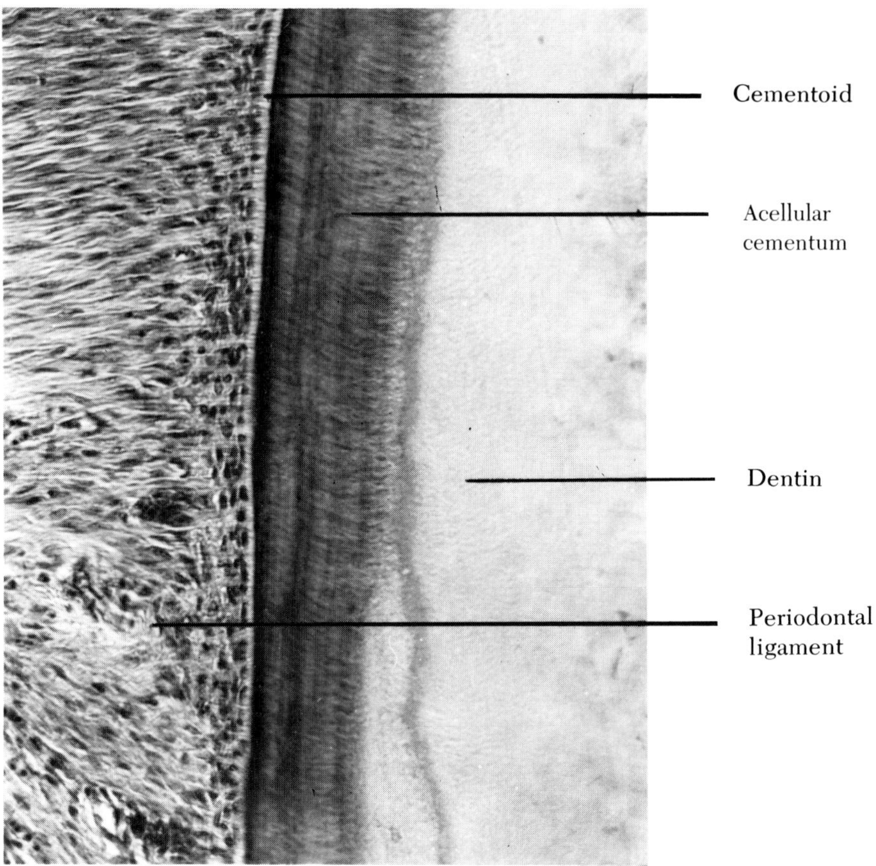

Fig. 7–5. Demineralized section of a tooth and its periodontal ligament. The outer surface of the cementum is the thin *cementoid* layer. It appears light in this section because it is less mineralized than the rest of the cementum. Cementoblasts are seen at the surface of the cementoid layer within the periodontal ligament.

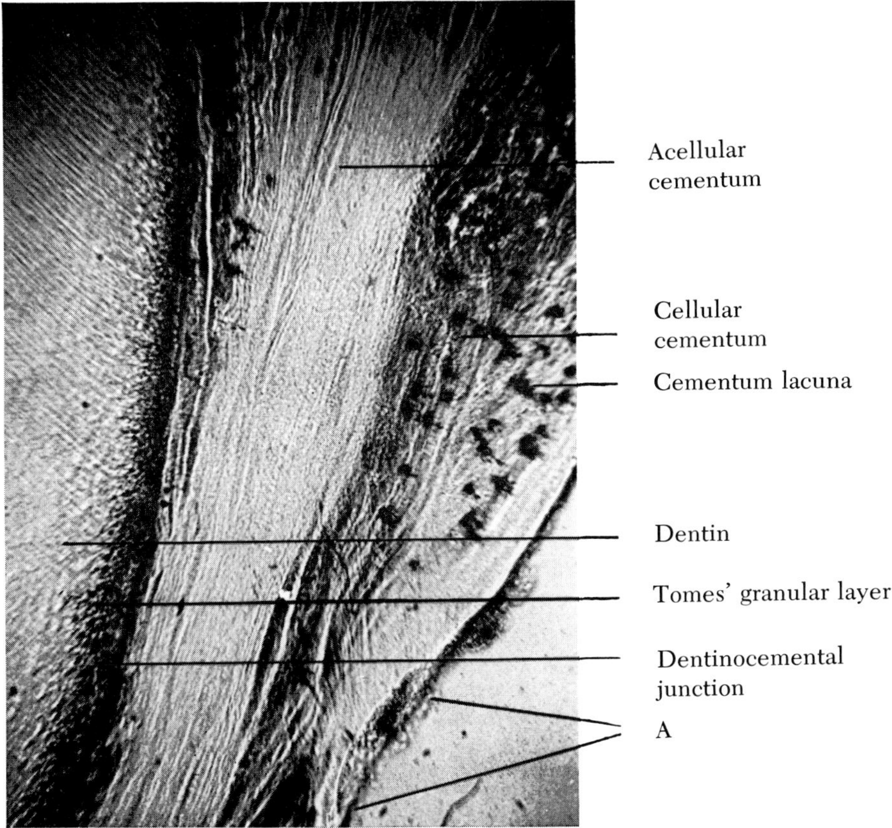

Fig. 7–6. Photomicrograph of an area of thick cementum on a tooth root, taken from an area similar to that shown at the tip of the lingual root of the tooth in Figure 7–1. A indicates the surface of the tooth root to which the periodontal ligament was attached.

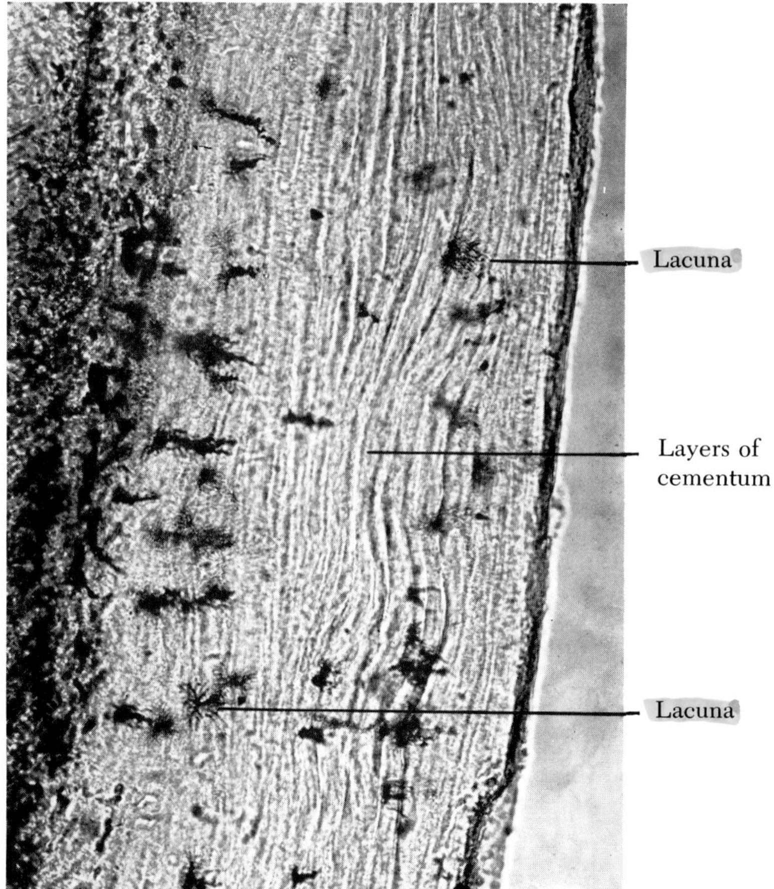

Fig. 7–7. Photomicrograph of an area of cementum seen with a higher power objective than the one used for Figure 7–6. Notice the canaliculi leading from the lacunae; and notice that they often are directed chiefly toward the outside surface of the root (to the right). The layer upon layer formation of cementum is clear.

jections of their cytoplasm. The space in the cementum which is occupied by the body of the cementocyte is called a *lacuna* (little space); and the spaces occupied by the cytoplasmic projections of the cementocyte are called *canaliculi* (little canals). Canaliculi of adjacent lacunae may join and thus connect neighboring lacunae. In cementum most of the canaliculi are directed toward the periodontal ligament (Figs. 7–7; 7–8).

Ordinarily cementocytes are not found throughout the entire cementum on the tooth root. Usually the thin cementum on the cervical portion of the root has no cementocytes (Figs. 7–1; 7–3; 7–5). In the apical portion of the root the cementum is usually relatively thick, and while in this region the cementum close to the dentin may have a few cementocytes, the outer layers often contain many irregularly distributed cementocytes (Figs. 7–1; 7–6; 7–7).

The surface of cementum shows different characteristics at different regions along the root. On some surfaces, the cementum has numerous projections (Fig. 7–9). Other areas may show numerous holes (canals) (Fig. 7–10).

Visible in the cementum by microscopic examination are *Sharpey's fibers* (Figs.

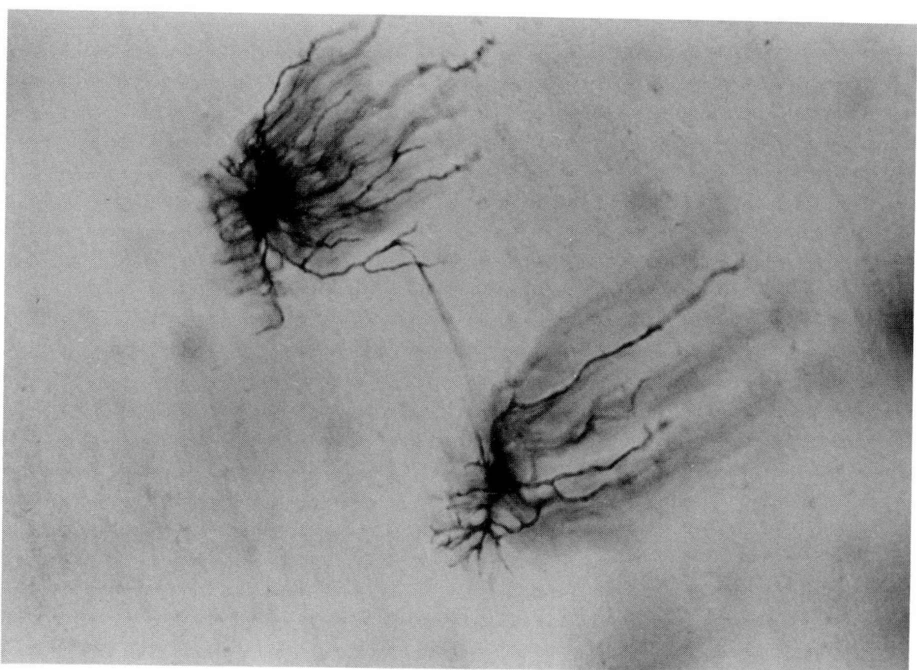

Fig. 7–8. Photomicrograph of the cementum of a ground tooth section showing high magnification of *lacunae* (spaces for body of cementoblast), and *canaliculi* (small canals, housing processes of cementocyts). Most of the hair-like canaliculi point toward the periodontal ligament, at the right here.

7–9; 7–11). These are the ends of bundles of fibers of the periodontal ligament which have become embedded in the cementum during its formation. They attach the periodontal ligament firmly to the tooth (Chapter 8).

CLINICAL IMPORTANCE OF CEMENTUM

The cementum is part of the mechanism by which a tooth is attached in the tooth socket. Just as the periodontal ligament is attached to the tooth by Sharpey's fibers embedded in the cementum, it is similarly attached to the tooth socket by Sharpey's fibers embedded in the bone (Figs. 7–11; 8–1). The result of this double attachment is that the tooth is literally suspended in its socket.

Cementum probably continues to be produced intermittently by cementoblasts of the periodontal ligament throughout the life of the tooth. Additions of cementum at the root apex compensate for the loss of crown length which results from attrition during years of use.

Cementum also repairs damage to the tooth root: it may replace lost areas of tooth root which have been resorbed following injury. While normal vertical pressures or light lateral pressures do not result in damage to the tooth root, a severe lateral pressure on a tooth may result not only in resorption of some areas of the bone of the tooth socket, but also in a localized resorption of the tooth root. Underlying dentin, as well as cementum, may be resorbed in some cases. When the cause of the resorption is removed, if the damage has not been too extensive, new cementum may be laid down over the damaged area, replacing both the lost cementum and the lost dentin.

The presence of *cementoid* (Fig. 7–5) on the outer surface of the root is an

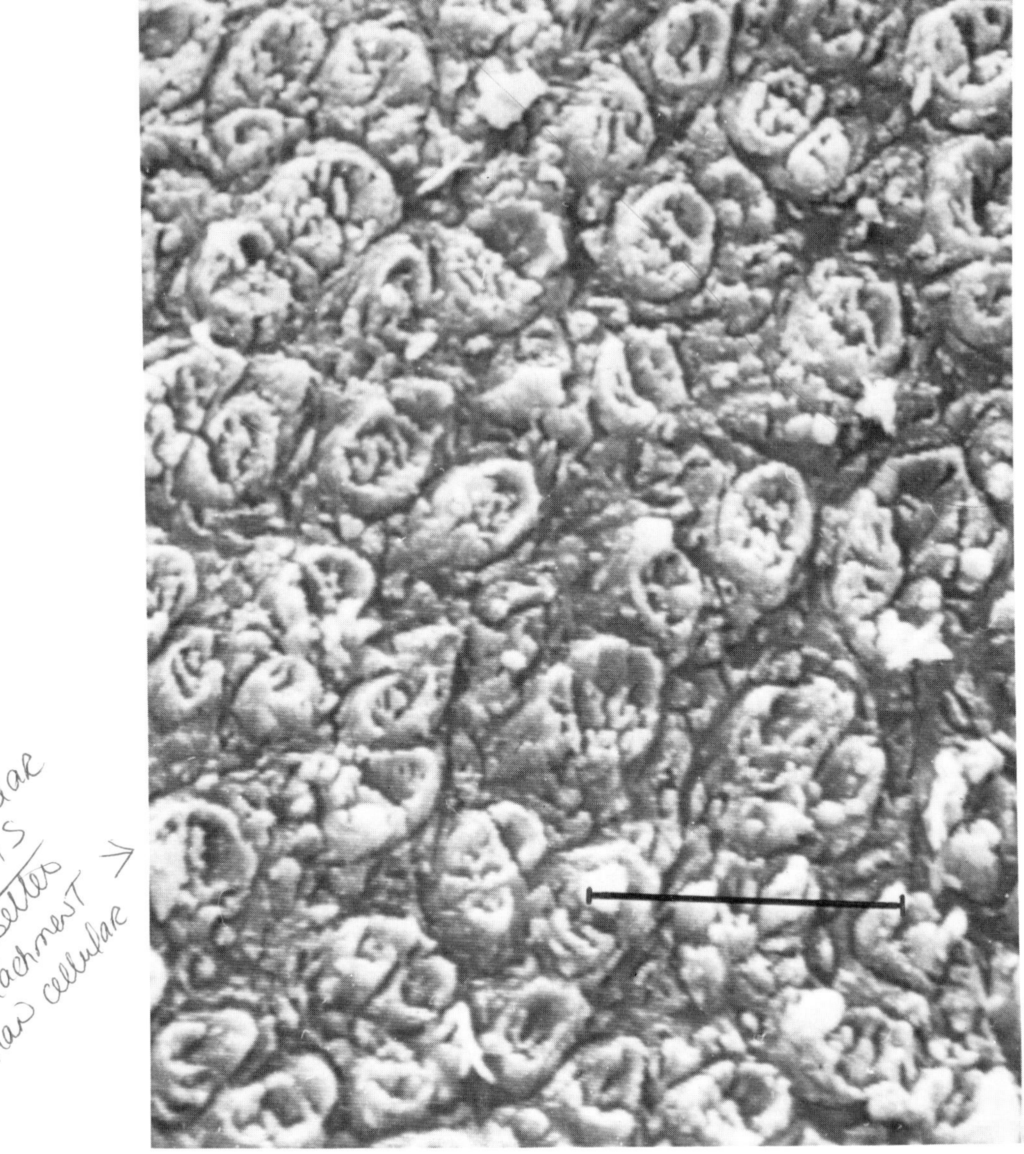

Fig. 7–9. Scanning electron micrograph of acellular cementum. Compare the difference in structure of cementum as seen here from the mid-root region to that in Figure 7–10. The many elevations are points of attachment of Sharpey's fibers. The length of the marker represents 20 μm. (Courtesy Dr. Dennis Foreman, College of Dentistry, The Ohio State University.)

important factor in the clinical success of orthodontic treatment. Cementoid, because it is only slightly mineralized, undergoes resorption less readily than bone. When the orthodontist establishes continued light lateral pressure on a tooth by the use of orthodontic appliances, the pressure is transmitted to the periodontal ligament and to the bone of the tooth socket, and the bone, not the tooth root, is resorbed. On the opposite side of the tooth socket, where the

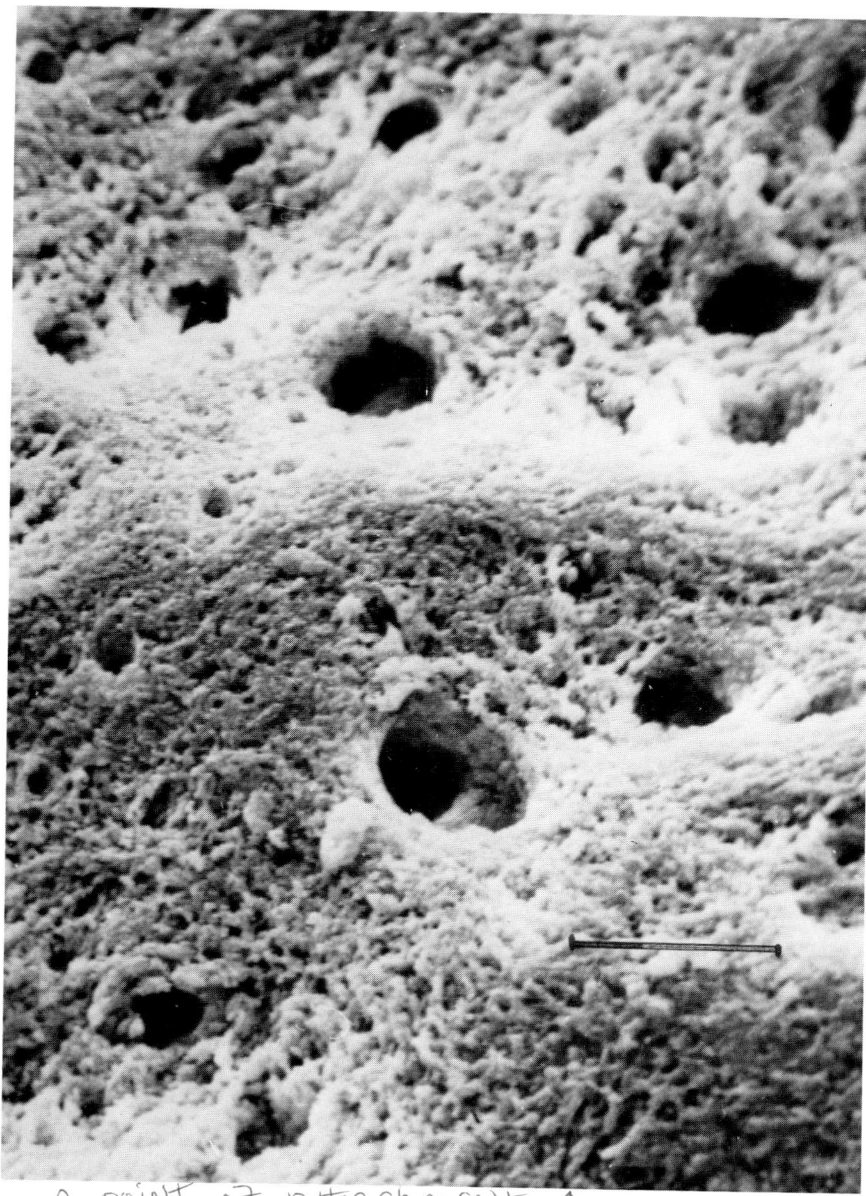

Fig. 7–10. Scanning electron micrograph of cellular cementum. Compare this region of the cementum with that seen in Figure 7–9. Here, the cementum is in the bifurcation region of a human molar. Numerous auxiliary canal orifices are visible. Some of these canals may communicate with the pulp cavity. The marker represents 20 μm. (Courtesy Dr. Dennis Foreman, College of Dentistry, The Ohio State University.)

periodontal ligament is under tension (pull) due to this lateral movement, addition of bone takes place, and there is thereby an actual change in the location of the tooth socket and in the position of the tooth (Chapter 9). The difference between the pressure used by the orthodontist and the pressure which causes damage to the tooth root lies chiefly in the difference in the severity of the pressure.

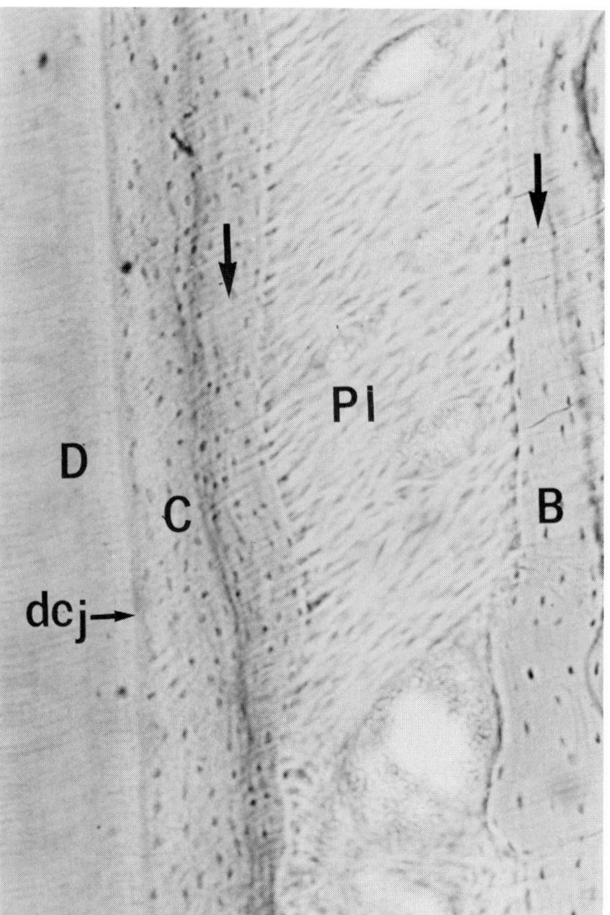

Fig. 7–11. High magnification of a section of a root and surrounding tissues. On close inspection, one can see the fibers of the periodontal ligament (Pl) passing into the cellular cementum (C) and surrounding bone (B) as embedded Sharpey's fibers (arrows). Dentin (D). Dentinocemental junction (dcj).

Cementum is sometimes formed in excessive amounts. Excessive cementum is variously called *hypercementosis*, *excementosis*, or *cementum hyperplasia*. It may occur on all or on only a few of the teeth in any mouth; and it may occur over the entire tooth root or only in localized areas (Fig. 7–1). The causes of excessive cementum formation are not fully known. A large amount of cementum sometimes is useful in that it may furnish additional attachment for periodontal ligament fibers. Again, it may be a handicap. If it occurs as a spicule protruding from the side of the root and interlocking in a resorbed area of the lamina dura (the bone of the tooth socket), or if it occurs as excessive cementum at the root apex producing a ball-shaped root end (Fig. 7–12), it may create a problem in extraction if for any reason the tooth must be removed.

Cementicles are small bodies of cementum which are sometimes found in the periodontal ligament (Fig. 8–14). They are usually regarded as of no clinical importance.

The external surface of cementum is as susceptible to caries as are the surfaces

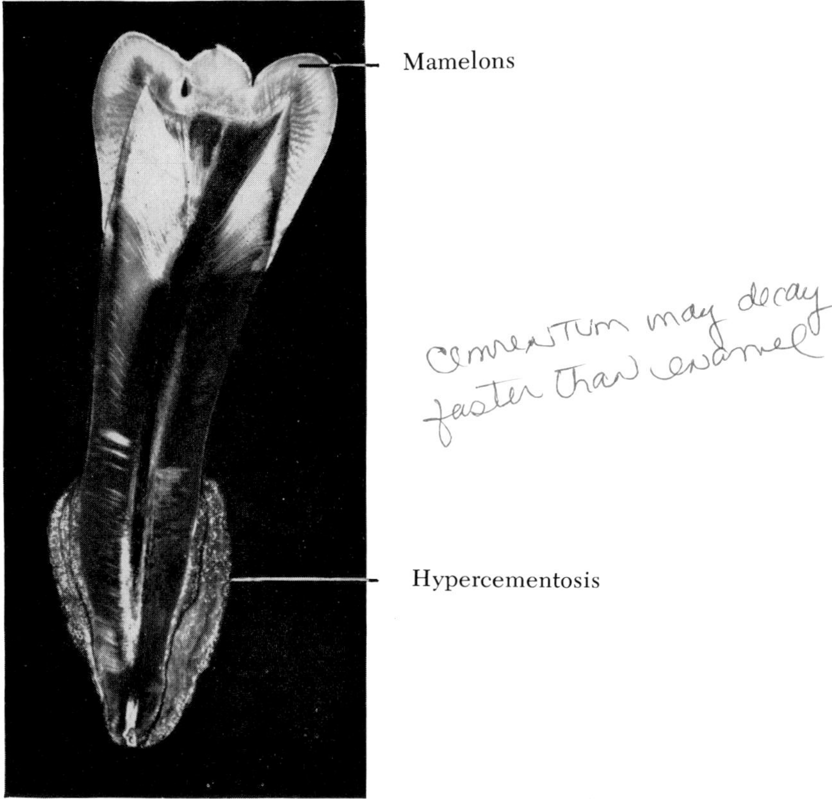

Fig. 7–12. Photomicrograph (low power) of a ground section of a mandibular incisor cut mesiodistally. Before this tooth was cut the apical half of the root looked like a round ball on the end of the tooth. This is hypercementosis. Notice, also, the conspicuous mamelons and the pit between the left and center mamelon.

of enamel and dentin.* If the gingiva migrates apically until the cementum becomes exposed to the oral evironment, the surface of the cementum is subject to the same caries activity that occurs at the surface of enamel.

*Interesting paper:
Hasen, S.P., Chilton, N.W., and Mumma, R.D., Jr., The Problem of Caries. 1. Literature review and clinical description. J. Am. Dent. Assoc. *86*:137, 1973.

Roots may resorb when premature orthodontics are used.
cementum is produced thru-out life, self repairing if cells are present,
cementoclast - will destroy ~~perio~~ cementum, comes from perio lig.
cementoblast - produce cementum, comes from perio. lig.

Chapter 8

PERIODONTAL LIGAMENT

LOCATION

The periodontal ligament (peri = around; odontos = tooth) is layer of connective tissue usually less than 0.25 mm in width which surrounds the root of a tooth, occupying the space between the tooth root and the bone of the tooth socket (Figs. 8–1; 9–1; 9–19). The periodontal ligament is also called *periodontal membrane.*

STRUCTURE OF THE PERIODONTAL LIGAMENT

The periodontal ligament is made up of cells, ground substance, fibrous types of intercellular substance, and tissue fluid. The most outstanding constituent is the fibrous intercellular substance which makes up the *fibers* of the periodontal ligament. Chemically, these fibers are *collagen.* They are physically constructed to withstand heavy forces, such as occur during mastication. Among these fibers are located *fibroblasts cells, blood vessels, nerves,* (Fig. 8–2) and in some areas small groups or strings of *epithelial cells,* and sometimes *cementicles.* In addition to these components there are often specialized cells which function in the formation of cementum (cementoblasts) and of bone (osteoblasts) (Fig. 8–3); and sometimes there are specialized cells associated with the resorption of cementum (cementoclasts) and of bone (osteoclasts). Other cell types present are *undifferentiated mesenchymal cells, macrophages,* and blood borne cells, *lymphocytes* being one type.

In width the periodontal ligament has been found to range from 0.12 to 0.33 mm. The width varies on different teeth and in different areas around the same tooth. Decreased function of the tooth seems to be accompanied by decreased width of the periodontal ligament (Fig. 8–4).

Bundles of periodontal ligament fibers are attached at one side of the periodontal ligament to the cementum covering the tooth root; and with the exception of certain fibers around the cervix of the tooth, bundles of fibers are attached at the other side of the periodontal ligament to the bone of the tooth socket (Fig. 8–1). This attachment takes place when the cementum and the bone are forming: ends of bundles of the periodontal ligament fibers become entrapped in the forming hard tissue. This attachment serves to hold the tooth firmly in the jaw. These entrapped heavy collagen fiber bundles of the periodontal ligament are referred to collectively as *Sharpey's fibers* (Figs. 8–5; 8–6; 8–7).

Although large bundles of fibers are attached to both cementum and bone, it need not necessarily follow that each fiber of each bundle extends uninterrupted from cementum to bone. Some individual fibers may extend from cementum or from bone toward the center of the periodontal ligament where possibly they

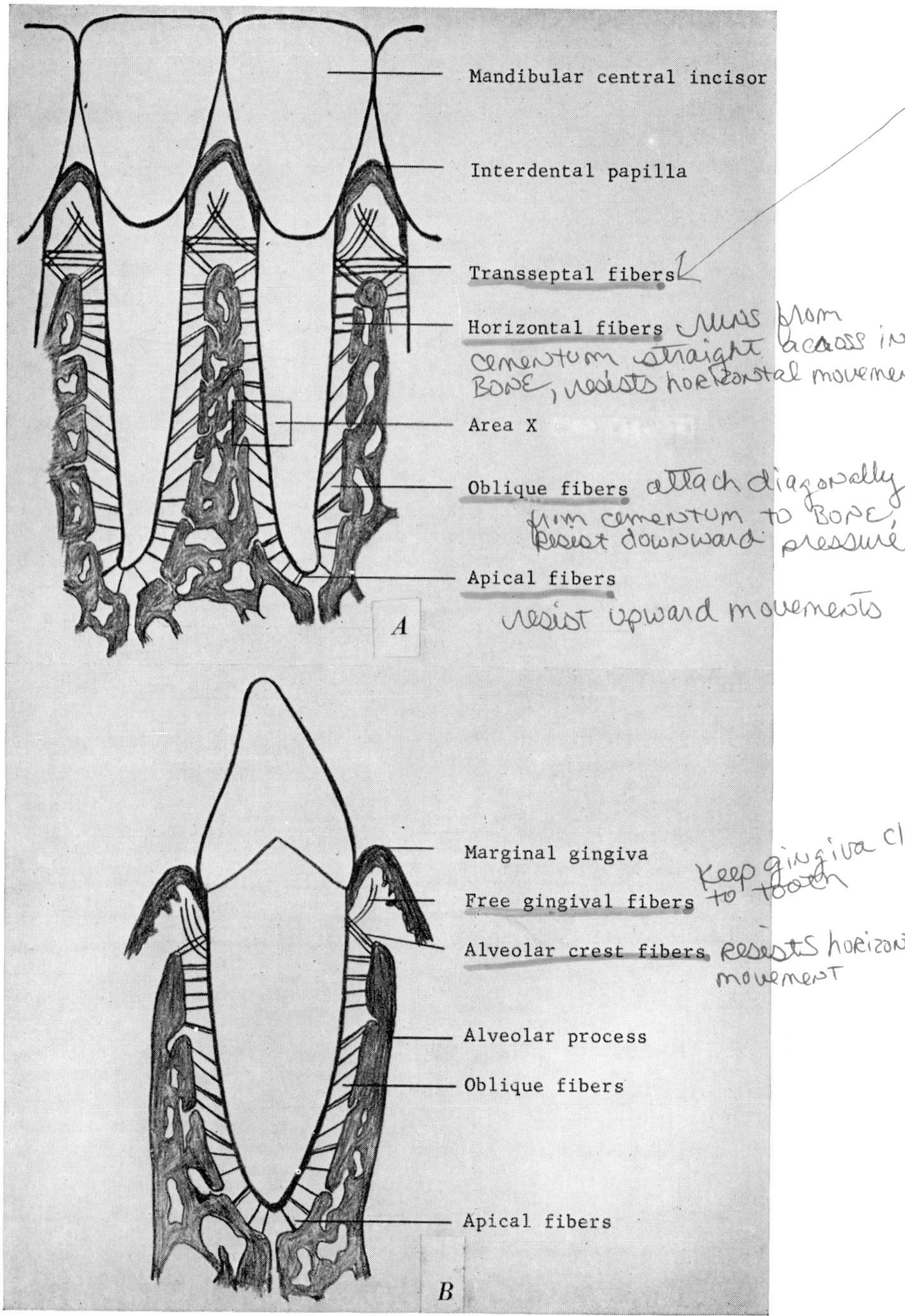

Fig. 8–1. Diagrammatic illustration of the arrangement of the periodontal ligament fibers around the tooth roots of the mandibular incisors. The width of the periodontal ligament is exaggerated in order to show the direction of the fibers. *A*. Facial view. *B*. Proximal view. Area X in Figure *A* is shown in histologic detail in Figure 8–2.

(NOT ATTACHED TO BONE)

→ transeptal fibers – from 1 cementum of a tooth across to cementum of another tooth,

interraticular fibers – only in between multirooted teeth, used to stabilize.

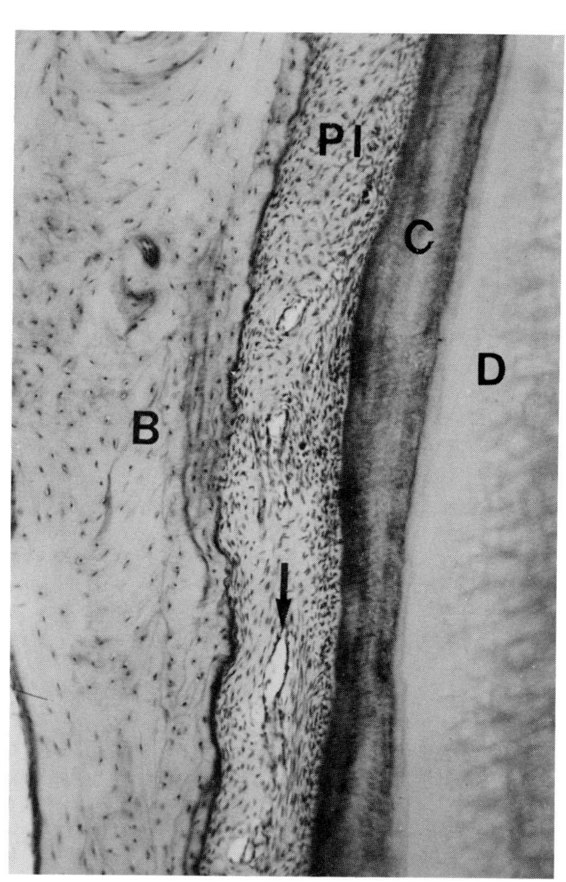

Fig. 8–2. This is a histologic section of area X in Figure 8–1. It shows the relation of the periodontal ligament (Pl) to the cementum (C), and to the surrounding bone of the socket (B). At this magnification the numerous cells appear as small dots, most are fibroblasts. Arrow points to blood vessel. Dentin (D).

ankylosis – when cementum of root is fused to BONE, very frequent, usually out of occlusion, & doesn't have perm. tooth under it.

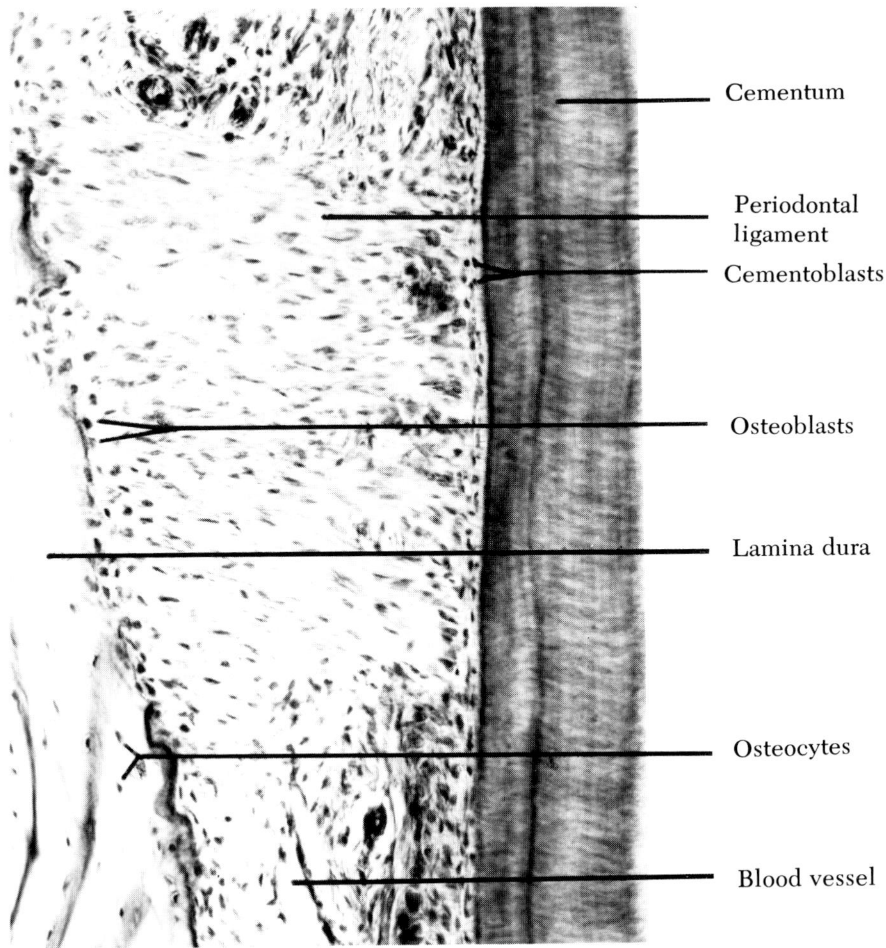

Fig. 8–3. Photomicrograph of a section of a human periodontal ligament and the adjacent cementum and lamina dura. Cementoblasts are seen along the surface of the cementoid layer of the cementum. Osteoblasts are clearly seen along the surface of the lamina dura. These cells are specialized connective tissue cells. The majority of cells seen scattered throughout the periodontal ligament are fibroblasts. These cells are located between the principal fiber bundles; here the fiber bundles appear white.

Epithelial rests – found in perio. lig.
(of Malazzae)

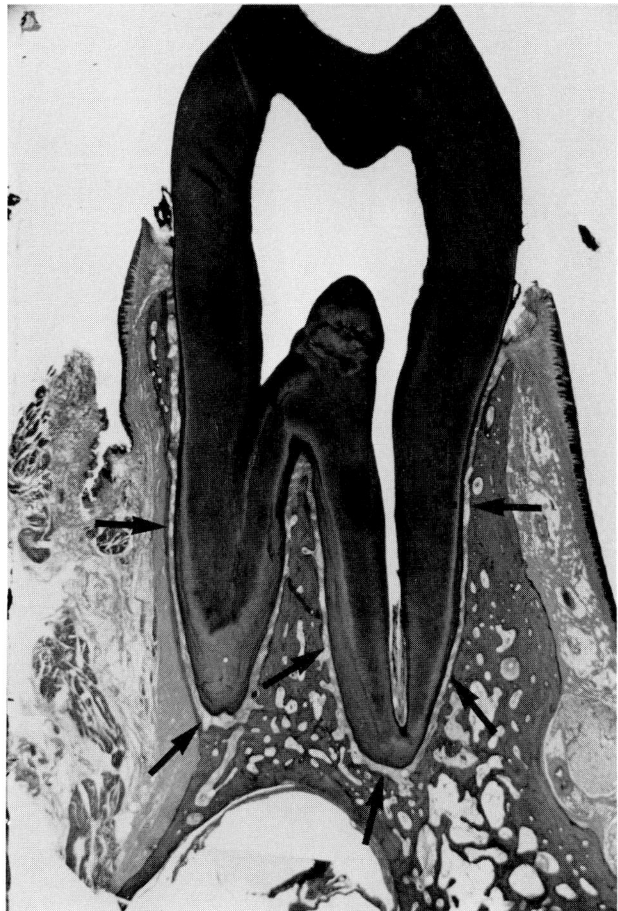

Fig. 8–4. Faciolingual section through a maxillary first premolar and its surrounding tissues. Notice the width of the periodontal ligament (arrows) around the roots. The pulp tissue and the enamel were lost during histologic processing.

terminate and where their ends are interwoven with ends of fibers from the opposite direction.

Around a nonfunctioning tooth (one which is not in occlusion with the teeth in the opposing arch) the periodontal ligament fibers are relaxed and wavy, with no definite orientation (Fig. 9–12); but around a tooth which is in firm function the fiber bundles are stretched straight and have a characteristic orientation on different areas of the tooth root (Figs. 8–7; 8–9). These large, well-oriented bundles of fibers are referred to as the *principal fibers of the periodontal ligament.*

PRINCIPAL FIBERS OF THE PERIODONTAL LIGAMENT

The principal fibers of the periodontal ligament around a heavily functioning tooth have such a clear and consistent arrangement that they have been classified into seven groups, each group being named according to its location and orientation: (1) the *free gingival fibers*, (2) the *transseptal fibers*, (3) the *alveolar crest fibers*, (4) the *horizontal fibers*, (5) the *oblique fibers*, (6) the *apical fibers*, and (7) the *interradicular fibers* (inter = between or among; radicular = root). Study the

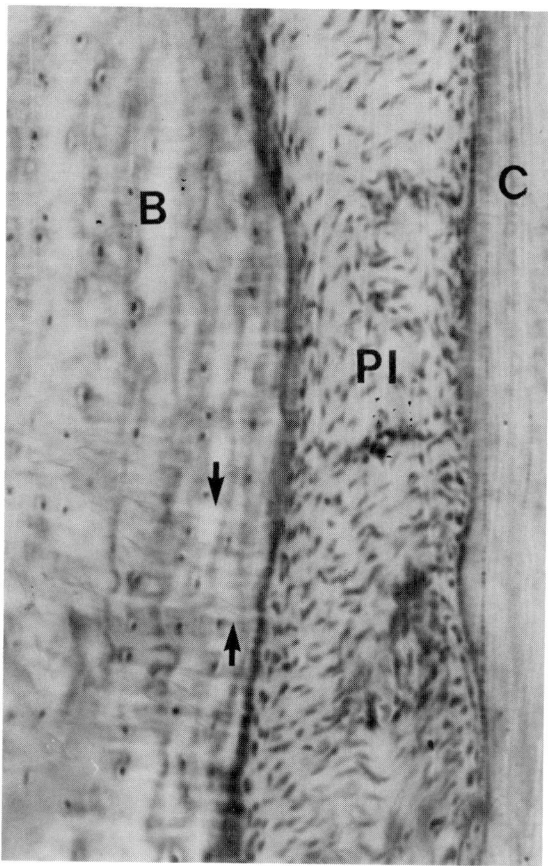

Fig. 8–5. Photomicrograph showing the relation of the periodontal ligament (Pl) to the cementum (C) and the bone of the socket (B). Of particular interest are the Sharpey's fibers embedded in the bone; here, the Sharpey's fibers appear as white horizontal lines (arrows).

position of these groups of fibers in Figures 8–1 and 8–4 as you read their description in the text.

1. *Free gingival fibers* are located around the cervical part of the root. Bundles of these fibers are embedded at one end in the cementum. The fibers extend from the cementum out into the gingiva which surrounds the neck of the tooth. In the gingiva the heavy bundles of fibers separate into individual fibers and intermingle with the connective tissue fibers of the gingiva. Examine Figures 8–1 and 11-6 for the location and arrangement of the free gingival fibers. Notice that a pressure applied on the incisal (or occlusal) part of the tooth would cause the free gingival fibers to be stretched taut with the result that this group of fibers would function to hold the gingiva firmly to the tooth surface.

2. *Transseptal fibers* are located just apical to the gingival fiber group and are on the mesial and distal sides of the tooth only. Bundles of these fibers are embedded at one end in the cementum of one tooth and at the other end in the cementum of the adjacent tooth. With the exception of the maxillary and mandibular central incisors, where the mesial sides of the right and left teeth are connected by these fibers, the transseptal fibers extend from the cementum on

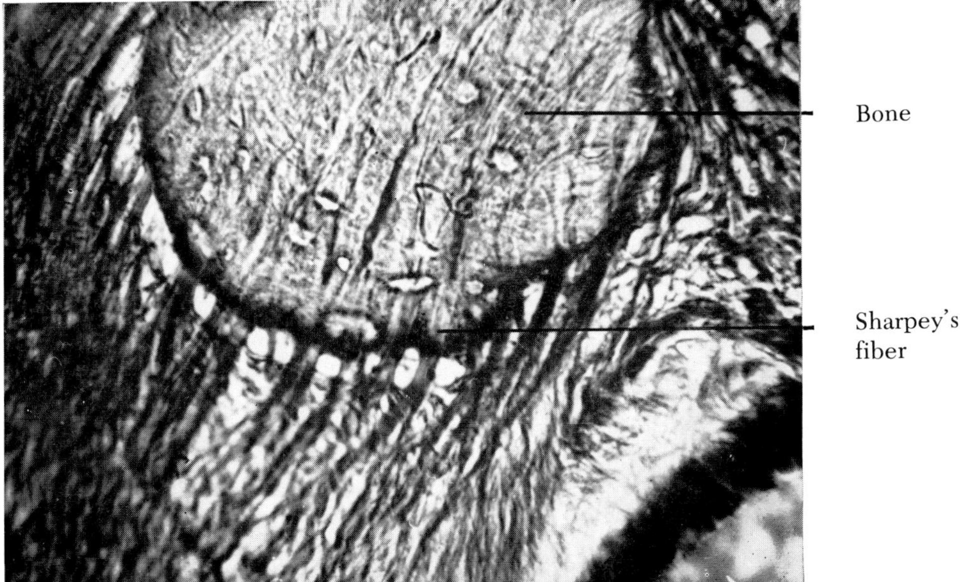

Fig. 8–6. Photomicrograph of an area of human bone in which numerous bundles of periodontal ligament fibers are embedded. The embedded ends of the fiber bundles are known as *Sharpey's fibers.* As seen here the strength of this attachment is impressive. (High power magnification.)

the mesial side of one tooth to the cementum on the distal side of the adjacent tooth. Notice in Figures 8–1 and 8–8 how they cross over the top of the bone between the teeth. These fibers help to maintain the teeth in their proper relationship to one another.

3. *Alveolar crest fibers* are located at the level of the alveolar crest (the margin of the bone which surrounds the tooth root). These fiber bundles are embedded on one side of the periodontal ligament in the cementum of the tooth root and on the other side of the periodontal ligament in the alveolar crest. They are of course found all around the tooth. Examine Figures 8–1 and 8–9 and notice how the arrangement of this group of fibers helps to resist horizontal movements of the tooth.

4. *Horizontal fibers* are located apical to the alveolar crest fibers. They are embedded in the cementum of the tooth root and in the bone of the tooth socket. They lie in a horizontal position relative to the jaw bone. They are of course all around the tooth root. Examine the arrangement of these fibers in Figures 8–1 and 8–9 and you will see how they function to resist horizontal pressures applied to the tooth crown.

5. *Oblique fibers* are located immediately apical to the horizontal group. They are attached to the cementum and to the bone of the tooth socket and they run in an oblique, or diagonal, direction. Look at the orientation of these fibers in Figures 8–1, 8–10 and 8–11: the end attached to the bone is always more toward the tooth crown than is the end attached to the cementum. Imagine a pressure applied vertically to the incisal (or occlusal) surface of the tooth. Such a pressure would stretch the oblique fibers taut and the tooth would be literally suspended in its socket (Figs. 8–10; 8–11). The result of such vertical pressure is a pull on, rather than a pressure on, both the cementum of the tooth root and the bone

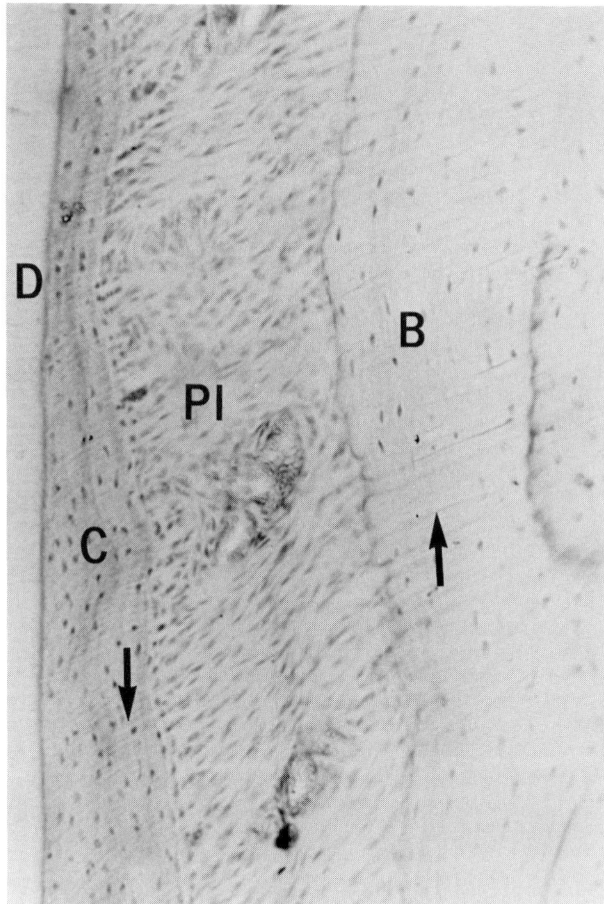

Fig. 8–7. Histologic section of the periodontal ligament (Pl) and its surrounding structures. Here, the ends of the collagen fiber bundles of the periodontal ligament are seen both in cementum (cellular) (C) and in the bone (B). In both cementum and bone these embedded ends are called *Sharpey's fibers* (arrows). The prominent structure in the periodontal ligament is an area of blood vessels and nerves. Dentin (D).

of the alveolus (tooth socket). This pull (tension) is fortunate, because continued pressure on bone ordinarily results in bone resorption. This group of strong oblique fiber bundles prevents the apex of the root from being jammed against the bottom of the socket.

At the transition between the oblique fibers and the radiating apical fibers there is a small region in which the fibers again extend in a horizontal plane. Although these fibers are usually not named in the arbitrary classification which has been given to the periodontal ligament fibers, they function with the previously described horizontal fibers in stabilizing the tooth.

6. *Apical fibers* radiate around the apex of the tooth. At approximately right angles to their attachment in the cementum they extend to their attachment in the bone at the bottom of the alveolus. As you can see by examining Figures 8–1 and 8–4 these apical fibers resist any force tending to lift the tooth from the

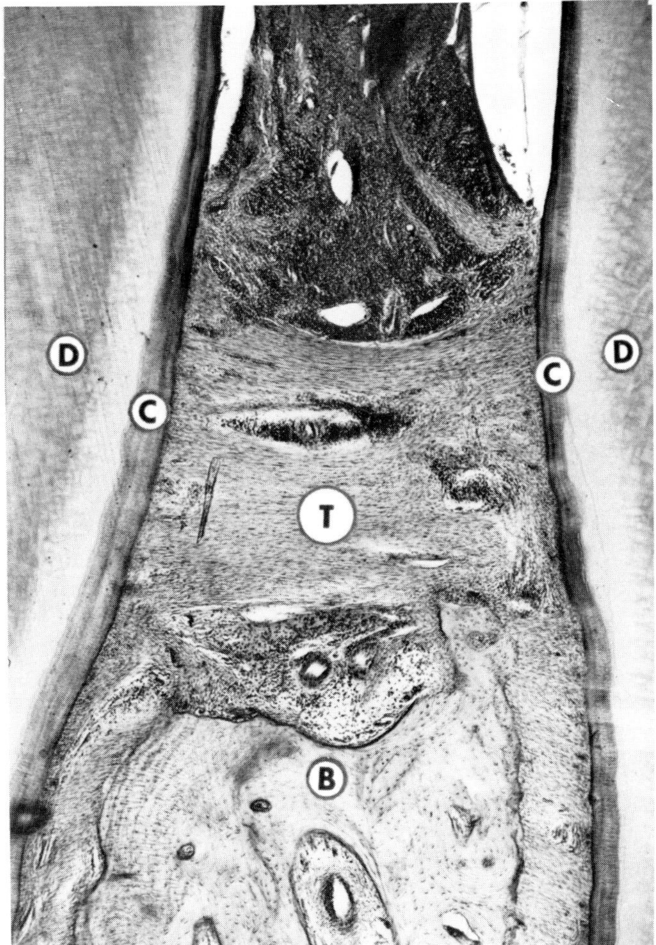

Fig. 8–8. Section cut through the lower permanent lateral and central incisors and their associated surrounding tissues. This is human tissue. Transseptal fibers bundles of the periodontal ligament are seen passing from the mesial cementum of the lower lateral incisor (left) to the distal cementum of the central incisor (right). These collagen fiber bundles cross over the top of the bone between the teeth. B-interdental bone; C-cementum; D-dentin; T-transseptal fiber bundles.

socket, and function with the fiber of other groups to stabilize the tooth against forces tending to produce a tilting movement.

7. *Interradicular fibers* are in the root furcation. They radiate from the crest of the interradicular septum to the cementum that lines the root furcation (Figs. 8–4; 9–19). They function in stabilizing the tooth.

Scattered among the principal fibers of the periodontal ligament are other smaller fibers which have no distinct orientation.

OTHER COMPONENTS OF THE PERIODONTAL LIGAMENT

Blood vessels of the peridontal ligament are branches of the superior or the inferior alveolar artery and vein. They enter the periodontal ligament at various locations: (1) at the fundus (bottom) of the alveolus, along with vessels which supply the tooth pulp; (2) through openings in the bone of the sides of the

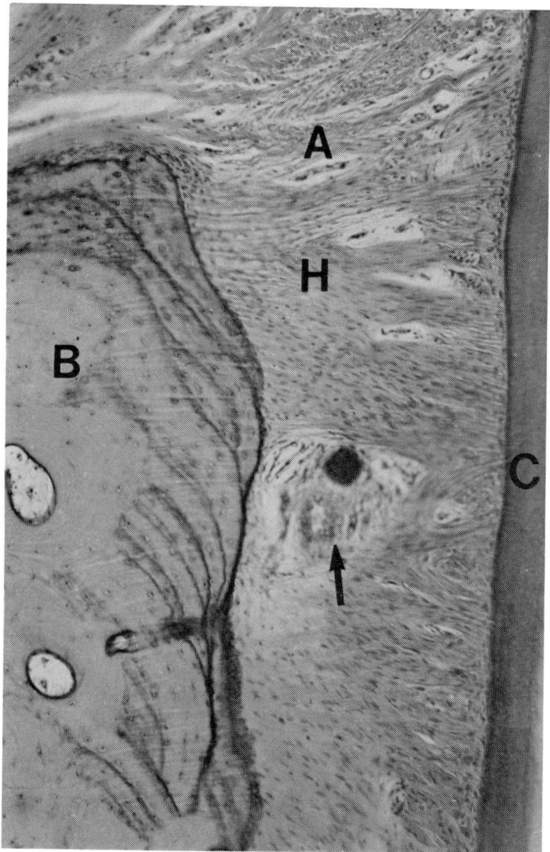

Fig. 8–9. Histologic section of the periodontal ligament in the region of the alveolar crest (A) and horizontal (H) fiber bundles. Sharpey's fibers (white lines) are seen in the crest part of the surrounding bone (B). The arrow indicates an area of blood vessels and nerves. Cementum (C).

alveolus, coming from the bone marrow spaces; and (3) from the deeper branches of gingival blood vessels which pass over the alveolar crest.

Lymphatic vessels follow the path of the blood vessels.

Nerves of the periodontal ligament generally follow the blood vessels. They are sensory nerves from the second division (in the maxilla) or the third division (in the mandible) of the fifth cranial nerve. They provide a sense of touch—that is, they enable the individual to be aware of a touch or tap given to the tooth.

Rests of Malassez are small groups of epithelial cells which are seen in microscopic examination of the periodontal ligament (Figs. 8–12; 8–13). They are sometimes called *epithelial rests*. At times such epithelial cells are seen microscopically as strings of cells rather than as round groups of cells in the periodontal ligament, in which case they are referred to as remains of *Hertwig's epithelial root sheath* (Fig. 3–32).* Whatever name is applied to these epithelial cells found in the periodontal ligament, they have come to be recognized as cells derived from the enamel organ which produced the tooth enamel at the time the tooth was

*Interesting paper: Valderhaug, J. and H.A. Zander: Relationship of "Epithelial Rests of Malassez" to Other Periodontal Structures. Periodontics, *5*:254, 1967.

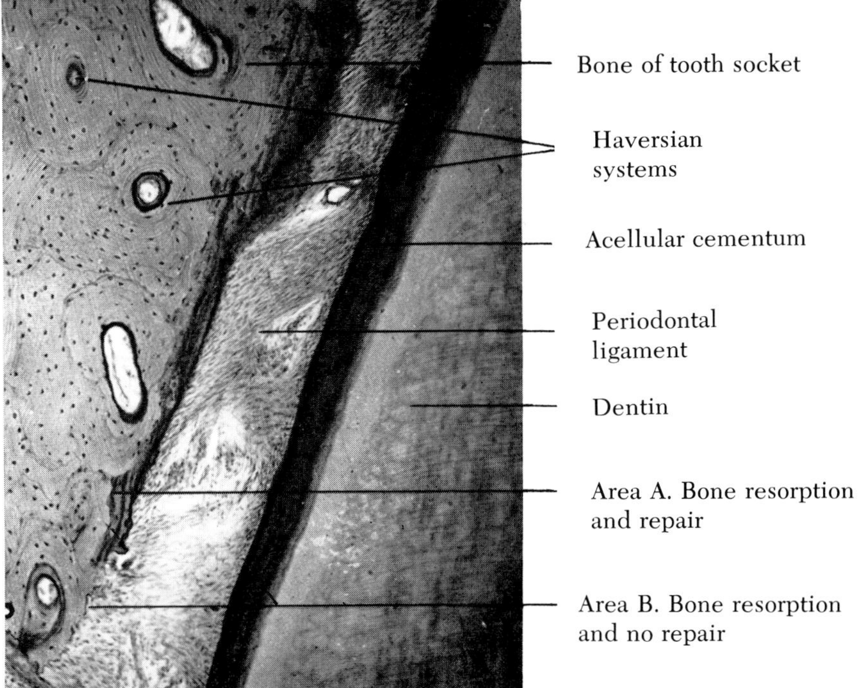

Fig. 8–10. Photomicrograph of a small area of tooth root with the associated periodontal ligament and lamina dura. The direction of the periodontal ligament fibers shows that the crown of the tooth was at the bottom of the pictured area. Notice the resorption of the alveolar bone at *area B*. At *area A* there has been bone resorption as far as the end of the pointer line; and then there was bone apposition (addition) on the surface of the resorbed area (repair).

forming (Chapter 3). Their presence may be important pathologically in the formation of certain tumors and cyst linings.

Cementicles are minute calcified bodies sometimes seen in microscopic examination of the periodontal ligament of older individuals (Fig. 8–14). Cementicles may be attached to the cementum, or they may be entirely separate from the tooth root. Their size varies but their shape is ordinarily spherical. Usually they are not considered to be of clinical importance.

Osteoblasts (osteo = bone; blasts = germ) are specialized connective tissue cells which are found at the surface of bone in locations where bone formation is occurring (Fig. 9–14). They may be seen in the periodontal ligament at the surface of the bone of the tooth socket in locations where bone is being laid down (Fig. 8–3). *Osteoclasts* (clast = break) are specialized connective tissue cells which border bone which is being resorbed. They may occur in the periodontal ligament next to the bone of the tooth socket in locations where bone resorption is taking place (Fig. 9–12). Similarly, *cementoblasts* (Figs. 8–3; 8–11) are specialized connective tissue cells which accompany cementum formation, and *cementoclasts* are specialized connective tissue cells which accompany cementum resorption. These cells occur in the periodontal ligament at the surface of the cementum where cementum formation or cementum resorption is taking place. See Chapter 9.

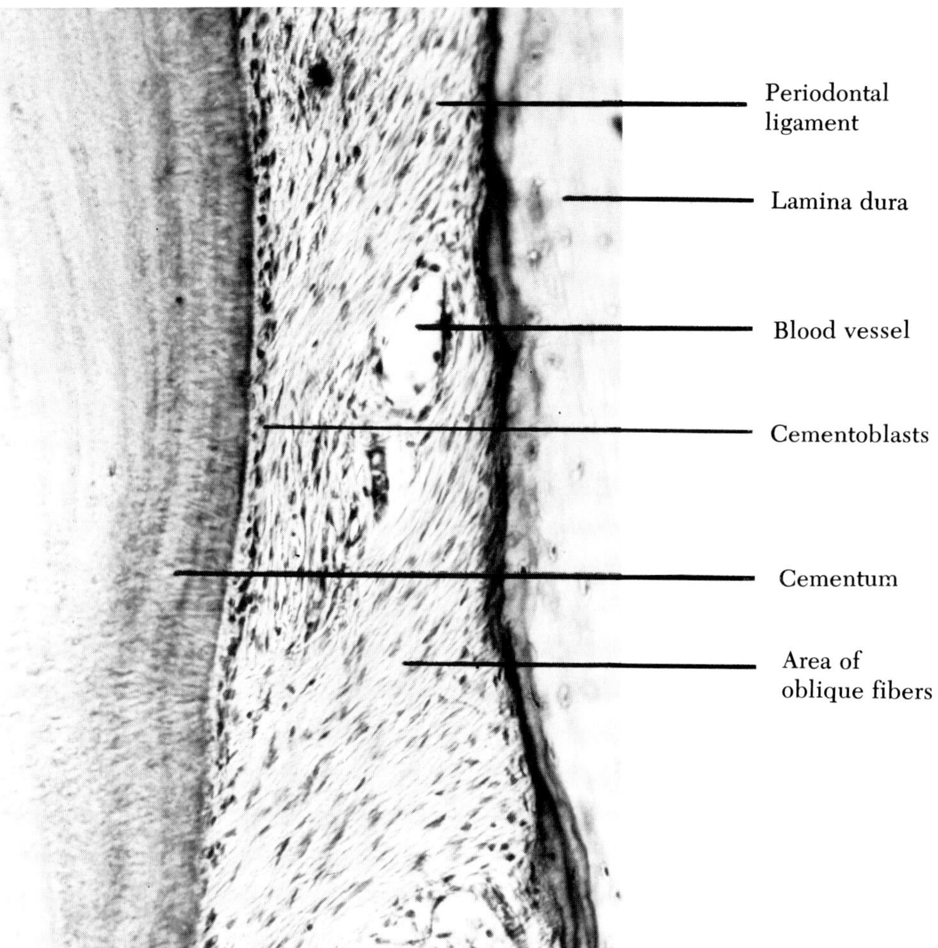

Fig. 8–11. Photomicrograph of a human periodontal ligament and adjacent tissues. This section was cut through the region of the *oblique* principal fiber bundles of the periodontal ligament. Note the more coronal attachment of these fiber bundles to the bone. Coronal part of the tooth is at the top.

FUNCTIONS AND CLINICAL IMPORTANCE OF THE PERIODONTAL LIGAMENT

The functions of the periodontal ligament may be described under five headings: (1) supportive, (2) formative, (3) resorptive, (4) sensory, and (5) nutritive.

The *supportive function* of the periodontal ligament results from the ingenious arrangement of its principal fibers. As you have seen, the fibers are so arranged that functional pressure on the tooth crown from any direction produces a tension (pulling) of certain fiber groups. Consequently, pressure on the tooth crown is transmitted to the bone of the tooth socket and to the cementum as a pull. Because of this fiber arrangement which suspends the tooth in its socket, the tooth is not pressed against the bone of the socket wall during the process of biting and chewing. These sturdy principal fibers of the periodontal ligament which separate the cementum of the tooth root from the wall of the socket by less than ¼ mm are able to withstand the heavy force produced by the powerful

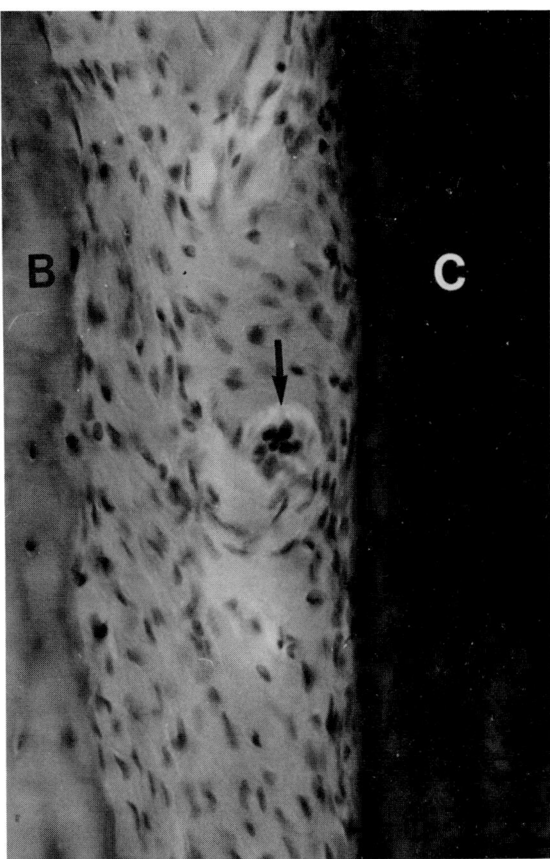

Fig. 8–12. Histologic section of the periodontal ligament and the associated bone (B) and cementum (C). The arrow indicates an epithelial rest of Malassez. Most of the other cells seen are fibroblasts.

jaw muscles in closing the jaws. A study of 53 young adults at the School of Denistry in Melbourne, Australia, showed the average biting force to be: for males, 19.6 kgf (kilograms force) (43 pounds) for anterior teeth and 29.3 kgf (65 pounds) for posterior teeth; for females 13.5 kgf (30 pounds) for anterior teeth and 21.3 kgf (47 pounds) for posterior teeth.*

A sudden excessive pressure applied to a tooth crown, such as in case of an accidental blow, may damage the periodontal ligament sufficiently to loosen the tooth.

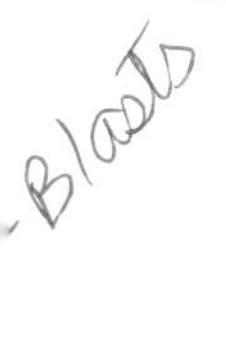

The *formative function* of the periodontal ligament is seen in both the developing tooth and in the adult functioning tooth. During tooth development cells of the periodontal ligament produce both the cementum of the tooth root and the bone of the tooth socket. In the functioning tooth cementoblasts of the periodontal ligament are able to produce cementum at any time during the life of the tooth; and its osteoblasts maintain the bone of the tooth socket by producing new bone following bone resorption (Fig. 8–10). The fibroblasts of the periodontal ligament produce the collagen and ground substance which are subject to a dynamic turnover, especially during orthodontic treatment. There is evidence that fibroblasts

*Atkinson, H.F., and W.J. Ralph: Tooth Loss and Biting Force in Man. J. Dent. Res., *52*(2):225, 1973.

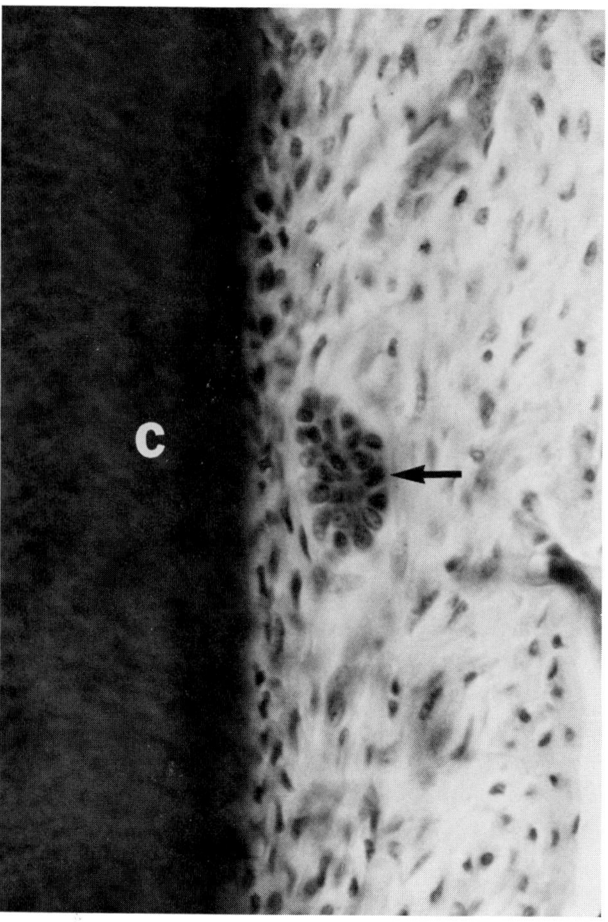

Fig. 8–13. Higher magnification of an epithelial rest (arrow) showing clearly the individual epithelial cells. Note the position of the epithelial rest near the cementum (C); this is the usual arrangement. Note also the numerous other cells scattered throughout the periodontal ligament.

may also play a role in the lysis (dissolution) of collagen fibers. When they perform this function, they are referred to as "fibroclasts."*

The *resorptive function* of the periodontal ligament accompanies the formative function. Whereas tension (pull) on the periodontal ligament fibers tends to stimulate cementum and bone formation, pressure stimulates bone resorption. Severe pressure produces rapid bone resorption, and sometimes may cause resorption of the more resistant cementum as well. If sufficiently severe, pressure may destroy areas of the periodontal ligament. More will be learned about the processes of bone formation and bone resorption in the discussion of bone and the alveolar process (Chapter 9).

The *sensory function* of the periodontal ligament is seen in the ability of an individual to estimate the amount of pressure in mastication and to identify which one of several teeth receives a slight tap with an instrument.

*Interesting paper: Ten Cate, A.R., Mills, C., and Solomon, G.: The Development of the Periodontium. A Transplantation and Autoradiographic Study. Anat. Rec. *170*:365, 1971.

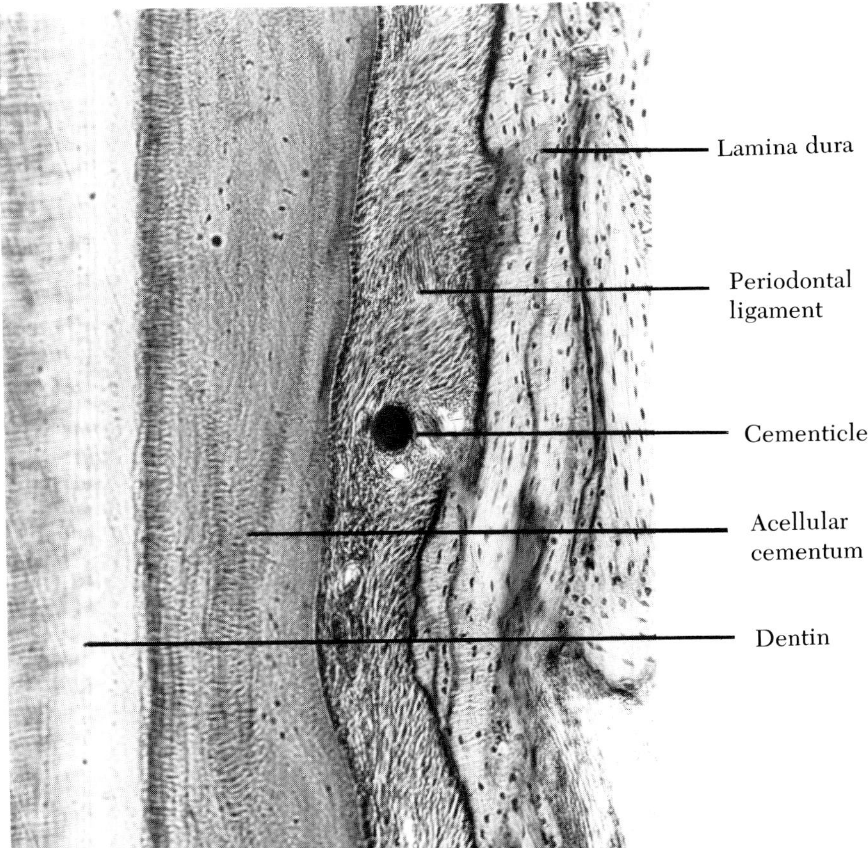

Fig. 8–14. Photomicrograph of a section through a human tooth and its periodontal ligament. A cementicle is seen surrounded by periodontal ligament tissue.

The *nutritive function* is served by the presence of blood vessels in the periodontal ligament.

It is obvious that without the periodontal ligament a tooth cannot be retained in its socket. Localized destruction of the periodontal ligament may be repaired by the formation of new tissue when the cause of the destruction is removed. Localized detachment from the cementum of the principal fibers of the periodontal ligament may be followed by fiber reattachment if removal of irritating factors permits the formation of new cementum. Extensive destruction of the periodontal ligament may result in the necessity for the removal of the tooth.

periosteum is tough
endosteum is fragile

Chapter 9

BONE AND THE ALVEOLAR PROCESS

BONE

The word *bone* is used to designate both an organ and a tissue. A *bone*, an organ, such as the mandible, for example, is composed of bone tissue; it contains in its center bone marrow, and it has closely associated with it blood vessels and nerves. Bone, a tissue, is one of the connective tissues. It is made up of (1) an organic matrix which mineralizes and (2) osteocytes (bone cells).

Gross Structure of a Bone (an organ)

Bones are solid-looking organs, but they are not solid structures throughout. The bone tissue of which bones are composed may be described in two classes: (1) *compact bone* and (2) *trabecular bone* (or *spongy bone*). The outside wall of a bone, the mandible, for example, is compact bone; but the mandible has a hollow center, the *bone marrow cavity*, into which *trabeculae* (bars or plates) of bone protrude. These trabeculae make up trabecular bone. In the spaces around the trabeculae in the bone marrow cavity is the *bone marrow*.

Examine Figure 9–1 which is a drawing of a cross section of a human mandible, and Figure 9–15 which is a drawing of a longitudinal section of a human mandible. Notice the compact character of the bone which makes up the outer wall of the mandible and the trabeculae which project into the marrow cavity. The number and size of the trabeculae in the marrow cavity of a bone are determined to a large degree by the functional activity of the organ: the greater the functional activity the greater the number of trabeculae.

Certain advantages result from this arrangement of bone tissue into compact and trabecular bone. For one thing, a large bone with trabeculae and bone marrow in its center is much lighter in weight than would be the same organ composed of solid bone tissue throughout. Also, the presence of the bone marrow makes available to the bone tissue nutrition from blood vessels which are located inside the organ as well as from blood vessels which lie on the outside surface.

The outside surface of all bones is covered by a thin connective tissue membrane called the *periosteum* (peri = around; osteum = bone). The inside surfaces of bones are covered with a much more delicate connective tissue membrane called the *endosteum* (endo = within) (Fig. 9–1).

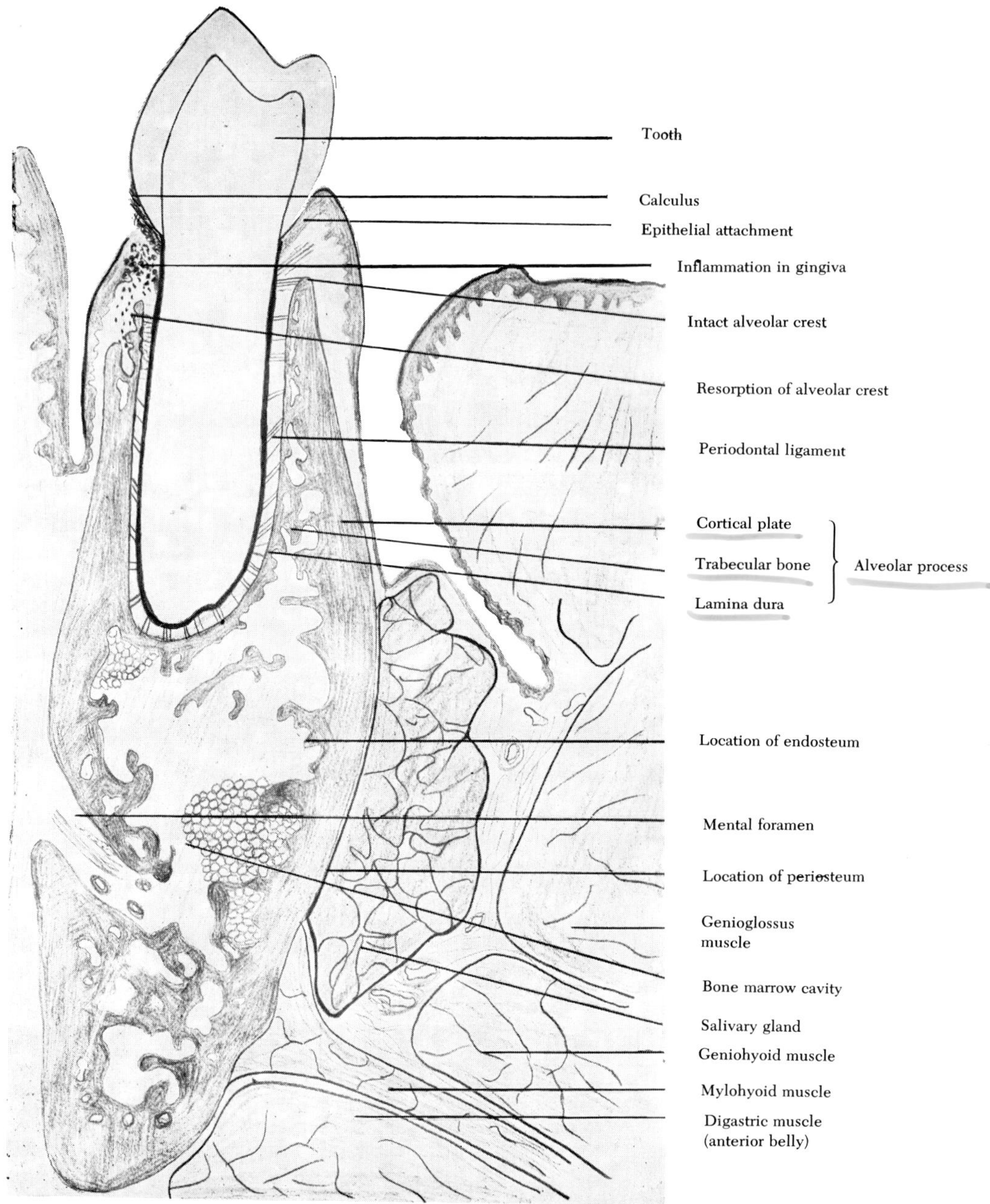

Fig. 9–1. Diagrammatic drawing of a faciolingual section of human mandible in the region of the second premolar (much enlarged). This section is not cut through the pulp cavtity of the tooth.

Microscopic Structure of Bone (a tissue)

Bone tissue consists of bone cells and a bone matrix which is made up of two kinds of intercellular substance, fibrous and ground substance. The intercellular substance becomes mineralized, which makes bone a hard tissue. Bone is about 50% mineral substance and about 50% organic substance and water. It has about the same hardness as cementum.

As is true for dentin and cementum, the fibrous type of intercellular substance is chemically *collagen;* the ground substance is a complex of mucopolysaccharides. The crystalline (inorganic) part of bone is similar to that of enamel, dentin and cementum-hydroxyapatite crystals.

The cells of the bone tissue, *osteocytes* (osteo = bone; cyte = cell), are distributed throughout the mineralized intercellular substance. The space in the bone matrix which is occupied by an osteocyte is called a *lacuna* (little space) (Figs. 9–2; 9–3). Lacunae are connected with one another by a system of *canaliculi* (little canals). These canaliculi extend not only from one lacuna to another, but some of them open into the various canals of bone where capillaries are located. Tissue fluids pass from the capillaries to the canaliculi and hence from one lacuna to another throughout the bone tissue.

Mature bone tissue is formed in thin layers, called *lamellae.* These lamellae have two different patterns of arrangement, and according to their pattern bone tissue is called either *Haversian system bone* or *lamellar bone.*

Haversian system

Haversian canal

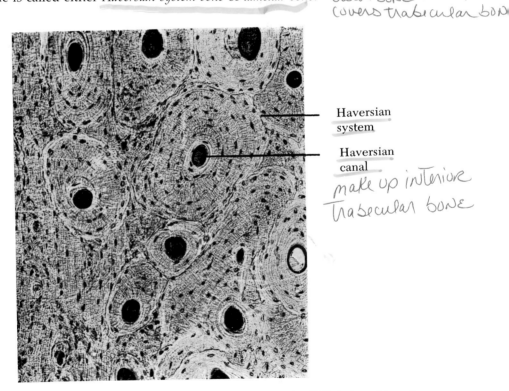

Fig. 9–2. Photomicrograph of a ground cross section of a dried, undecalicified piece of bone from a human clavicle. Cross sections of several Haversian systems are present. The concentric lamellae and lacunae of the Haversian systems are clear. In the center of each Haversian system is the Haversian canal. (Compare with Figures 9–3 and 9–6).

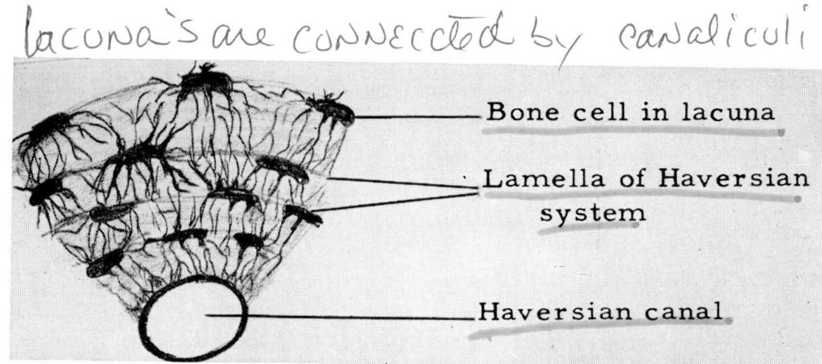

Fig. 9–3. Diagrammatic drawing of a sector of an Haversian system cut in cross section. This is greatly enlarged. The diameter of an Haversian system is something more or less than 0.1 mm.

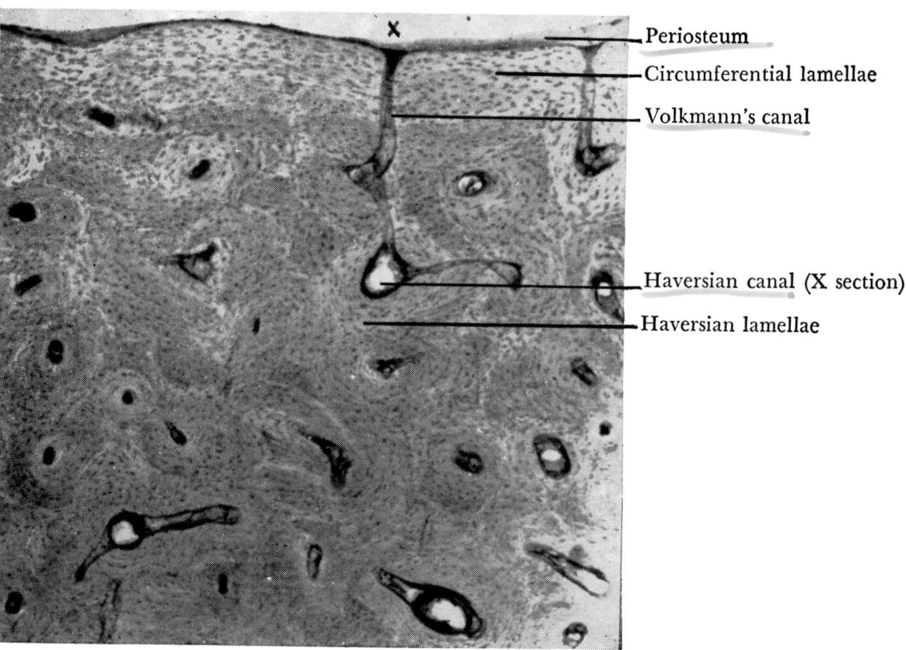

Fig. 9–4. Photomicrograph of a ground cross section of a human femur. (Low power magnification.) At the top of the picture is the bone surface with a portion of the periosteum still adhering to it in some places. The bone lamellae at the surface have a circumferential arrangement. Beneath the circumferential lamellae are Haversian systems where the lamellae are in concentric layers. In the center of each Haversian system is a Haversian canal. In several places a Volkmann's canal enters an Haversian canal. Near the bottom of the picture Volkmann's canals are entering an Haversian canal from two directions. In the upper right two Volkmann's canals are entering from the outside of the organ. The one marked x is seen in higher magnification in Figure 9–5.

In *Haversian system bone* the lamellae are arranged in concentric circles around a very small central canal which is called an *Haversian canal.* The canal contains capillary-like blood vessels surrounded by a loose, soft tissue, referred to as *perivascular connective tissue.* A series of concentric lamellae with the included Haversian canal is called an *Haversian system* (Figs. 9–2; 9–4; 9–5). An Haversian system may have from 4 to 20 concentric lamellae and may measure somewhat more or less than 0.1 mm in diameter.

In *lamellar bone* the lamellae are not arranged in small concentric circles. Lamellar bone makes up the outside surface of most bones, the lamellae following the surface, or circumference, of the bone (Figs. 9–4; 9–5; 9–6). In this location the lamellar bone is sometimes given the additional names of *circumferential bone,* or *subperiosteal bone* (subperiosteal = beneath the periosteum). Lamellar bone also often makes up the surfaces of the trabeculae of trabecular bone; and in this location it may be called *subendosteal bone* (beneath the endosteum). Both patterns of arrangement of lamellae, i.e., Haversian system bone and lamellar bone, are found in all mature human bones.

Regardless of the arrangement of bone lamellae, bone tissue contains osteocytes which lie in lacunae and connect through canaliculi. This system of connected bone cells (Figs. 9–2; 9–6) is the means by which nutrients are distributed throughout the bone tissue. In an Haversian system some of the canaliculi open into the Haversian canal, providing a pathway by which nutrients from the blood vessels contained in the canal may reach the osteocytes of the Haversian system.

Bone is a vascular tissue; it contains many blood vessels. Arteries and veins enter and leave a bone in various places both from the outside surface and from the bone marrow cavity. The canals in a bone through which blood vessels pass into the bone tissue from the outside of the organ or from the bone marrow cavity are called *Volkmann's canals* (Figs. 9–4; 9–5; 9–6). Branches of the blood vessels contained in Volkmann's canals enter the smaller Haversian canals.

It seems remarkable that blood vessels should enter bones and be distributed throughout bones in the way that they are; but actually, in the embryonic development of the body, the larger blood vessels are formed and are in place before bone formation begins. As bone is formed it simply surrounds and encloses any blood vessels located in the area. Therefore we find blood vessels entering and leaving bones at various points.

Bone marrow, which occupies the centers of bones in the spaces around the trabeculae, is a soft tissue (Fig. 9–1). There are two types of bone marrow: (1) *red marrow* (Fig. 9–7), which is found in most of the bones of young individuals and has the function of producing red and white blood cells; and (2) *yellow marrow* (fat marrow), which does not have a blood-forming function. In adults most red marrow becomes converted into yellow marrow. Only certain locations in the adult skeleton retain the red type of marrow which continues to perform the function of hemopoiesis (hemo = blood; poiesis = creation).

Periosteum and Endosteum

The outside surface of a bone is covered by a more or less tough connective tissue membrane called the *periosteum.* A thinner, more delicate connective tissue membrane, called the *endosteum,* covers the inner surface of compact bone and the trabeculae in the bone marrow cavity, and lines the Haversian canals and

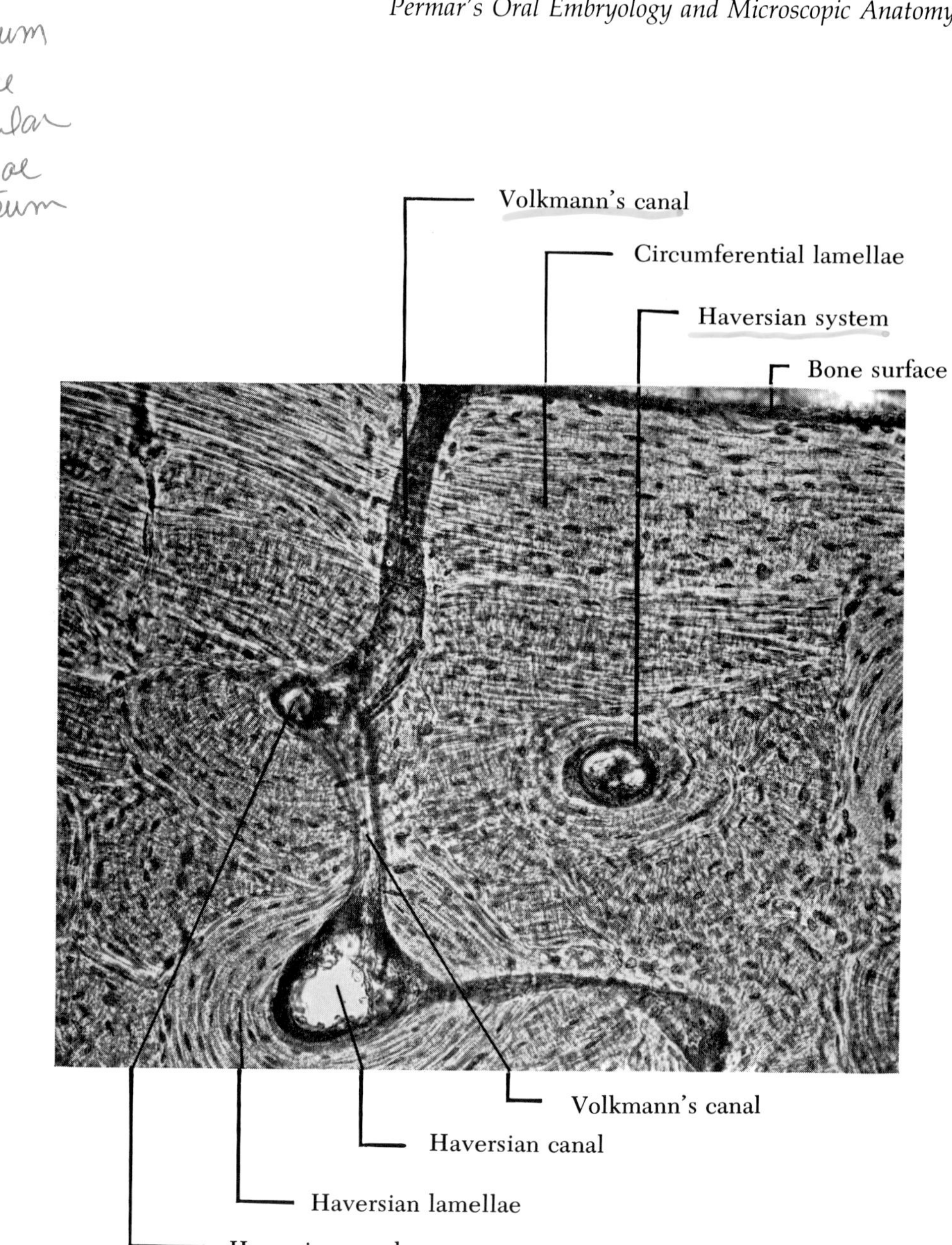

Fig. 9–5. This photomicrograph of a ground section of bone is a higher magnification of the area marked x in Figure 9–4. The surface of the bone is seen in the upper right. A Volkmann's canal cuts through the surface circumferential lamellae and enters an Haversian canal slightly at left of center. The Volkmann's canal continues (toward the bottom of picture) to a second Haversian canal (note the concentric bone lamellae around the canal). The Volkmann's canal then turns right (across bottom of picture). By such a route blood vessels and nerves supply bone tissue.

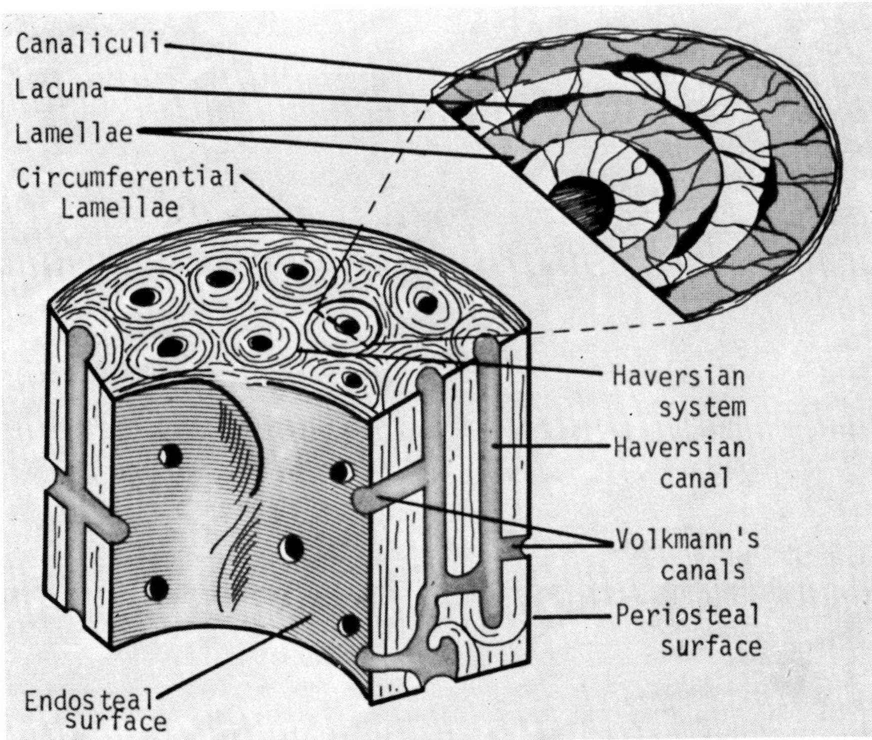

Fig. 9–6. Diagrammatic illustration of a piece of long bone cut in such a way that there is seen a cross section and a longitudinal section of the organ and also the wall of the bone marrow cavity. The holes in the marrow cavity wall are openings of canals that carry blood vessels between the bone marrow and the bone tissue. On the longitudinal surface of the bone, canals are seen to lie longitudinally in the organ and to have horizontal branches from one long canal to another and from long canals to the marrow cavity. Looking at the crosscut surface we see cross sections of the long canals each surrounded by several bone lamellae. Each canal (Haversian canal) and its several lamellae (Haversian lamellae) constitute an *Haversian system.* On this same surface are seen the circumferential lamellae that constitute the outer surface of the organ.

An enlargement of half of a cross section of a single Haversian system shows the Haversian canal surrounded by several Haversian lamellae. Between the lamellae are *lacunae* that in the living bone housed *osteocytes.* The lacunae are connected with one another and with the Haversian canal by numerous *canaliculi.*

the Volkmann's canals. These two membranes, the periosteum and the endosteum, function both in the formation and in the resorption of bone tissue.

The periodontal ligament which surrounds the root of a tooth and separates it from the bone of the tooth socket is a specialized periosteum. It functions on one side in the formation and resorption of the bone comprising the tooth socket and on the other side in the formation and resorption of the cementum covering the tooth root.

Growth of Bone

Bone growth includes both *bone formation* and *bone resorption.*

Bone formation is the conversion of relatively unspecialized connective tissue into bone matrix and bone cells, and the subsequent mineralization of the bone

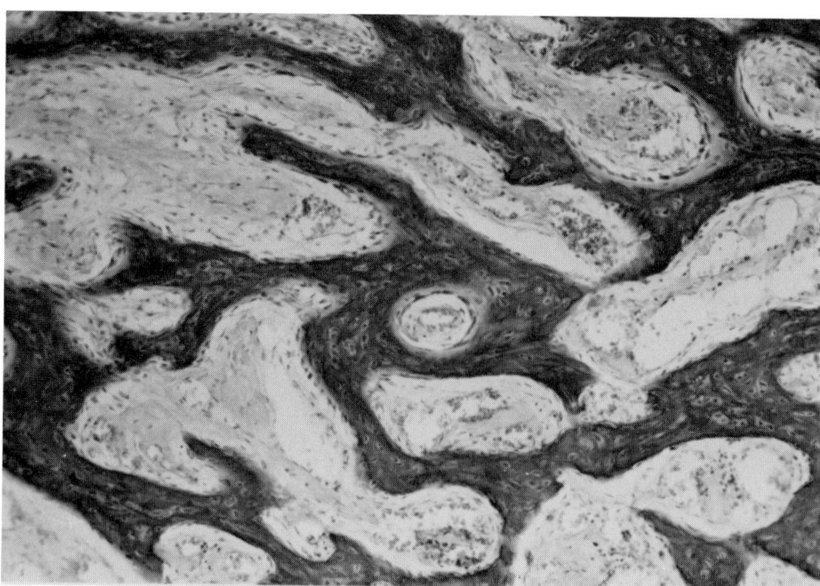

Fig. 9–7. Section from a developing human mandible showing the early appearance of red bone marrow tissue. The soft marrow tissue is enclosed within the forming bone trabeculae.

matrix. Bone matrix is composed of two kinds of intercellular substance: fibrous and ground substance. It arises as a result of a chemical change which takes place in the intercellular substances of unspecialized connective tissue. The bone cells are certain cells of this same connective tissue which are entrapped in the forming bone matrix. In a growing bone the connective tissue which forms the new bone is the periosteum, or the endosteum, as the case may be, depending

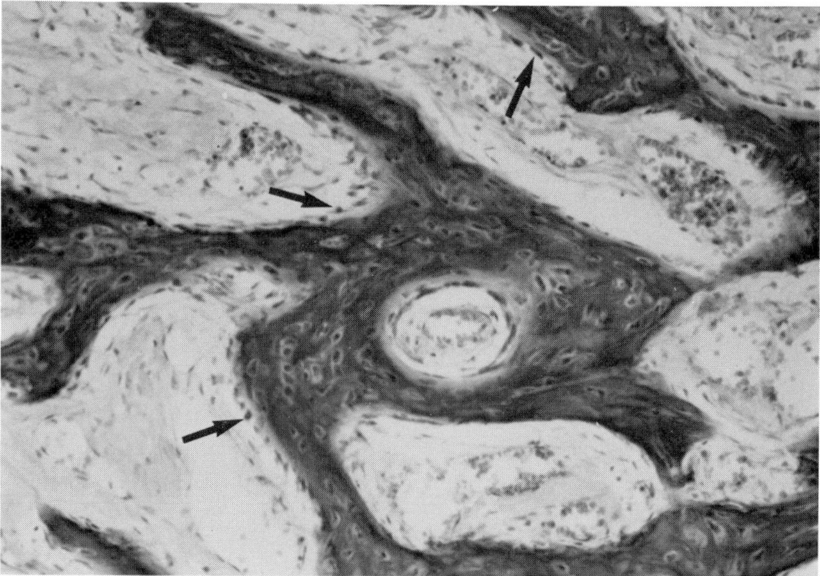

Fig. 9–8. Photomicrograph of a section of forming bone in the area of the mandible. This represents intramembranous bone formation. Osteoblasts (arrows) appear at the surface of the forming bone.

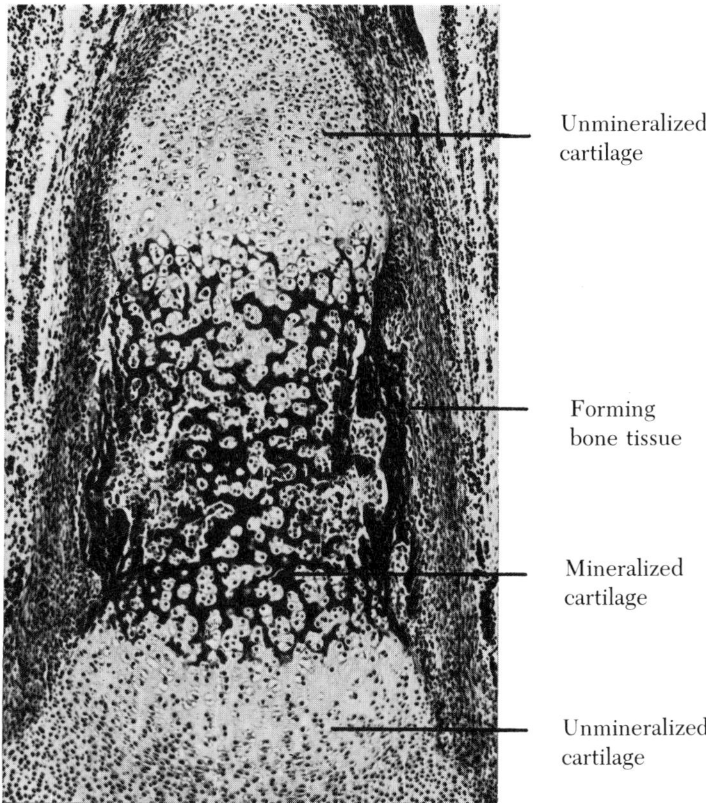

Fig. 9–9. Photomicrograph of a section of a developing bone from the foot of a human fetus. This is endochondral bone formation. The ends of the organ are cartilage that is not yet calcified. The center portion has areas of mineralized cartilage (dark in the picture). The unmineralized cartilage will gradually calcify and be resorbed and will be replaced by bone tissue. Forming bone tissue is present at the outer surface of the mineralized cartilage.

on whether the new bone is being added to the outside or to the inside of the organ. The intercellular substance of the part of the periosteum (or endosteum) which lies against the bone surface is chemically changed into the bone matrix. Some of the cells of the periosteum (or endosteum) next to the bone surface become specialized and are called *osteoblasts* (osteo = bone; blast = germ) (Figs. 9–8; 9–10; 9–11). As the new bone matrix is formed, some of these osteoblasts become surrounded by it and so become cells of the bone tissue, *osteocytes* (Figs. 9–3; 9–14). Because the osteoblasts in the periosteum (or endosteum) are not completely isolated cells but have their cytoplasm connected with other osteoblasts by numerous thin projections, the osteocytes likewise are not isolated cells but have their cytoplasm connected with other osteocytes by the same thin projections (Fig. 9–6). The spaces in the bone matrix occupied by the osteocytes are the lacunae; and the spaces occupied by the numerous cytoplasmic connections are the canaliculi.

In the embryonic development of certain bones the formation of bone tissue is preceded by the formation of a cartilage model which resembles in shape the bone that is to be formed and which serves as a pattern for the future bone. This cartilage predecessor of the bone mineralizes and then is gradually removed

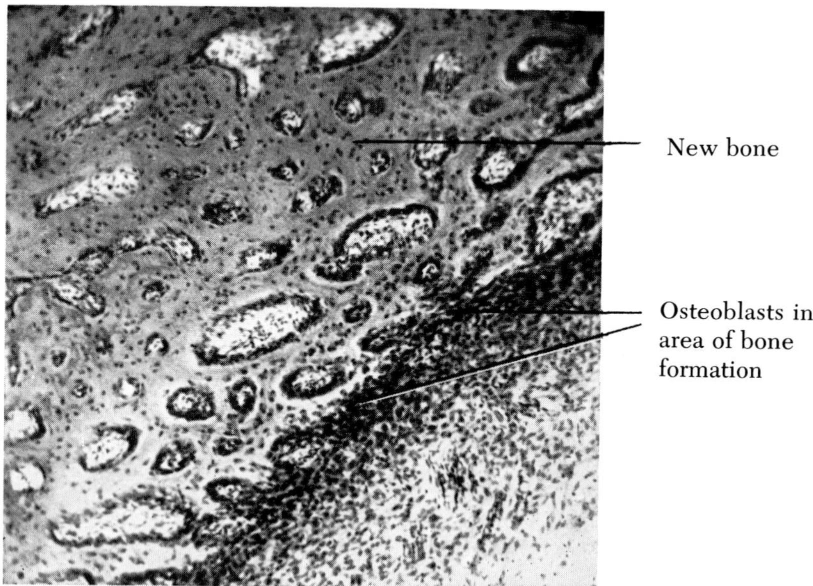

Fig. 9–10. Photomicrograph of a section of forming bone in the area of the mandible in a kitten fetus. This is intramembranous bone formation. Osteoblasts are numerous. The connective tissue from which the bone is forming is in the lower right corner. (Medium power magnfication.)

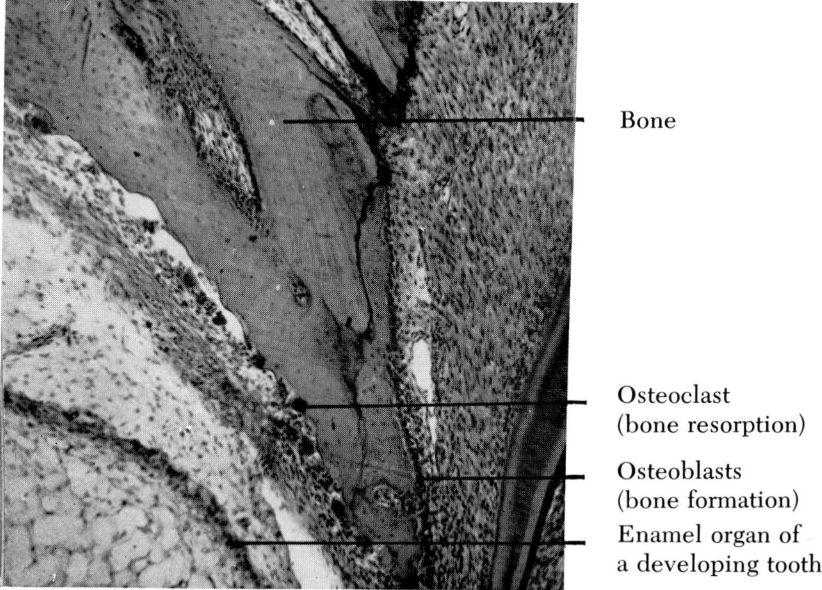

Fig. 9–11. Photomicrograph of a small area of kitten mandible in the region of developing teeth. The large triangular piece of bone shows bone resorption on one side *(left)* and bone formation on the other side *(right).* In the area of bone resorption are a large number of osteoclasts on the bone surface. Resorption in this area is probably due to the presence of a developing tooth, the enamel organ of which is seen in the lower left. On the right side of the triangular bone the presence of numerous, closely packed osteoblasts on the bone surface are associated with formation of bone tissue in this area. (Low power magnification.)

by resorption. As the mineralized cartilage is resorbed, bone tissue is formed to replace it. Bones which arise in this way, with a cartilage structure preceding the development of bone tissue, are said to be formed by *endochondral formation* (Fig. 9–9). Examples of bones formed in this manner are the long bones of the arms and legs.

In the embryonic development of other bones, the bone tissue is formed without a preceding cartilage pattern, and these bones are said to be formed by *intramembranous formation* (Figs. 9–8; 9–10). Examples of bones formed in this manner, with no preceding cartilage structure, are the mandible and the maxillae. The process of the conversion of unspecialized connective tissue into bone and the final microscopic structure of bone tissue are the same whether or not bone formation has been preceded by cartilage.

At first glance bone appears to be a permanent and unchanging tissue. Actually, bone is in a state of constant change. Bone tissue formation continues practically throughout the life of the bone, but the organ does not thereby become indefinitely heavier and greater in mass. The density and size of a bone are limited by the fact that the formation of bone tissue in one place is compensated for by the resorption of bone tissue in another.

Bone resorption is the removal of both the mineral materials and the organic matrix of bone. Resorption of bone should not be confused with demineralization of bone (or other hard tissues) such as occurs when the tissue is removed from the body and taken to the laboratory to be placed in a weak acid solution. In this laboratory procedure, called demineralization, the mineral material is removed and the organic material remains. In bone resorption, the organic matrix and the mineral material are both removed, and nothing of the bone remains.

Bone resorption occurs just beneath the periosteum or endosteum. A specialized type of cell called an *osteoclast* (clast = break) is associated with the resorption of bone tissue (Figs. 9–11; 9–12). Osteoclasts are multinucleated cells (contain more than one nucleus), the nuclei ranging from 2 or 3 dozen to a dozen or more in a single cell (Fig. 9–13).

Bone formation and bone resorption are processes that occur intermittently in all bones throughout the life of an individual. The intramembranous bone (Fig. 9–8) and the endochondral bone (Fig. 9–9) that form in the early development of the individual are gradually resorbed and are replaced by mature bone. With growth and function the mature bone undergoes an endless process of resorption in one place and apposition (formation) in another (Fig. 9–14). Haversian systems are partially or wholly resorbed and then replaced by other Haversian systems or by lamellar bone. Lamellar bone is resorbed and replaced by Haversian system bone or by new lamellar bone. This turnover is rapid during the growth of the individual and occurs more slowly later in life. After full individual growth is attained, however, the processes of bone change may occur rapidly in places where function or trauma stimulate resorption or apposition.

Bone formation and bone resorption are taking place continuously in some areas of the bone tissue that surrounds the teeth. They occur in response to certain stimuli. In the tooth socket the stimuli which govern bone formation and bone resorption are: (1) tension (pull) on the periodontal ligament fibers attached to the bone, and (2) pressure on the periodontal ligament and on the bone. Tension on the periodontal ligament fibers induces bone formation; pressure induces bone resorption.

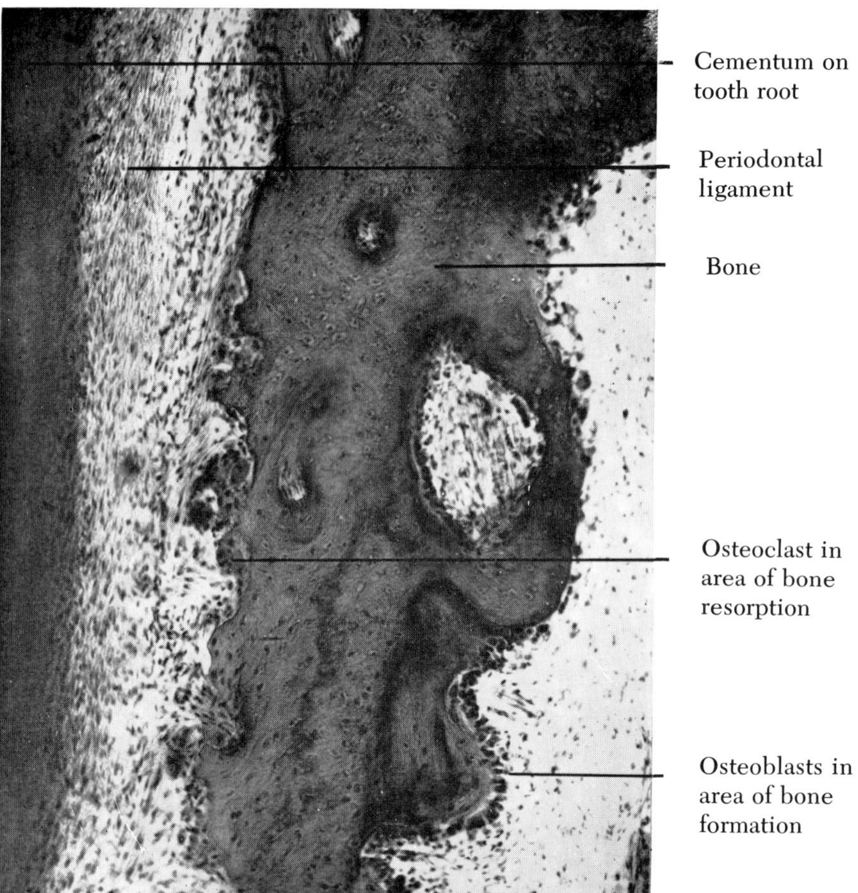

Fig. 9–12. Photomicrograph of an area of tooth root, periodontal ligament, and alveolar bone (lamina dura). This was a tooth not in function: notice the lack of orientation of periodontal ligament fibers. There is bone resorption on the bone surface next to the periodontal ligament. Notice the osteoclasts. On the outer surface of the bone (to the right) the presence of osteoblasts indicates bone formation. (Medium power magnification.)

THE ALVEOLAR PROCESS

The *alveolar process* is defined as that part of the mandible and maxillae which surrounds and supports the teeth (Figs. 9–15; 9–16). The alveolar process supports the tooth roots on the facial and on the palatal and lingual sides; it extends between the teeth, separating them on the mesial and distal sides; and it extends into the furcation of the roots of multirooted teeth (Figs. 9–1; 9–17; 9–18). The occlusal border of the alveolar process, located near the cervix of the tooth, is referred to as the *alveolar crest.*

The alveolar porcess may be described as being composed of the *lamina dura** and the *supporting bone.* The lamina dura is the bone of the wall of the tooth socket. The supporting bone is made up of (1) the *cortical plate,* which is the outside wall of the mandible and the maxillae and (2) the *trabecular bone* which is located between the lamina dura and the cortical bone in many areas (Figs.

*Also called *alveolar bone, true alveolar bone, alveolar bone proper,* and *cribriform plate.*

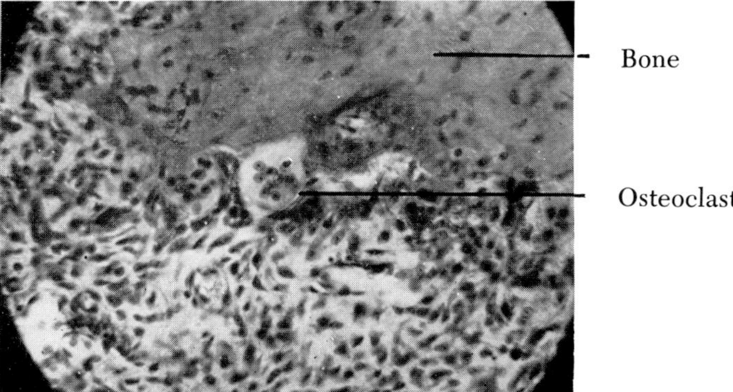

Fig. 9–13. Photomicrograph (high power magnification) of osteoclasts in the area of bone development of a kitten mandible. Bone development of course includes bone resorption as well as bone formation and the presence of osteoclasts indicates that this is an area of resorption. Bone is at the top of the picture; bone-forming connective tissue is at the bottom. The osteoclast in the center of the picture distinctly shows the presence of nine nuclei.

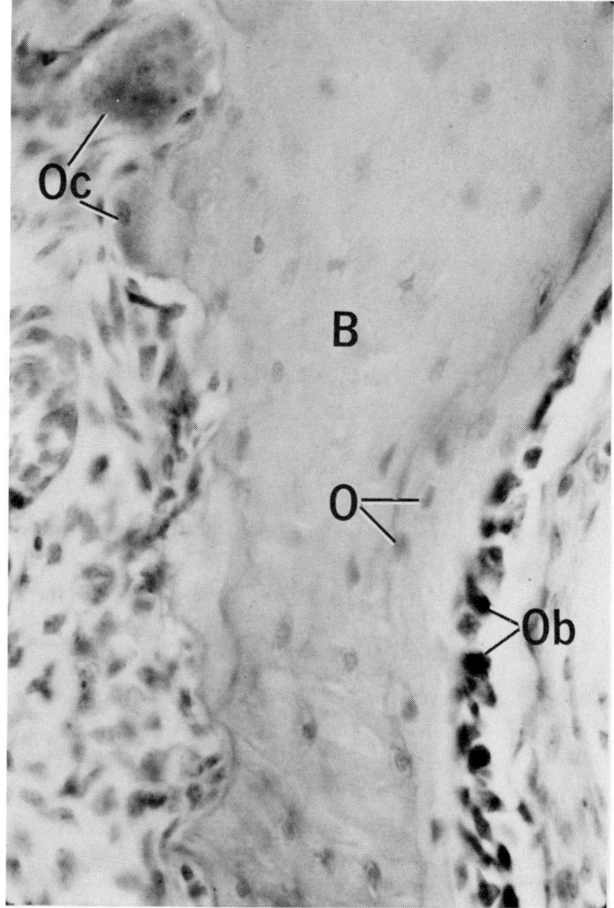

Fig. 9–14. Higher magnification of an area of bone (B) showing resorption on the left side by *osteoclasts* (Oc) and formation on the right side by *osteoblasts* (Ob). *Osteocytes* (O).

overgrowth OR loss of lamina dura indicates disease state

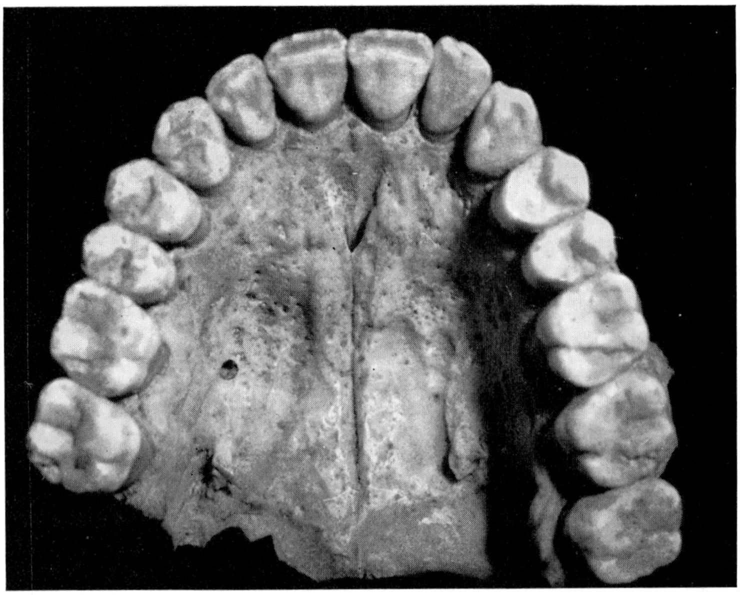

Fig. 9–15. A human maxilla. The palatal part of the alveolar process merges without a distinct line into the bone of the palate. The alveolar process extending between the teeth is seen clearly. The alveolar crest is the edge of the alveolar process around the cervix of the tooth. Notice the attrition of the incisal edges of the anterior teeth.

9–18; 9–19). In some areas the the alveolar process is thin and contains little or no trabecular bone: the lamina dura and the cortical plate are fused. This kind of thin alveolar process is found, among other places, on the facial surfaces of mandibular anterior teeth.

Clinical Aspects of Bone Reaction in the Alveolar Process

The trabecular bone and the lamina dura which support a tooth react in different ways to changes in tooth function. When a tooth is in strong masticatory function, the trabecular bone in the alveolar process and the trabecular bone beneath the alveolus* of the tooth are composed of numerous heavy bone trabeculae. If the tooth is removed from function by loss of opposing teeth, these supporting trabeculae become less numerous and smaller. If the tooth in question is again placed in occlusion by the replacement of the lost teeth in the opposing arch, more trabecular bone will again form around the tooth which has resumed masticatory function.

The lamina dura, which is the wall of the tooth socket, does not respond by resorption to loss of masticatory function of the tooth. However, the lamina dura may respond by resorption to various stimuli such as trauma due to faulty occlusion, or periodontal disease, or pressures produced during orthodontic treatment, or pressures produced by mesial drift (see Chapter 12). Also, addition of bone tissue to the lamina dura at the base of the alveolus may be a factor in the continued occlusal movement of a tooth as attrition on the occlusal or incisal surface takes place. This addition to the lamina dura and the addition of ce-

*Pronounced ăl vē′ ō lŭs (the tooth socket)

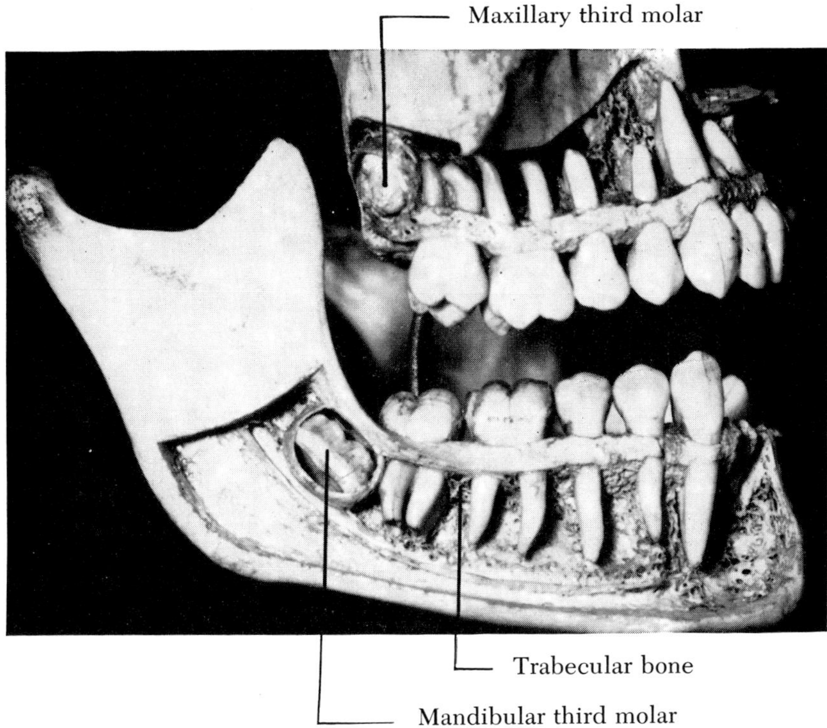

Fig. 9–16. A human maxilla and mandible with the facial parts of the alveolar process removed excepting near the cervical border. In the mandible some trabecular bone remains among the tooth roots. Notice the location and position of the developing mandibular and maxillary third molars. The crown of the mandibular third molar is nearly completed in the ramus of the mandible. Its occlusal surface is directed mesially and occlusally. It is surrounded by a bony crypt. The maxillary third molar is directed buccally and distally.

mentum to the root may partially compensate for loss of crown length due to attrition.

Inflammation and swelling of the soft tissues around a tooth may result in damage to the periodontal ligament and resorption of the crest of the alveolar process (Figs. 9–1; 9–11; 9–13). The presence of calculus in the gingival sulcus has the potentiality to set off a series of events: the calculus produces inflammation and swelling of the adjacent soft tissues. This condition involves and damages the periodontal ligament fibers around the neck of the tooth. Damage to the periodontal ligament results in resorption of the bone to which the fibers are attached. Continued inflammation produces continued bone resorption. Eventually so much damage may be done to the periodontal ligament and to the lamina dura that removal of the tooth becomes necessary.

Good oral hygiene and prompt dental care will prevent such serious involvement because of the following consequential reactions: (1) Removal of the calculus may be expected to result in the elimination of the inflammation and swelling. (2) Elimination of the inflammation and swelling permits repair of the periodontal ligament. (3) At the same time there will be an arrest of the resorption of the bone of the alveolar crest. (4) Additional cementum may be produced on the tooth root in the affected area with an accompanying reattachment of the previously damaged periodontal ligament. (5) Repair of some of the resorbed

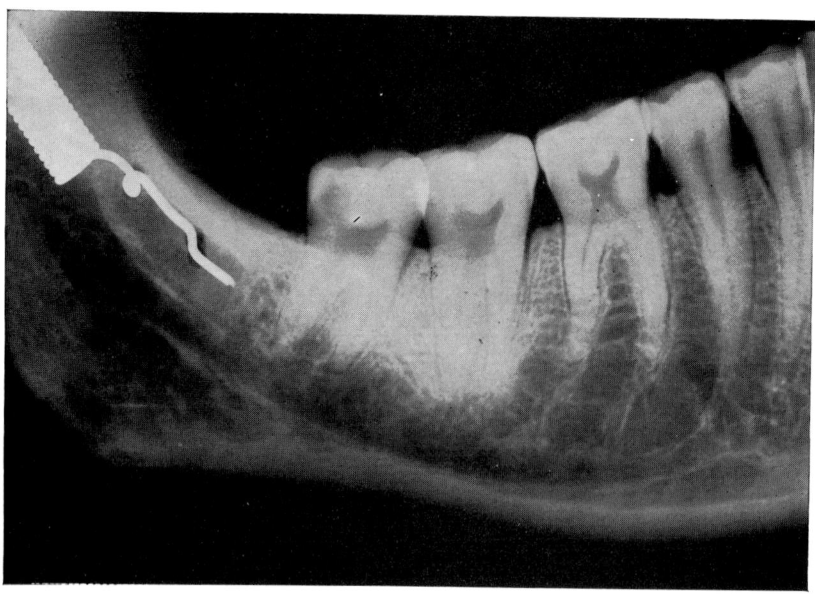

Fig. 9–17. Radiograph of a human mandible similar to that in Figure 9–16. The third molar is erupted and the roots appear to be fully formed. The trabeculae in the interradicular bone (between the roots) and the interdental bone (between the teeth) have a characteristic orientation: many are positioned horizontally. The space occupied by the periodontal ligament is seen here most clearly on the distal side of the distal root of the first molar. In the ramus of the mandible and extending beneath the tooth roots is the mandibular canal. The locations where branches from the mandibular nerve extended from the mandibular canal to the apical foramina of the first molar roots are visible in the bone pattern. (The white object at the left is a spring that attached the mandible to the temporal bone of the prepared skull.) (Courtesy Dr. Richard C. O'Brien, College of Dentistry, The Ohio State University.)

areas of the lamina dura may occur, and some bone construction may possibly take place on the alveolar crest. It is probable that the alveolar crest will occupy a position apical to that of the original position—that is, there will not be enough bone replacement on the alveolar crest to make it as high as it was originally.

Teeth are sometimes, either by accident or by design, subjected to pressure on the crown from a horizontal direction (Figs. 9–18; 9–19). If the pressure is continued and is not so severe as to damage the periodontal ligament, it will produce an adaptive response in the lamina dura. On the side of the tooth socket toward which the tooth is pushed the periodontal ligament and the lamina dura are subjected to pressures, and bone resorption occurs. On the side of the tooth socket away from which the tooth is pulled the periodontal ligament fibers are subjected to tension, and additional bone of the lamina dura is formed. The result of this bone resorption and bone formation is a change in the location of the tooth socket and also, of course, in the location of the tooth.

Such a change in the position of a tooth may be a result of change in occlusal pressures. Or it may be a consequence of treatment applied by the orthodontist to improve unsatisfactory tooth alignment. The orthodontist places appliances on a patient's teeth and adjusts them at intervals so that proper pressures and tensions are maintained. Teeth being treated actually change location in the mouth. The success of this treatment is due to three factors: (1) Bone is resorbed more easily than cementum. (2) The area of the lamina dura toward which the

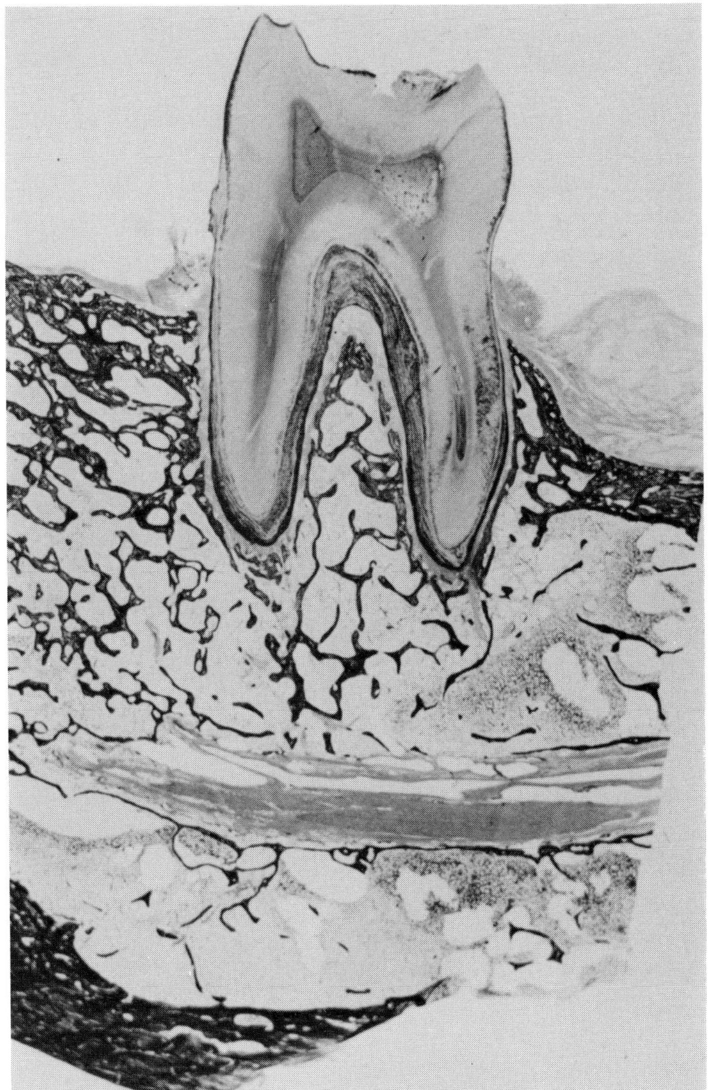

Fig. 9–18. Histologic section through a mandibular first molar and its alveolar process. For a detailed description, see diagram of this section in Figure 9–19. Enamel of the tooth was lost during histologic preparation.

tooth is moved is resorbed. (3) The area of the lamina dura away from which the tooth is moved is built up.

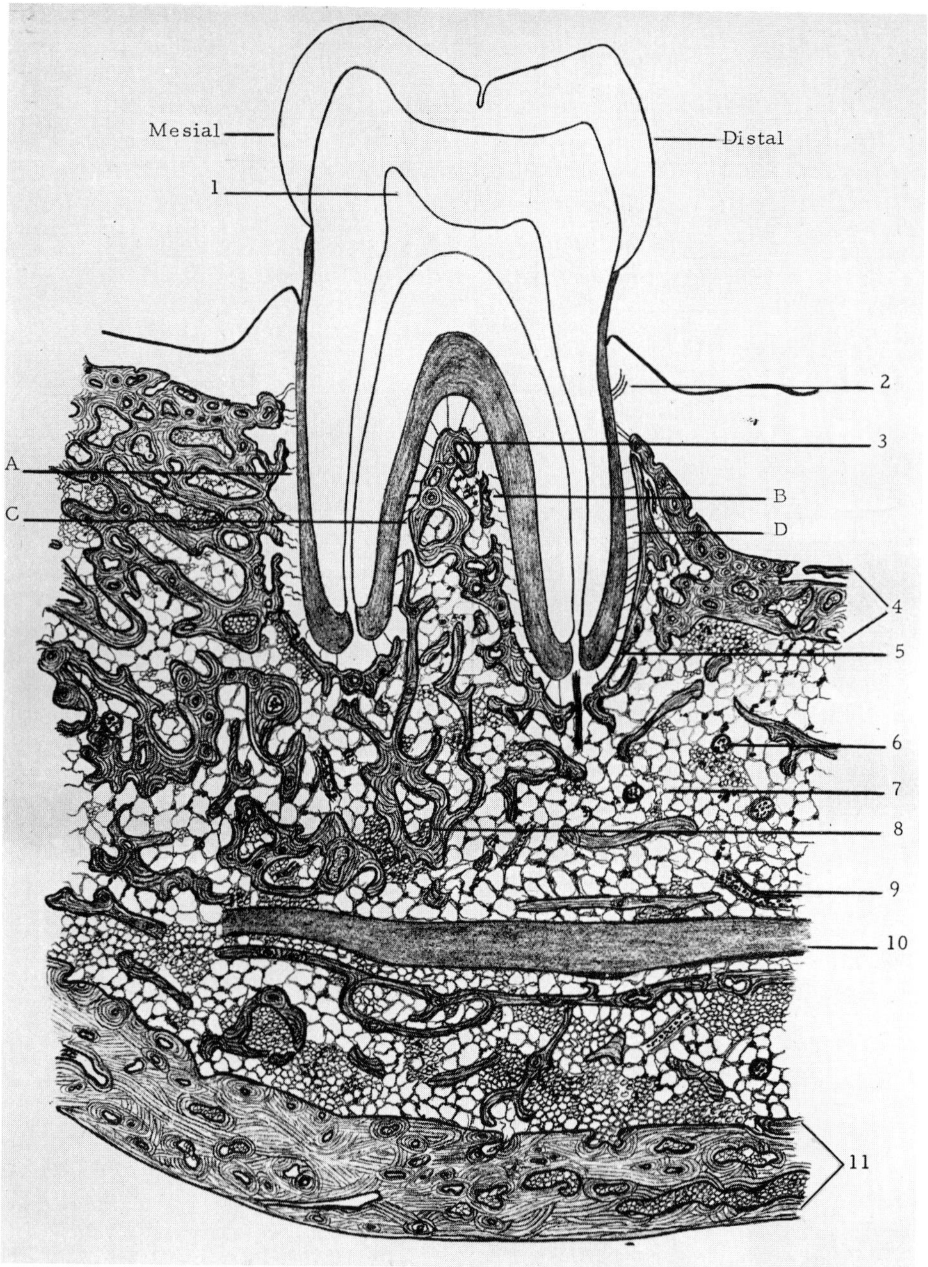

Fig. 9–19. Diagrammatic drawing of a section of a human mandible bearing an isolated first molar tooth, cut mesiodistally. 1. Pulp horn. 2. Gingival fibers of periodontal ligament. 3. Bone of interradicular septum (between the roots). 4. Cortical bone on ridge of mandible. 5. Lamina dura bone near apex of distal root. 6. Cross section small blood vessel. 7. Fat marrow. 8. Trabecular bone scattered throughout bone marrow cavity. 9. Longitudinal section blood vessel. 10. Inferior alveolar nerve. 11. Cortical bone on inferior surface of mandible. *A*, *B*, *C*, and *D* indicate different areas of the periodontal ligament. *A*, the periodontal ligament on the mesial side of the mesial root; and *B*, the periodontal ligament on the mesial side of the distal root. At both *A* and *B* the principal fibers have a wavy appearance and there is evidence of resorption of the lamina dura bone. *C*, the periodontal ligament on the distal side of the mesial root; and *D*, the periodontal ligament on the distal side of the distal root. At *C* and *D* the principal fibers are straight and there is no evidence of resorption of the lamina dura. It may be inferred that this tooth was undergoing a slight movement in a mesial direction: the slight pressure on the mesial side of the each root resulted in relaxed periodontal ligament fibers and in bone resorption in the lamina dura. On the distal side of each root the fibers are straight and there is no evidence of bone resorption. The interradicular fibers of the periodontal ligament radiate from the crest of the interradicular septum to the cementum that lines the root furcation.

Table 9–1. Comparison of the Four Mineralized Tissues

	Enamel	Dentin	Cementum	Bone
Embryonic tissue origin	lining epithelium*	mesenchyme	mesenchyme	mesenchyme
Matrix forming cell	ameloblast	odontoblast	cementoblast	osteoblast
Growth mechanism	appositional	appositional	appositional	appositional
Organic material				
fibrous	enamelins*	collagen	collagen	collagen
ground substance	mucopoly-saccharide	mucopoly-saccharide	mucopoly-saccharide	mucopoly-saccharide
Tissue fluid	present	present	present	present
Internal cellular elements	none*	cell processes	(cellular) cells and processes (acellular) none	cells and processes
Internal cellular space	none*	tubules	(cellular) lacunae and canaliculi (acellular) none	lacunae and canaliculi
Internal vascular canals	none	none	none	present*
Adjacent "free" surface environment	saliva*	pulp (connective tissue)	periodontal ligament (connective tissue)	periosteum and endosteum (connective tissue)

*Denotes differences

Chapter 10

THE ORAL MUCOUS MEMBRANE AND THE SALIVARY GLANDS

MUCOUS MEMBRANES

Definition

A mucous membrane is the lining of a body cavity that opens to the outside of the body. Mucous membranes are found lining the oral cavity, the nasal cavity and sinuses, the trachea, the stomach and intestines, the urinary bladder, the uterus.

Histologic Structures of Mucous Membranes

Histologically a mucous membrane is a modified skin. It is made up of two layers: (1) a surface layer of *epithelial tissue* and (2) an underlying layer of *connective tissue* (called *lamina propria)*. Mucous membranes are structurally less thick and tough than the skin; and whereas the skin is kept slightly moist by secretions from oil glands and sweat glands which empty onto the surface, mucous membranes are kept very moist by secretions from mucous glands, serous glands, or other secretory cells which empty onto the surface. The epithelium of a mucous membrane is protective in function, and in some areas it is also secretory and absorptive in function. The connective tissue of a mucous membrane underlies the epithelium and contains blood vessels, nerves, and sometimes glands.

Mucous membranes in different parts of the body differ in a number of ways, and in each location their structure seems to be excellently suited to perform the functions required. In places where the mucous membrane is normally protected from wear and tear it is very thin and delicate, but in areas which are subjected to functional friction it is thicker and resistant to injury.

Protected cavities such as the nasal cavity, the stomach, and the intestines are lined by delicate types of mucous membranes. *In the nasal cavity* the epithelial part of the mucous membrane is composed of pseudostratified columnar cells (Fig. 1–3D). Many of these columnar cells have *cilia*—tiny hair-like projections—on their exposed ends, while others, called *goblet cells*, secrete mucus* which keeps the surface of the mucosa* moist. The connective tissue part of the nasal mucous membrane is likewise thin and delicate and contains nerves and blood

**Mucus* (noun) is a viscous, watery secretion that covers a *mucous* (adjective) membrane. *Mucosa* (noun) is another name of mucous membrane.

vessels and mucous and serous glands which open onto the surface of the mucosa. This moist, ciliated mucous membrane of the nasal passage functions as a dirt-catcher and helps to prevent the dust which is inhaled with the air from reaching the lungs.

Lining the stomach is a mucous membrane which is somewhat thicker than that of the nasal cavity, and which is arranged in many folds and wrinkles. The epithelium of the stomach mucosa is made up of simple columnar cells which are without cilia and which have a secretory function (Fig. 1–3C). The underlying connective tissue contains many glands.

In many respects resembling the stomach mucosa, the *mucosa of the small intestine* has an epithelium composed of simple columnar cells some of which are goblet cells that secrete mucus and others of which have the function of absorbing food materials from the intestine. The connective tissue contains many glands.

Contrasted with the protected, delicate mucous membranes of the nasal cavity, the stomach, and the intestines is the more sturdy *mucosa that lines the oral cavity.* The lining of the mouth is constantly subjected to rubbing and scraping, not only by the process of mastication of food but also by the presence of the teeth in the mouth; and here again the structure of the mucous membrane is suited to its usage.

THE ORAL MUCOUS MEMBRANE

Histologic Structure of Oral Mucous Membrane

The mucous membrane lining of the mouth is heavier and more resistant to injury than the mucous membranes of more protected cavities. Its histologic structure enables the oral mucosa to withstand the wear and tear of ordinary oral function and to resist bacterial infection. Like all mucous membranes, the oral mucosa is composed of a combination of epithelial tissue and connective tissue. The surface epithelial tissue is attached to the underlying connective tissue by a basement membrane (Fig. 1–3).

The *epithelial portion of the oral mucosa* is stratified squamous in character—that is, the epithelial cells are mostly flat in shape and are several layers deep (Fig. 1–3E). As in all stratified squamous epithelium, the basal layer of epithelial cells, which rests upon the connective tissues, is composed of cuboidal rather than flat cells; and it is in this basal layer that most of the cell division takes place. As new epithelial cells are produced by mitosis in the basal layer, some of the basal cells and the cells superficial to them are forced outward and eventually they reach the surface.

Different things happen to these surface epithelial cells in different parts of the mouth. In areas of the mouth where the mucosa is relatively protected, such as on the inside of the cheeks and lips and on the under side of the tongue, the surface epithelial cells are sloughed off into the saliva as new epithelial cells are produced in the basal layer. A scraping from the inside of the cheeks spread onto a glass slide and examined under the microscope will be seen to contain squamous epithelial cells.

In some other parts of the mouth where the oral mucosa is subject to considerable wear and tear, such as the hard palate and the gingiva, the surface epithelial cells are not sloughed off (Fig. 10–1). Instead, they lose their nuclei

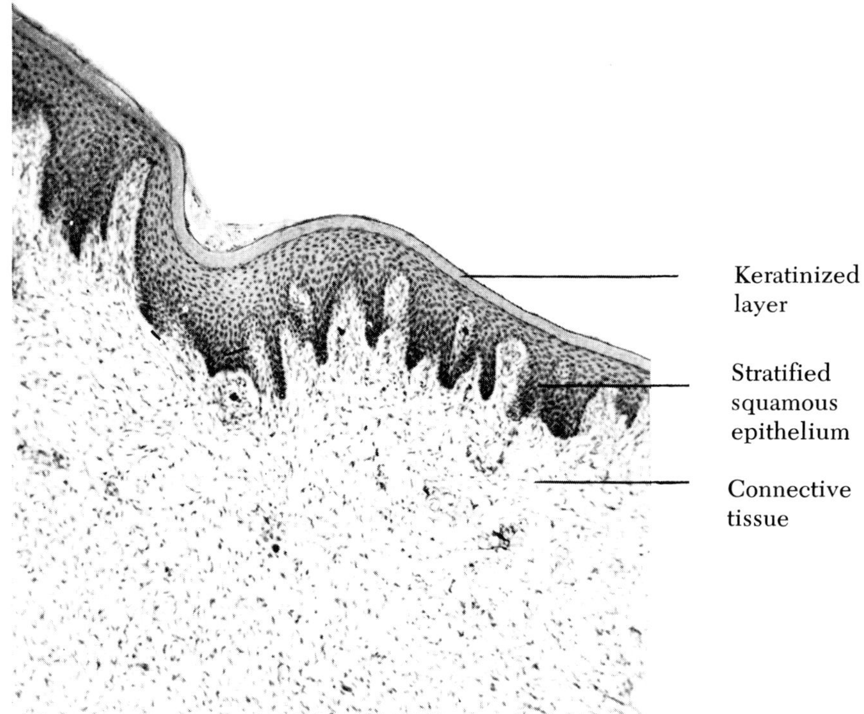

Fig. 10–1. Photomicrograph of a section of human gingiva. (As seen under low power magnification.)

and their cell boundaries and form a noncellular, tough, protective layer on the surface of the stratified squamous epithelial cells. This tough layer is called the *keratin* layer*, and epithelium on which such a layer occurs is called *keratinized* epithelium* (Figs. 10–1; 10–2). The keratin layer wears with use, of course, but it is continuously replaced by the aging cells beneath it.

The *connective tissue portion of the oral mucosa* is composed chiefly of fibrous connective tissue in which are blood vessels and nerves. It is separated from the overlying stratified squamous epithelium by a thin basement membrane. In most places the junction between the connective tissue and the epithelium is an irregular boundary with projections of connective tissue extending like fingers up into the epithelium, but not reaching the surface. In some areas of the oral mucosa these projections are characteristically much longer and more numerous than in other areas (Fig. 10–3). This irregularity of contact surfaces between the two tissues serves to increase the area from which the epithelium can receive nourishment from the underlying connective tissue.

The connective tissue of the oral mucosa varies in thickness in different parts of the mouth; and it also varies in the nature of its attachment to the underlying tissue. In some areas of the mouth the connective tissue of the oral mucosa is attached firmly to underlying bone, as in the part of the gingiva which is attached to the periosteum of the alveolar process. In other areas of the mouth the connective tissue of the oral mucosa rests upon a looser type of connective tissue called the *submucosa*, which contains larger blood vessels, nerves, glands, and fat tissue. Such an attachment of oral mucosa to submucosa is seen in the cheek.

*Pronounced kĕr′ a tĭn īzed.

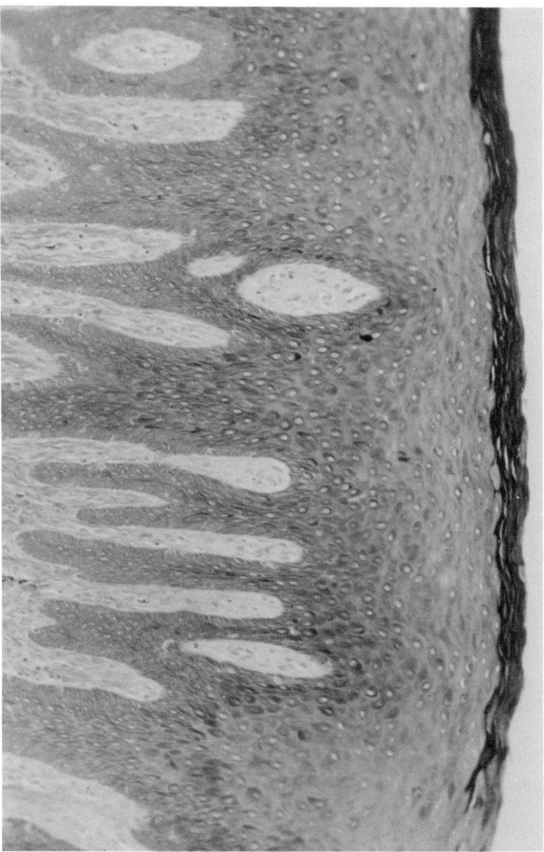

Fig. 10–2. Higher magnification of a section of human gingiva. The strata arrangement of the epithelial cells, including the keratin layer (dark layer at right) are clearly seen. The underlying lighter staining connective tissue interdigitates with the epithelium.

The character of the submucosa varies in different parts of the mouth, and its nature helps to determine the character of the mucosa which it supports.

For convenience in discussion an attempt has been made to classify the different areas of oral mucosa. The classification divides the oral mucosa into three categories: (1) the *masticatory mucosa,* (2) the *lining mucosa,* and (3) the *specialized mucosa.* If you will carefully examine someone's mouth and observe the mucosa in different places, such a division will seem logical.

Masticatory mucosa
- Gingiva
- Hard palate

Lining mucosa
- Lips and cheeks
- Floor of mouth
- Under side of tongue
- Soft palate
- Alveolar mucosa

Specialized mucosa
- Dorsum of tongue

The *masticatory mucosa* is the name given to the mucous membrane of the

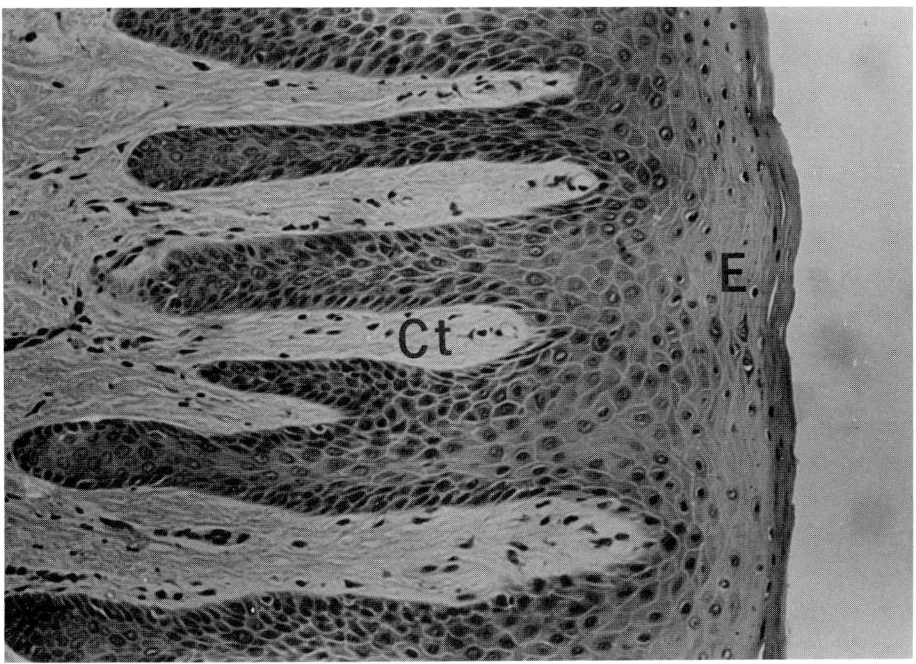

Fig. 10–3. Histologic section of human gingiva showing the interdigitation between the epithelium (E) and the connective tissue (Ct). The dark surface layer of the epithelium is keratin. Notice the fibrous nature of the connective tissue.

gingiva and the *hard palate*. These are the areas of the oral mucosa most used during the mastication of food. The epithelium of the masticatory mucosa is usually keratinized.

Looking into a person's mouth you will see that the necks of the teeth and the bone in which the teeth are set are covered with a firm mucous membrane which fits close around the teeth and is tightly attached to the bone. This part of the oral mucosa is called *gingiva* (Figs. 10–4; 10–5). The gingiva is usually keratinized, is firm, and has a stippled appearance. Except for a narrow zone around the necks of the teeth the gingival mucosa is attached firmly to the underlying tissue. If you will examine the facial side of the upper and lower jaws, you will notice that several millimeters rootward from the margin of the gingiva there is a scalloped line which divides the *gingival mucosa* from the alveolar mucosa (Figs. 10–4; 10–5). The *alveolar mucosa* may be distinguished from gingiva because it is redder, shiny, and loose-fitting. Figure 10–6 shows clearly the scalloped junction between the gingival mucosa and the alveolar mucosa.

The mucosa covering the *hard palate* is usually well keratinized (Fig. 10–7). It is attached directly to the bone of the roof of the mouth only in the area of the *palatine raphe*,* which is the anteroposterior elevation in the center of the hard palate that you can feel with your tongue. On either side of the palatine raphe the palatine mucosa has a *submucosa* between it and the bone. In the anterior part the submucosa in the hard palate contains much fat tissue, and in the posterior part it contains large salivary glands of the mucous type. The ducts

*Pronounced rā′ fē (fr. Greek) *raphe* = a seam or suture.

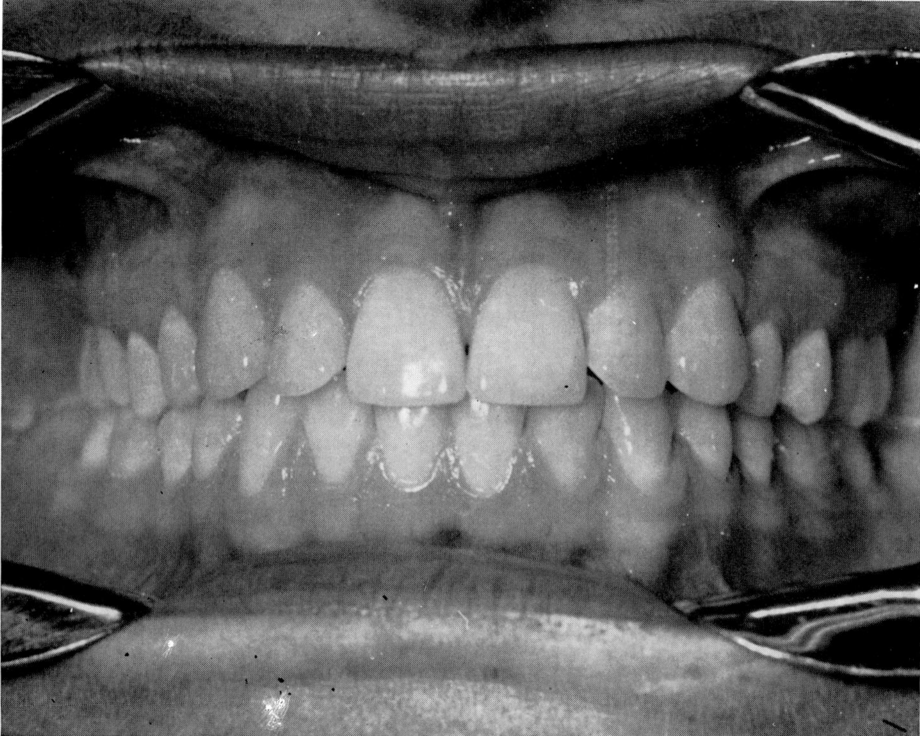

Fig. 10–4. The subject of this photograph was a young woman twenty-two years old. The gingival margin fits snugly against the enamel of the tooth crowns, and the interdental papillae fill the interdental spaces (the space between the teeth cervical to the areas of contact). The alveolar mucosa is clearly seen in the maxillary vestibule; it is seen less clearly in this picture in the mandibular vestibule.

of these glands open onto the surface of the palate mucosa. These small openings usually are not visible to the naked eye.

Notwithstanding the presence of the fat tissue and gland tissue in the submucosa of the hard palate, the oral mucosa in this area is firmly attached to the underlying bone structure. This is accomplished by strands of connective tissue which extend from the mucosa through the submucosa and attach firmly to the bone of the roof of the mouth.

Lining *mucosa* is located in those areas of the oral cavity where the mucous membrane might logically be regarded as functioning as a lining organ rather than as a masticatory organ. Such nonmasticatory areas are the floor of the mouth and the underside of the tongue (Fig. 10–8), the alveolar mucosa (Fig. 10–6), the soft palate, and the inside of the cheeks and lips. In none of these areas is the mucosa firmly attached to underlying bone, and ordinarily the epithelium in these areas is not keratinized.

Examine someone's mouth and ask the person to lift his tongue (Fig. 10–8). The floor of the mouth and the underside of the tongue are covered with lining mucosa, the epithelium of which is nonkeratinized, shiny, and thin enough that blood vessels located in the underlying connective tissue are clearly visible. The fold of mucosa extending lengthwise in the center of the undersurface of the tongue is the *lingual frenum.* Comparison of this frenum in a number of indi-

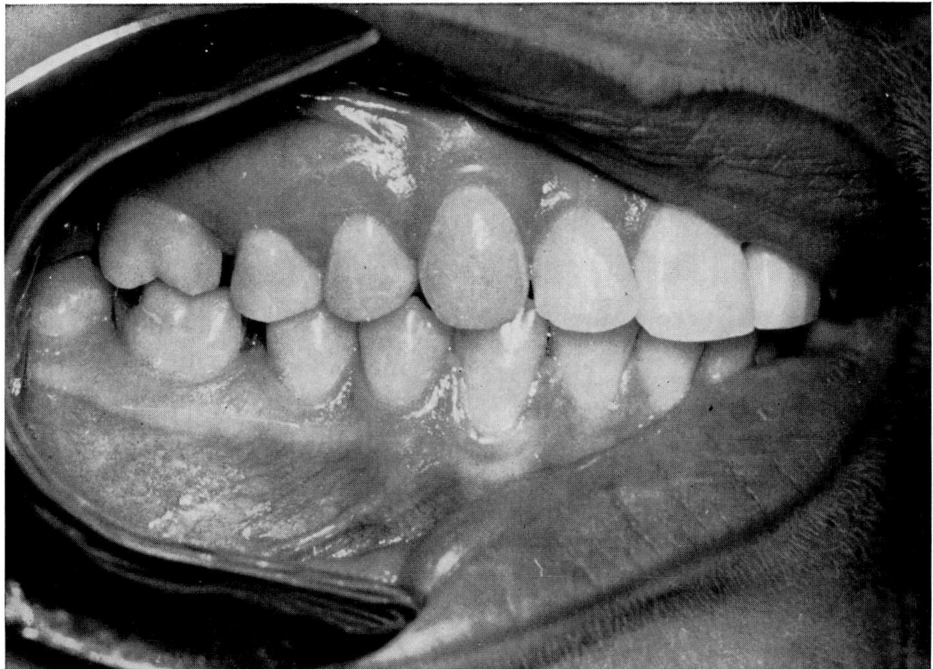

Fig. 10–5. The subject is the same as in Figure 10–4. The line between the gingiva and the alveolar mucosa of the lower jaw is clear. Notice the loose-fitting appearance of the alveolar mucosa and the minute blood vessels which are close to the surface. The gingiva is firm, light in color, and has a stippled (pitted) surface texture.

viduals will reveal that it varies considerably in size and extent. At the lower end of the lingual frenum, where the undersurface of the tongue is attached to the floor of the mouth, is a nearly horizontal fold of tissue extending to the right and left of the frenum. This horizontal fold is the *plica sublingualis.** Along the crest of the plica sublingualis are small openings of ducts, usually invisible to the naked eye, which lead from the sublingual salivary glands and empty into the mouth beneath the tongue. In the center of the plica sublingualis, one on either side of the base of the lingual frenum, are the larger openings of *Wharton's ducts* which carry the salivary secretions from the submandibular glands, and also from the sublingual glands, to the oral cavity. If you have ever opened your mouth and been surprised by having two thin streams of saliva shoot out from beneath your tongue, you now know where they came from.

Now, continuing your examination of the mouth, pull the lower lip down and out and the upper lip up and out, and then pull the cheeks back at the corners of the mouth. Notice the alveolar mucosa which lines the *oral vestibules.*† The epithelium of this mucosa is nonkeratinized, shiny, red, and partially transparent to underlying blood vessels. It is clearly demarcated from the paler gingiva mucosa by a scalloped line (Figs. 10–5; 10–6).

The *soft palate,* which begins distal to the maxillary third molar teeth, is a mass

*Pronounced pli′ kȧ sŭb lĭng guăl ĭs.
†The maxillary and mandibular *oral vestibules* are the spaces between the facial surfaces of the teeth and their supporting bone and the oral surfaces of the cheeks and lips. A finger inserted in the mouth between the teeth and the cheek or lip is in the *vestibule.*

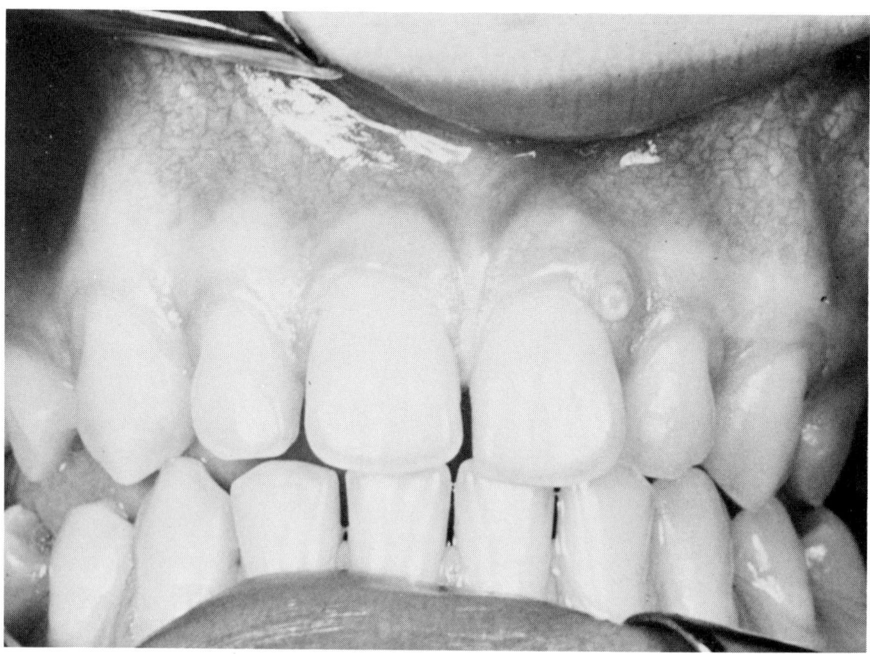

Fig. 10–6. This subject has a clear scalloped line between the *gingiva* (masticatory type of mucosa), and the *alveolar mucosa* (lining type of mucosa) in the upper facial area. On close inspection, small blood vessels are seen in the thinner and nonkeratinized alveolar mucosa.

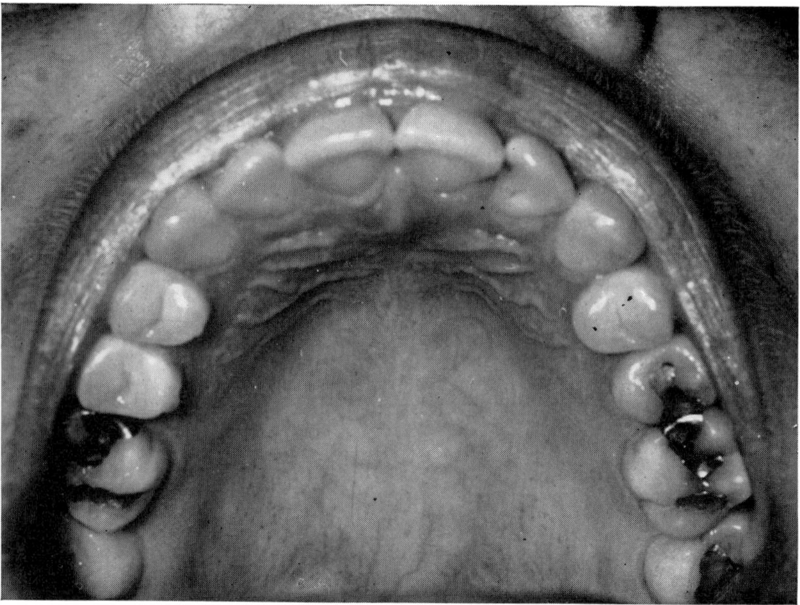

Fig. 10–7. The subject is the same as in Figure 10–4. The hard palate is well keratinized; the palatine rugae* (the horizontal ridges behind the anterior teeth) are distinct. The palatine raphe, distinguished with difficulty in this photograph, extends from anterior to posterior in the center line. Notice how the gingiva fits snugly around the palatal sides of the teeth.
*Plural, pronounced rōō' jē; singular is *ruga,* pronounced rōō' ġa.

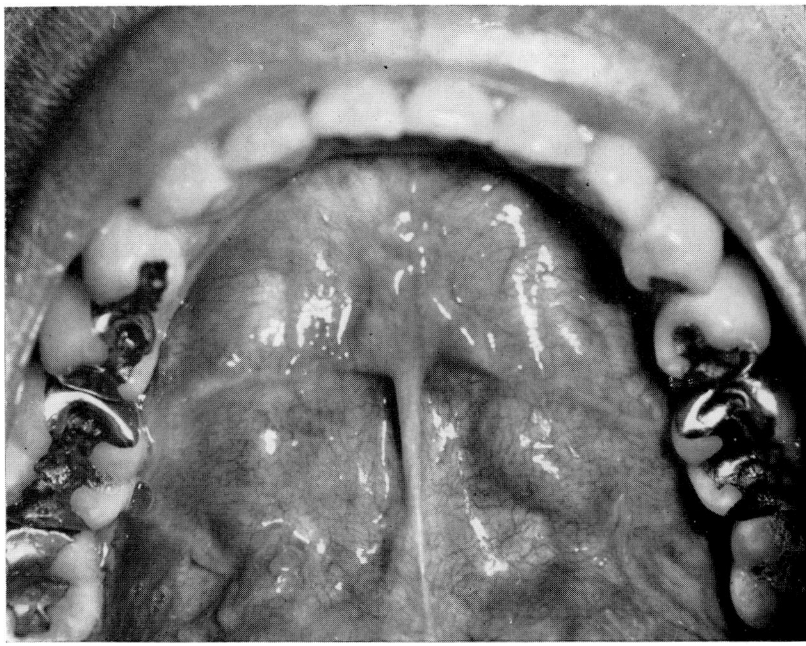

Fig. 10–8. The subject is the same as in Figure 10–4. This is a photograph of the floor of the mouth and part of the under surface of the elevated tongue; the mandibular anterior teeth are at the bottom of the picture. The *lingual frenum*, which tends to hold the tongue to the floor of the mouth, divides the area into right and left halves. The horizontal fold (the *sublingual fold*, or *plica sublingualis*), lying where the base of the tongue meets the floor of the mouth, bears the openings of the ducts from the sublingual and submandibular glands.

where soft & hard palate meets is the vibrating line. post dam.

of flexible muscle covered on the oral surface with oral mucosa. The epithelium of this mucosa ordinarily is not keratinized. Numerous salivary glands lie beneath the mucosa of the soft palate and empty onto its surface.

In the cheeks and lips there is a thick submucosa which contains fat tissue and also many salivary glands whose minute duct openings are scattered over the surface of the mucosa. Occasionally you may see what appears to be a pea-sized bubble just beneath the surface. This condition is due to a stoppage in one of these small salivary ducts which has resulted in an accumulation at this point of the secretion from a salivary gland. This bubble is called a *mucocele*.*

If you will examine the cheek mucosa inside the corners of the mouth of several individuals you will often find an area which has a few, or numerous, small yellowish spots which are called *Fordyce's spots*. These spots are openings onto the oral mucosa of sebaceous glands, which, of course, are usually thought of as being restricted to the skin on the outside of the body. They occur here, it is said, as a result of the narrowing of the wide embryonic mouth during early face development—*i.e.*, in the filling in of the angle between the maxillary process and the mandibular arch at either corner of the mouth some skin glands are entrapped. However near fact this explanation may be, it does not account for the presence of sebaceous glands on the red margin of the upper lip, and their usual absence on the lower lip; their presence on areas of cheek mucosa above,

*Pronounced mū' kō sēl.

below, and behind the area of narrowing of the embryonic mouth; their seeming absence in human fetuses; nor their greater number in adults than in children.

Specialized mucosa is the term applied to the mucous membrane located on the dorsum (top side) of the tongue. The mucosa in this area is distinctly different from other oral mucosa. Examine someone's tongue and you will see that the mucosa of its upper surface is formed into innumerable small *papillae* (hills). These papillae are of several kinds, different in size and shape, and some of them bear microscopic organs which supply the sense of taste.

Filiform papillae (thread-like) (Figs. 10–9; 10–10) cover the top surface of the tongue and give it a velvety appearance. The epithelium covering the tips of the filiform papillae is usually heavily keratinized (Fig. 10–11). In the human tongue the keratinization is not sufficient to impart the sandpaper-like quality you feel in the keratinized papillae on a kitten's tongue if the kitten licks your hand.

Fungiform papillae (mushroom-shaped) (Figs. 10–9; 10–12) are larger and less numerous than the filiform. They are scattered among the filiform papillae. Due to their thinner epithelium they appear redder in color than the filiform papillae. They may be clearly seen by careful examination of the tongue.

Foliate papillae are located along the lateral borders of the posterior part of the tongue. In the human tongue these papillae are not well developed (Fig. 10–14).

Circumvallate papillae (also called *vallate papillae*) (Figs. 10–9; 10–13) are located well back on the tongue between the body and the base of the tongue. They are relatively large, conspicuous structures, 8 to 10 in number, arranged in a V-shaped line with the point of the V directed toward the throat. Each papilla is surrounded by a trench, or trough, into the bottom of which open ducts leading from the salivary glands beneath (Von Ebner's glands). The saliva from these glands floods the trench around the papilla and serves as a solvent for food substances.

Now along the lateral surfaces of these papillae are groups of specialized epithelial cells called *taste buds*. When food substances, in solution in the saliva from Von Ebner's glands, come in contact with the taste buds, the individual experiences a sensation of taste.

Fungiform, foliate, and circumvallate papillae all contain organs of taste, but they are more conspicuous on the circumvallate papillae.

Figure 10–14 is a photomicrograph of a section of rabbit tongue in the area of the foliate papillae, showing taste buds along the sides of the papillae. These rabbit papillae are, of course, different in shape from human circumvallate papillae, but the taste buds are very like those of the circumvallate papillae of the human tongue, and they are more easily studied in the rabbit tongue. Figure 10–15 is a higher magnification of the taste buds seen in the center of the picture in Figure 10–14. Notice the fine detail of their construction.

THE SALIVARY GLANDS

Histology and Function of Salivary Glands

Salivary glands may be classified as *duct* glands, as *exocrine*, and as either pure *serous*, pure *mucous*, or *mixed* (sero-mucous) glands.

Salivary glands produce a colorless, slightly sticky fluid called *saliva* which is

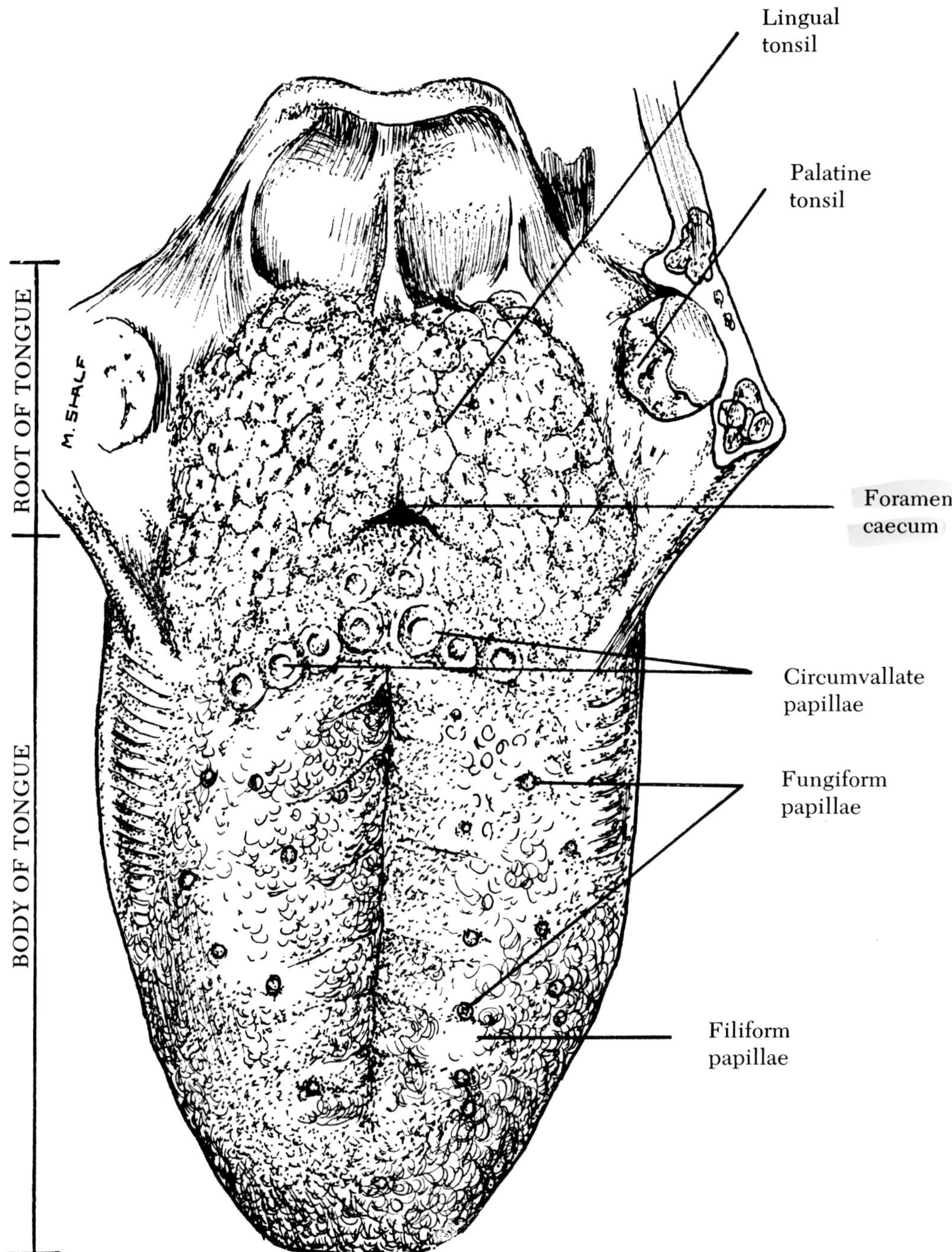

Fig. 10–9. Diagrammatic drawing of the dorsum of the human tongue. The division between the body and root is indicated, as are the locations of the kinds of papillae, the foramen caecum, and the lingual tonsil.

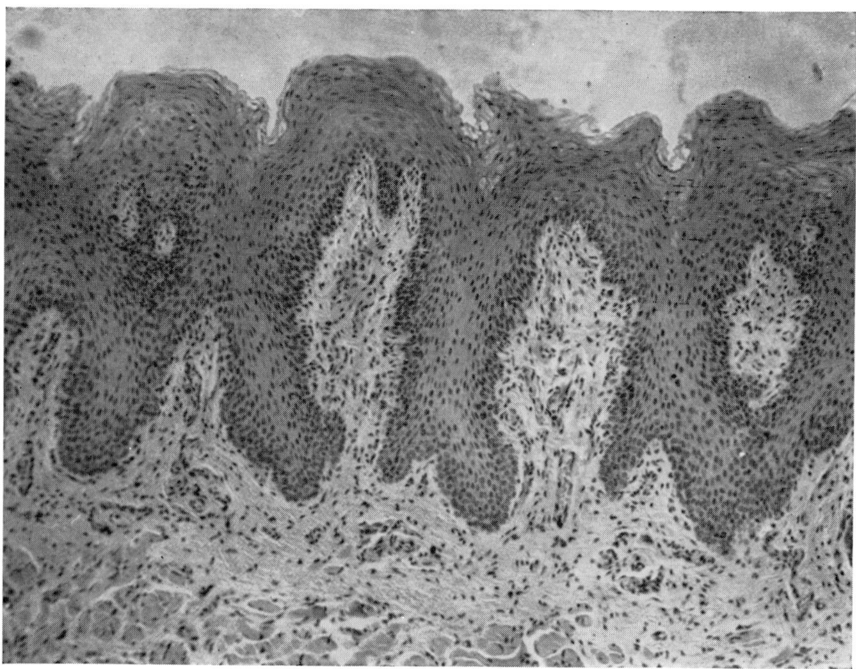

Fig. 10–10. Photomicrograph of a vertical section through the upper surface of a human tongue. These are filiform papillae. In this section the surface of the epithelium does not appear to be heavily keratinized.

discharged into the oral cavity through ducts that open onto the surface of the oral mucosa.

In embryonic development the salivary glands are formed from the epithelium that lines the early oral cavity. In certain areas cells of the embryonic oral epithelium grow downward into the underlying connective tissue (Fig. 10–16A and B), and as they multiply the epithelial cells of this downgrowth become modified and very specialized and form the salivary glands. Some of the cells develop into the secretory cells of the glands, and others develop into the ducts of the glands. The secretory cells secrete saliva. There are two types of secretory cells: *serous cells* and *mucous cells* (Fig. 10–18). Salivary glands are made up of serous cells, of mucous cells, or of a combination of the two kinds of secretory cells plus the ducts which connect them. The secreted product of serous cells contains an enzyme called amylase (ptyalin) which contributes to the breakdown of starches. A secreted product of the mucous cells is mucin which acts as a lubricant to the oral cavity. Besides these substances the salivary glands secrete other materials among which are proteins and salts which act as buffers and prevent the saliva from becoming suddenly acid or alkaline. Also, saliva contains some antibacterial factors which inhibit the growth of some bacteria. In addition to these products of the salivary glands, saliva which has been lying in the mouth contains various sorts of debris such as epithelial cells sloughed off the oral mucosa, degenerating white blood cells, and bacteria.

The total amount of saliva produced by the salivary glands varies greatly in different individuals, but an approximate amount is about 3 pints a day.

Functions of saliva may be enumerated: (1) it assists in the mastication of food; (2) it serves as a solvent; (3) it contributes to the digestion of carbohydrates;

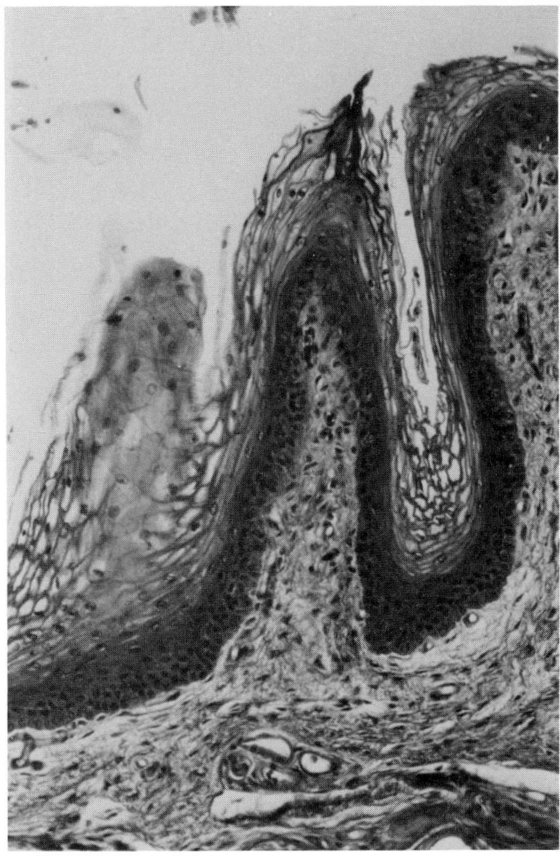

Fig. 10–11. Histologic section of a filiform papilla showing heavy keratinization. The dark area is the rest of the epithelium. Notice the core of connective tissue underlying the epithelium.

(4) it lubricates food and oral tissues; (5) it acts as a buffer; (6) it cleanses the mouth by flushing out debris; (7) it acts to inhibit the growth of some microorganisms.

Distribution of Salivary Glands

Salivary glands may be described in two groups: *(A) major salivary glands and (B) minor salivary glands*. The major salivary glands are (1) *parotid*, (2) *submandibular (submaxillary)*, and (3) *sublingual*. The minor salivary glands vary in size and are widely distributed beneath the oral mucous membrane.

The *major salivary glands* are, or course, paired organs. The *parotid glands* are flattened organs located under the skin of the face in front of and below each ear. They are the largest of the salivary glands, and in adult human beings their secretory cells are all serous in type (Fig. 10–17). The parotid gland is the gland involved in epidemic parotitis, commonly known as mumps. The main duct of each parotid gland, the *parotid duct (Stensen's duct)*, opens into the oral cavity on the wall of either cheek opposite the second maxillary molar tooth. If the tongue is passed over this area a small prominence may be felt at the point where the duct opens into the mouth.

The *submandibular glands* are located beneath the posterior part of the tongue.

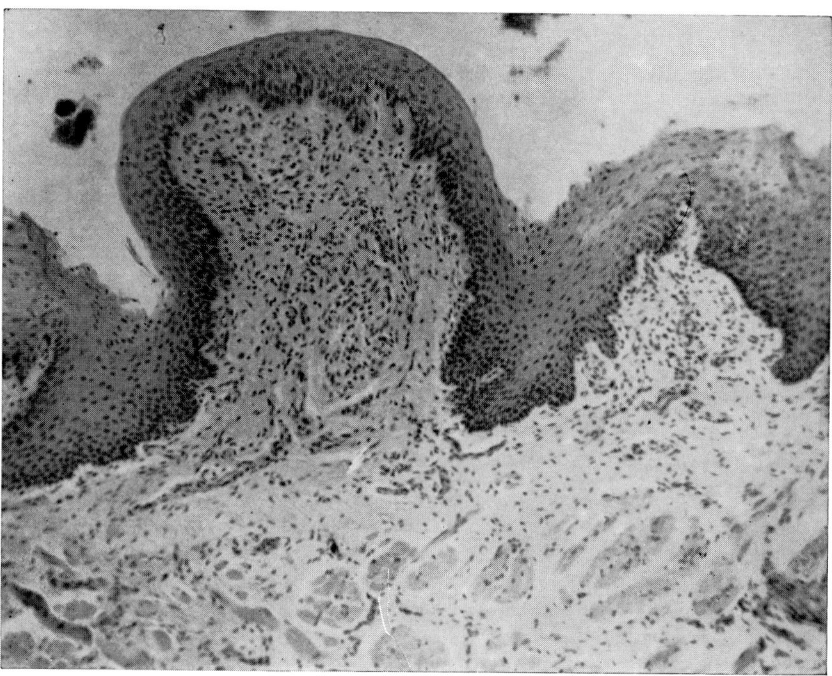

Fig. 10–12. Photomicrograph of a vertical section through the upper surface of a human tongue. This is a fungiform papilla. Examine someone's tongue and locate some papillae of this type.

They lie in a depression on the inner surface of either side of the mandible just anterior to the angle of the jaw. The secretory cells which make up these glands are a combination of serous and mucous cells, the serous being the more numerous (Figs. 10–18; 10–19). The secreted product of these glands is a mixture of serous and mucous substances. The main ducts which carry the products of the submandibular glands to the oral cavity open into the mouth beneath the tongue, one on either side of the center line. You can see the openings easily as two small prominences in this area (Fig. 10–8). These ducts are known as the *submandibular ducts (Wharton's ducts,* Fig. 10–16A).

The *sublingual glands* are located beneath the mucosa in the floor of the mouth anterior to the submandibular glands. They are composed of a mixture of serous and mucous types of cells, but are predominantly mucous in character (Fig. 10–20). The main ducts which carry the products of this pair of glands are several in number, and all open beneath the tongue. Some open along the crest of the plica sublingualis, while others join the submandibular ducts and share the same openings. Examine carefully the area under the tongue in a human mouth.

The *minor salivary glands* may be described according to their location in the oral cavity. Beneath the mucous membrane of the cheeks and lips are numerous small glands which are a mixture of mucous and serous secretory cells, the mucous cells being the more numerous. The minute duct openings of these small glands are scattered over the surface of the cheek and lip mucosa. Larger salivary glands made up entirely of mucous cells lie beneath the mucous membrane of the roof of the mouth and have minute duct openings distributed over the entire surface of the hard and soft palate. The tongue has glands in its

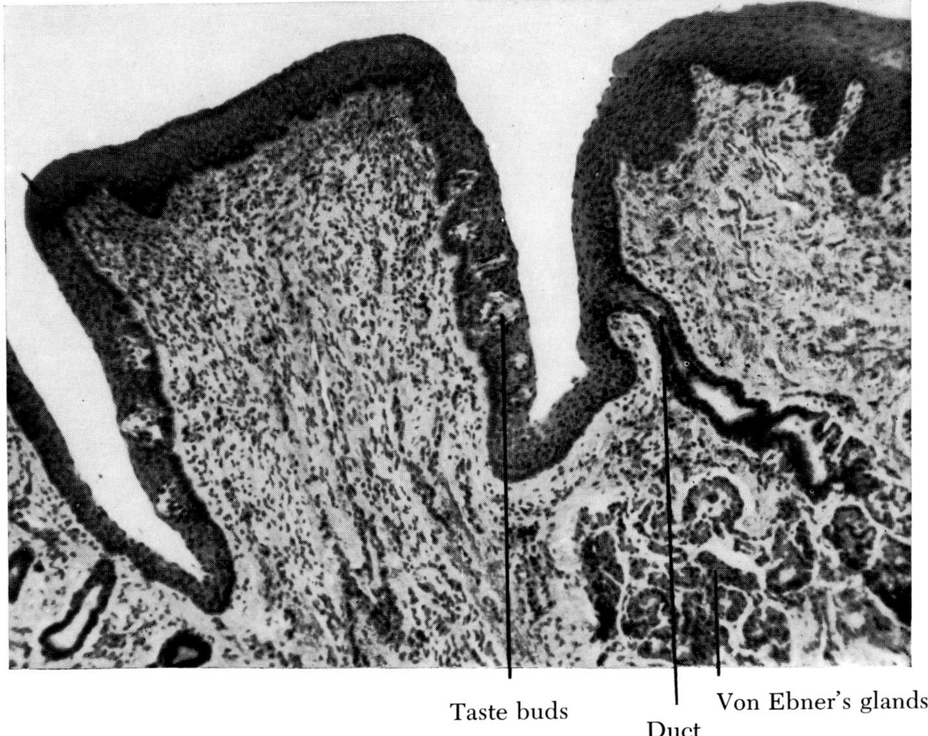

Fig. 10–13. Photomicrograph of a vertical section through the dorsum (upper surface) of a human tongue. This is a circumvallate papilla. The papillae may be from 2 to 3 mm in diameter. Taste buds are located along the side surface; a duct from Von Ebner's salivary glands empties into the base of the trench around the papilla. This section is cut through the length of the duct, but it is a little to one side of the duct opening, so you cannot see in this illustration exactly the point at which the duct opens into the trench.

anterior part which are mixed in character (contain both serous and mucous cells). In the posterior part of the tongue are the pure serous *Von Ebner's glands* whose ducts empty into the trenches of the circumvallate papillae (Fig. 10–13). There are also pure mucous glands in the root of the tongue and in the floor of the mouth (Fig. 10–21).

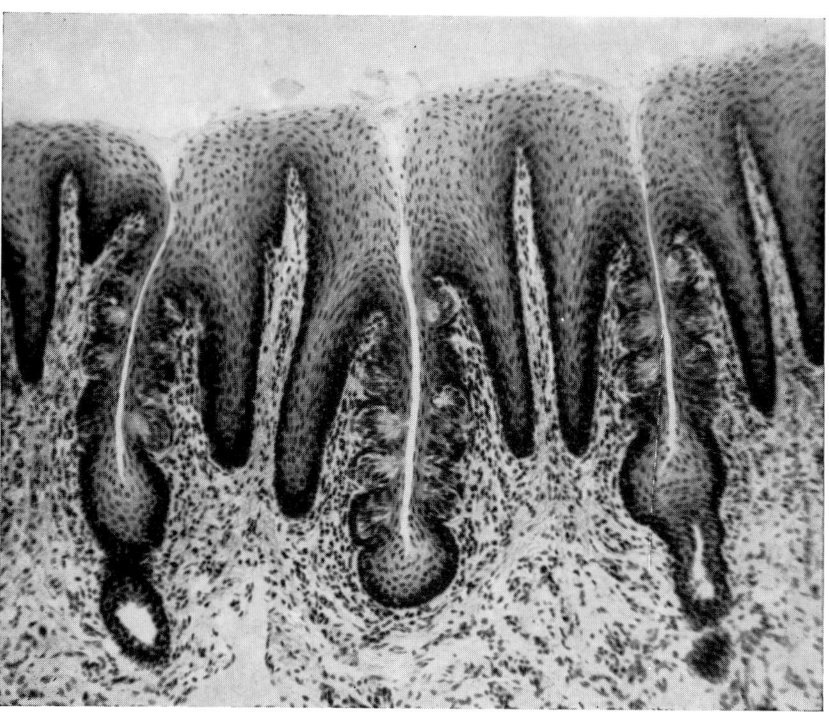

Fig. 10–14. Photomicrograph of a section through the side of a rabbit tongue. These are foliate papillae. They are a different shape and are better developed in a rabbit than in man. The taste buds are clearly seen in the epithelium along the sides of the papillae. (See Figure 10–15 for an enlargement.)

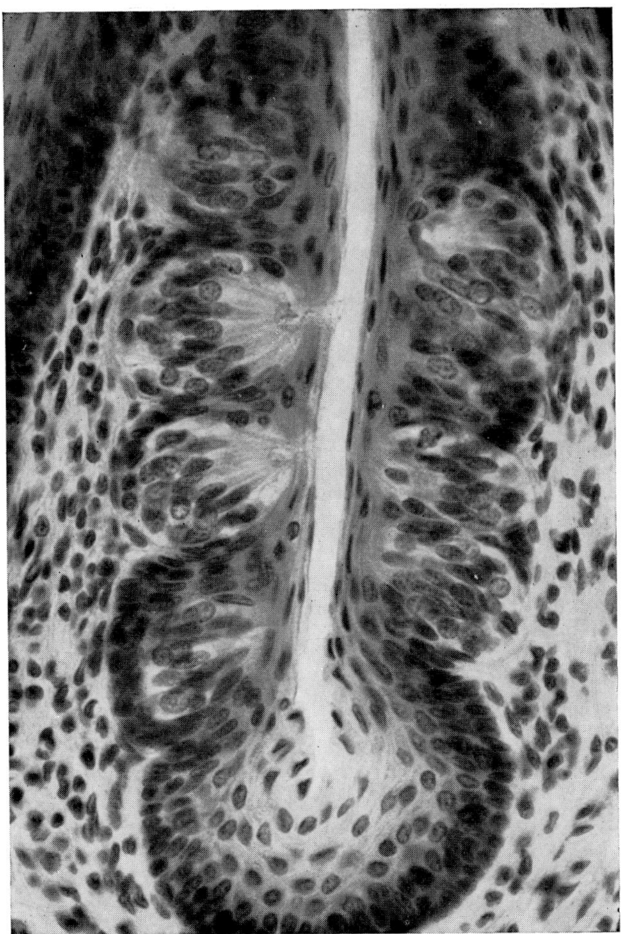

Fig. 10–15. Photomicrograph at a higher magnification of the taste buds seen in the center of the picture in Figure 10–14. On the left of the vertical space between the two papillae are two taste buds cut exactly through their centers. Notice the little porelike opening to the surface.

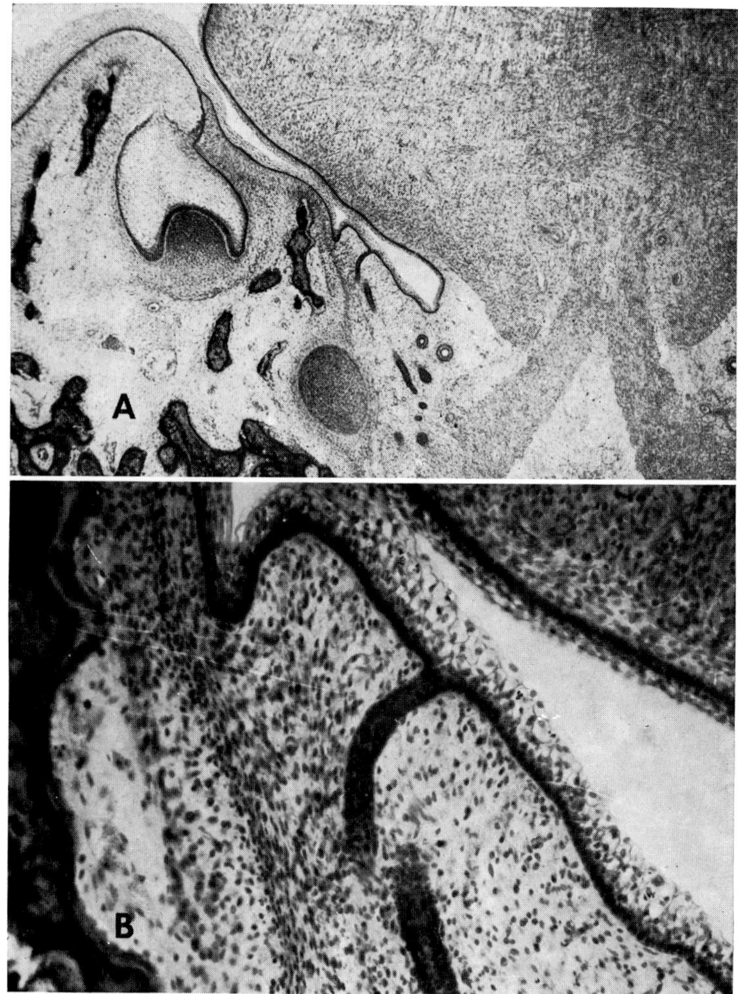

Fig. 10–16. Photomicrograph of a frontal section of one side of the lower jaw of a five-month-old human fetus. *A*. The tongue is on the right and the tooth germ of a posterior tooth is on the left. From the oral epithelium under the tongue a slender growth of epithelial cells curves downward into the connective tissue. This is the beginning of the development of a salivary gland and its secretory duct. The two small circles beneath the tongue are cross sections of two salivary gland ducts, parts of the larger *Wharton's duct*. *B*. A higher magnification of the area under the tongue.

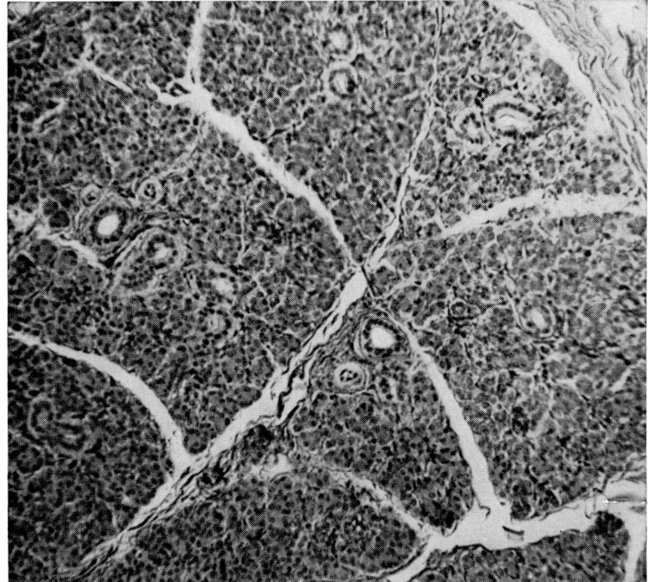

Fig. 10–17. Photomicrograph of a section of human parotid gland. The secretory cells are all serous in type. In several places are seen cross sections of the ducts of this gland: they appear here as circular openings lined with cuboidal epithelial cells. These small ducts coalesce into larger ducts, which empty the gland secretions into the mouth at openings located on the inside of the cheek.

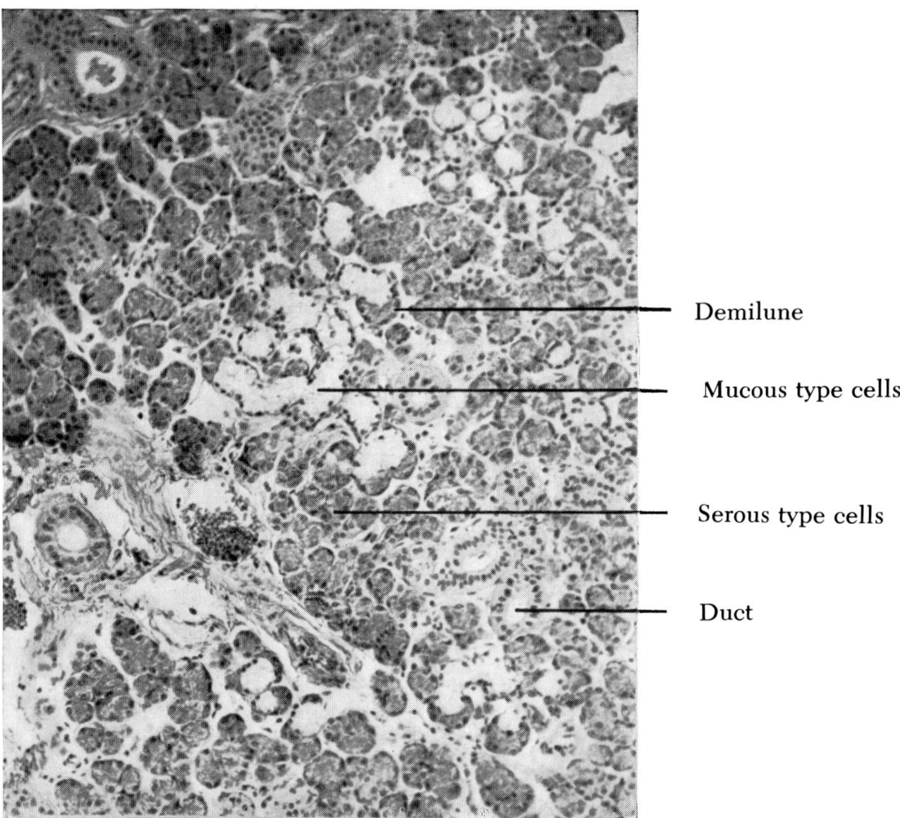

Fig. 10–18. Photomicrograph of a section of human submandibular gland. The secretory cells are of both serous and mucous types, the serous type being the more numerous. In the center of the picture are seen groups of light colored mucous type cells, which in some cases have serous cells capping them on one side. Because in histologic sections these capping cells have a new-moon shape, some imaginative histologists have called them *demilunes* (half-moons). Cross sections of ducts are seen in the section.

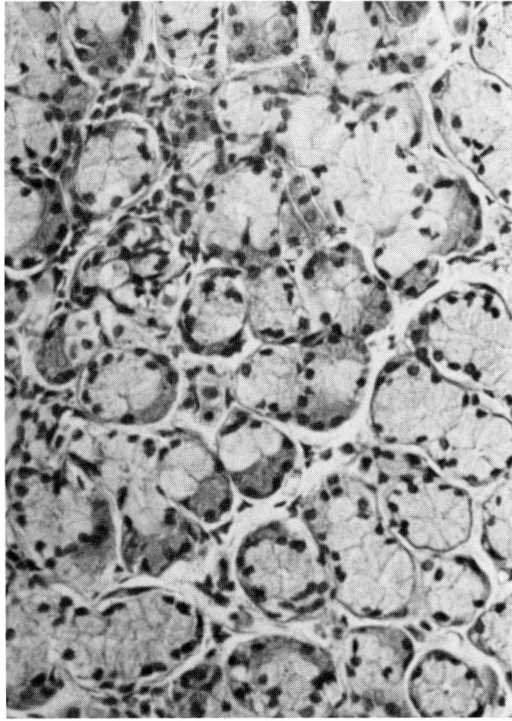

Fig. 10–19. Higher magnification of a section of a human submandibular gland. The darker cells here are serous cells of demilunes; the lighter staining cells are mucous cells.

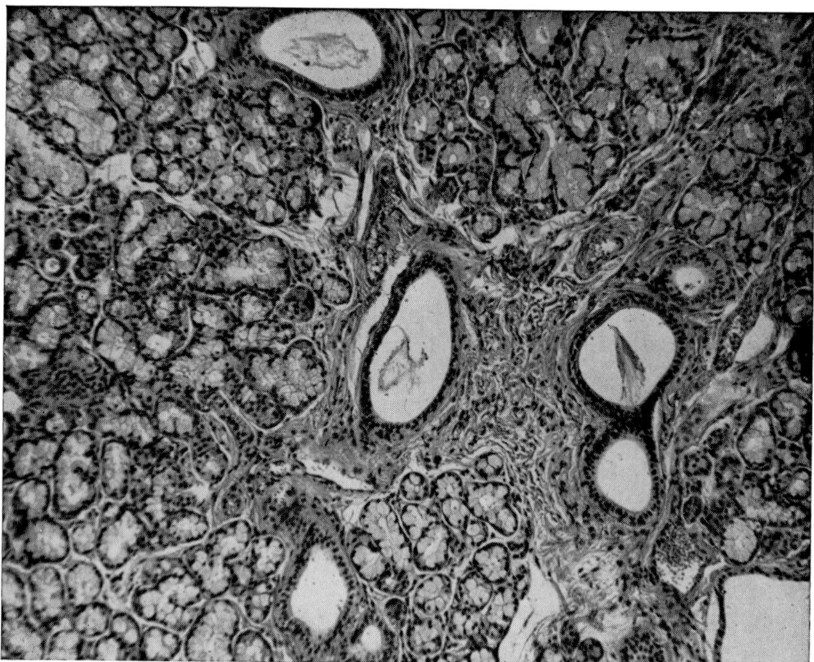

Fig. 10–20. Photomicrograph of a section of human sublingual gland. Most of the secretory cells here are of the mucous type. The darker stained serous type cells are sparingly scattered in the gland, often in the form of demilunes. Cross sections of ducts are also seen here.

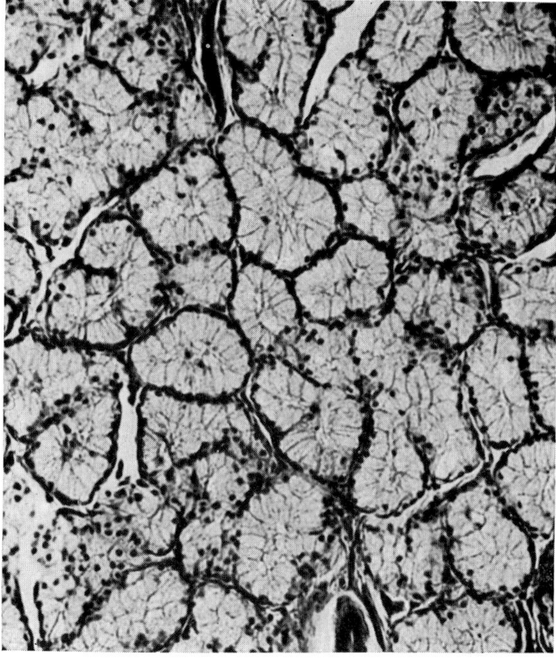

Fig. 10–21. Photomicrograph of a section of a minor sublingual gland from the floor of the mouth. All of the secretory cells here are of the mucous type.

Chapter 11

THE GINGIVA

LOCATION

Gingiva is the part of the oral mucosa that is firmly attached to the alveolar process and to the cervical parts of the teeth and that surrounds the cervices of the teeth.

Gingiva on the facial side of the maxillae and mandible in the premolar and molar regions is called *buccal gingiva,* and in the incisor and canine regions, *labial gingiva.* Gingiva on the inside of the mandibular arch is called *lingual gingiva,* and on the inside of the maxillary arch, *palatal gingiva.*

CLINICAL APPEARANCE

To study the clinical appearance of the gingiva, stand before a mirror or use a classmate as a subject. Pull out and down on the lower lip, and out and up on the the upper lip. Below the crowns of the mandibular teeth and above the crowns of the maxillary teeth you see that the oral mucous membrane is firm and has a stippled, or finely pitted, surface. This is gingiva (Fig. 11–1). In people who have a fair skin the color of the gingiva is a slightly grayish pink. In dark complexioned individuals the gingiva frequently is either spotted with brown or is fairly even grayish brown all over due to the melanin which occurs in some of the cells of the epithelium. Around the facial surface of the anterior teeth, four or five millimeters from the cervical margin, the gingiva ends in a scalloped line and the oral mucosa beyond this line is red, shiny, and loosely attached to the underlying tissue. Examine also the gingiva around the buccal side of the mandibular and maxillary posterior teeth. The color and surface textures here are the same as in the anterior region, and a scalloped line marks the apical border.

Now examine the lingual side of the mandibular arch. The gingiva is firmly attached to the underlying hard tissue, while oral mucosa beneath the tongue is loose, shiny, and redder in color than the gingiva. Examine the palatal side of the maxillary arch. On the maxilla the palatal gingiva blends without a distinct line into the oral mucosa of the hard palate (Fig. 11–2).

Look again at the facial and at the lingual and palatal surfaces of the mandibular and maxillary arches. The position and shape of the gingival margin depend largely on the age of the individual. In a young person the gingiva covers the cervical part of the enamel of the tooth, so that the *clinical crown* (the part of the tooth exposed in the oral cavity) is smaller than the *anatomic crown* (the part of

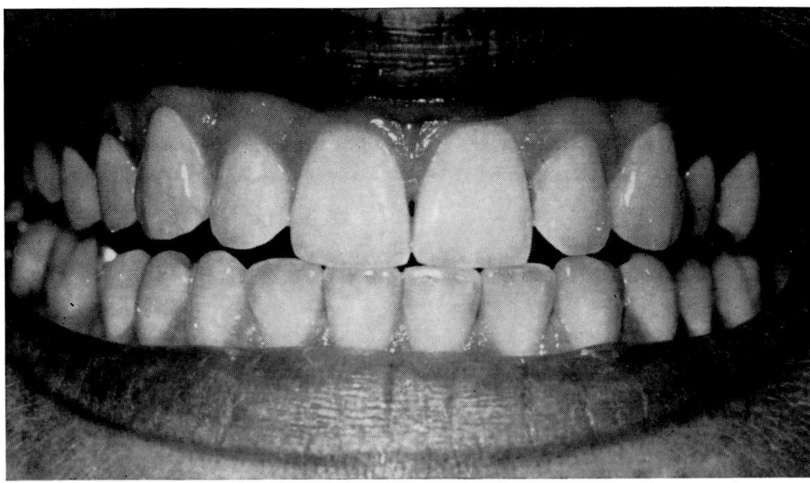

Fig. 11–1. The subject of this photograph was a young woman aged twenty-two years. The gingiva is firm and stippled in appearance; the interdental papillae fill the interproximal spaces; the gingival margin is still on the enamel on all teeth, making the clinical crowns slightly smaller than the anatomic crowns.

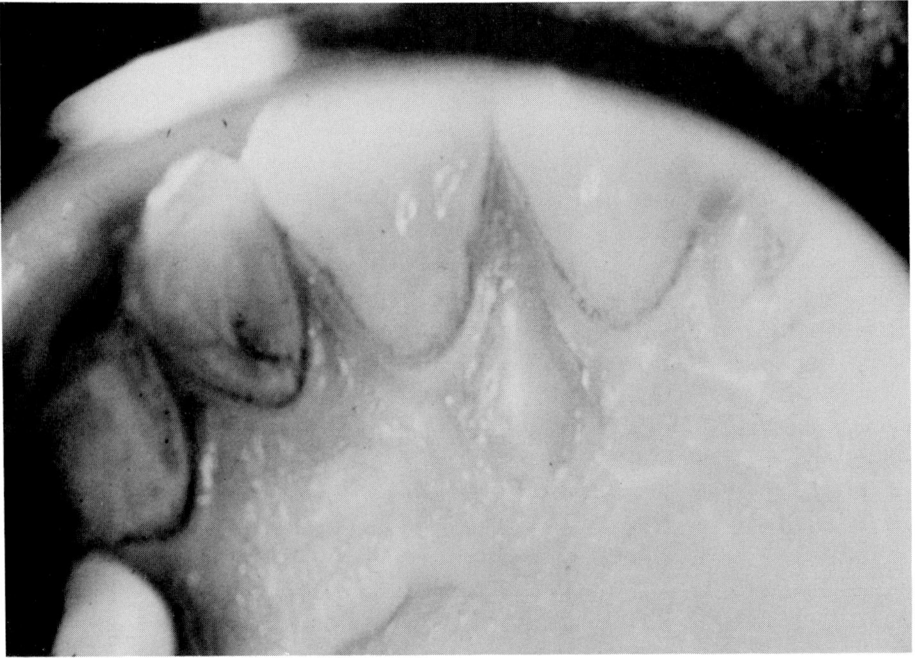

Fig. 11–2. Palatal side of the maxillary arch. The palatal gingiva blends without a distinct line into the oral mucosa of the hard palate. The structure just lingual to the central incisors is the *incisive papilla.* Notice the calculus at the cervical area of the crowns.

the tooth that has an enamel surface); and between the teeth a triangular wedge of gingiva, the *interdental papilla*, fills the interproximal space (Fig. 11–1).*

Between the teeth, where the interdental papilla meets or nearly meets the point of tooth contact, there is an indentation, or depression, on the crest of the papilla. This depression is called a *col.*† (The word *col* usually refers to a pass between adjacent peaks of a mountain chain. In this case, the facial and lingual points of the interdental papilla represent the adjacent mountain peaks, and the depression between them is the col.) This hidden col can be a sheltered reservoir for entrapped food. When adjacent teeth are not in contact or when a tooth is missing, there is no interdental papilla and no col.

Now consider a person thirty or thirty-five years of age. The interdental papillae may not extend to the areas of tooth contact, and most or all of the tooth enamel probably is uncovered: the clinical crown and the anatomic crown are often about the same.

Now examine a person fifty or sixty years old and compare what you see here with what you saw in the very young person and in the younger adult. In the middle aged or older person you will probably find that not only do the interdental papillae fail to fill the spaces that exist between the teeth cervical to the contact areas (the interproximal spaces), but on some or all surfaces of the teeth cementum can be seen around the cervix (Fig. 11–3). The gingival margin in this older person is located so far rootward that some of the root cementum is exposed in the oral cavity, and the clinical crown of the tooth is larger than the anatomic crown.

This age change in the position of the gingiva on the tooth is a condition that

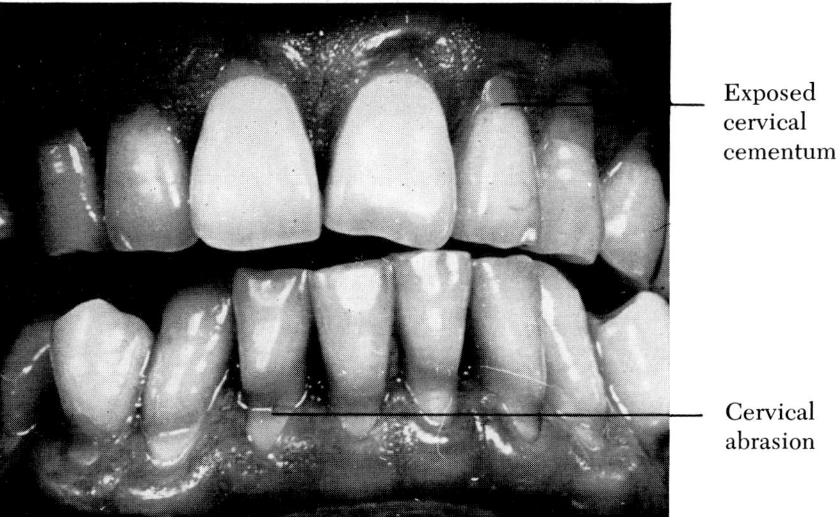

Fig. 11–3. Clinical photograph of maxillary and mandibular anterior teeth with associated gingiva. The subject was sixty years old. Notice the stippled gingiva; the position of the interdental papillae; the exposed but undamaged cementum on the left maxillary lateral incisor and on the right maxillary central incisor. Notice the exposed and deeply cut cementum on the mandibular anterior teeth. This is cervical abrasion.

*Valuable reference:
Carranza, F.: *Glickman's Clinical Periodontology*, 6th ed. Philadelphia, W.B. Saunders Co., 1984.
†Pronounced kōl.

is to be expected, just as it is expected that with age hair will become gray and skin will become wrinkled. Of course, diseases of the tissues around the teeth may produce pathologic changes with gingival recession at any age. What we are discussing here are usual and expected age changes.

HISTOLOGICAL STRUCTURE

Gingiva is a masticatory type of oral mucous membrane (Chapter 10). As is true for other areas of the oral mucous membrane, the gingiva is composed of connective tissue and epithelial tissue. The connective tissue (called *lamina propria*) is of the fibrous type, while the epithelial tissue, which is of course on the surface, is stratified squamous in character and is usually keratinized (Fig. 10–1). This keratinization causes the color of the gingiva to be grayish pink rather than red if it is not pigmented, or grayish brown rather than reddish brown if pigmenation is present; and the finger-shaped projections of the connective tissue into the epithelium (Fig. 11–4) probably produce the pitted condition of the surface of the epithelium in some places. The gingiva does not have a submucosa, but rest directly on the underlying hard tissue; and ordinarily the gingiva contains no salivary glands (Fig. 11–5).

The connective tissue of the free gingiva does have in it several particularly oriented sets of collagen fibers. Certain groups of periodontal ligament fibers penetrate the gingiva: the transseptal fibers, the free gingival fibers, and the

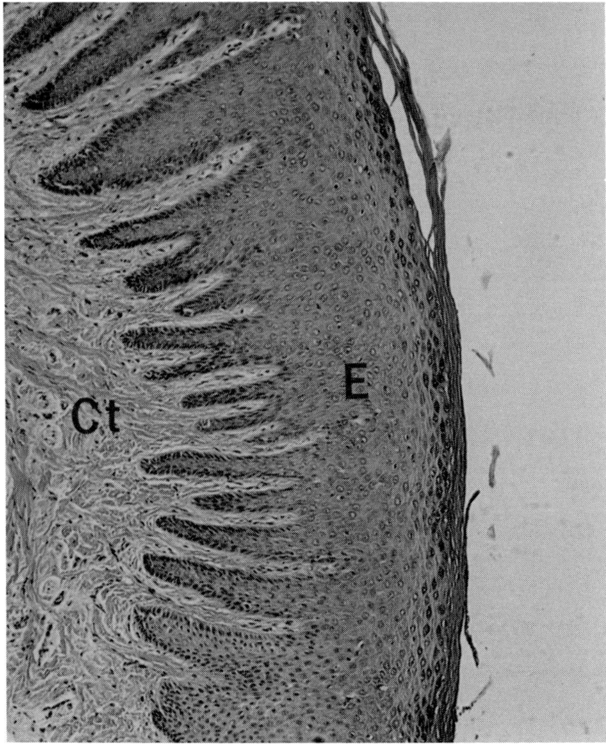

Fig. 11–4. Section of the human gingiva showing the interdigitation between the keratinized stratified squamous epithelium (E) and the fibrous connective tissue (Ct). A portion of the keratin (above) has pulled away from the adjacent epithelial cells.

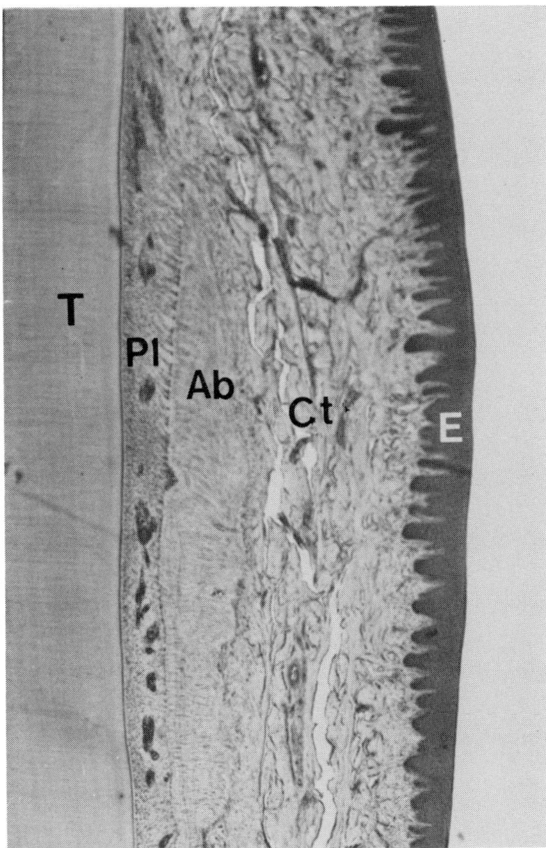

Fig. 11–5. Histologic section through a portion of the gingiva and its underlying structures. Scanning from the right, the following are seen: (E) epithelium and the connective tissue (Ct) of the gingiva; (Ab) alveolar bone (bone of tooth socket); (Pl) periodontal ligament; (T) tooth. Compare to Figure 11–6.

alveologingival fibers (see Chapter 8 and Figures 8–1; 11–6; 11–7). A group of fibers located in the connective tissue of the gingiva, but which are not periodontal ligament fibers, encircle the tooth like a ring, not attached either to cementum or to bone. These are the *circular fibers* of the gingiva.

THE GINGIVAL SULCUS

Around all teeth beneath the coronal border of the gingiva there is a space, or crevice, called the *gingival sulcus* (Fig. 11–6). A small dental instrument can be inserted into this space as far as the bottom *of the gingival sulcus.* This border of the gingiva which is not attached to the tooth surface is called the *free gingiva.* The inner wall of the sulcus is, of course, the tooth surface; and the outer wall is the stratified squamous *epithelium of the gingival sulcus,* which is continuous coronally over the *gingival margin* with the stratified squamous epithelium of the outer surface of the gingiva, and is continuous apically with the *attachment* (or *junctional*) *epithelium* (Figs. 11–6; 11–8).

The depth of the gingival sulcus has been reported to vary from 0 to 6 mm. The preferable depth is usually considered to be near zero. The depth of the

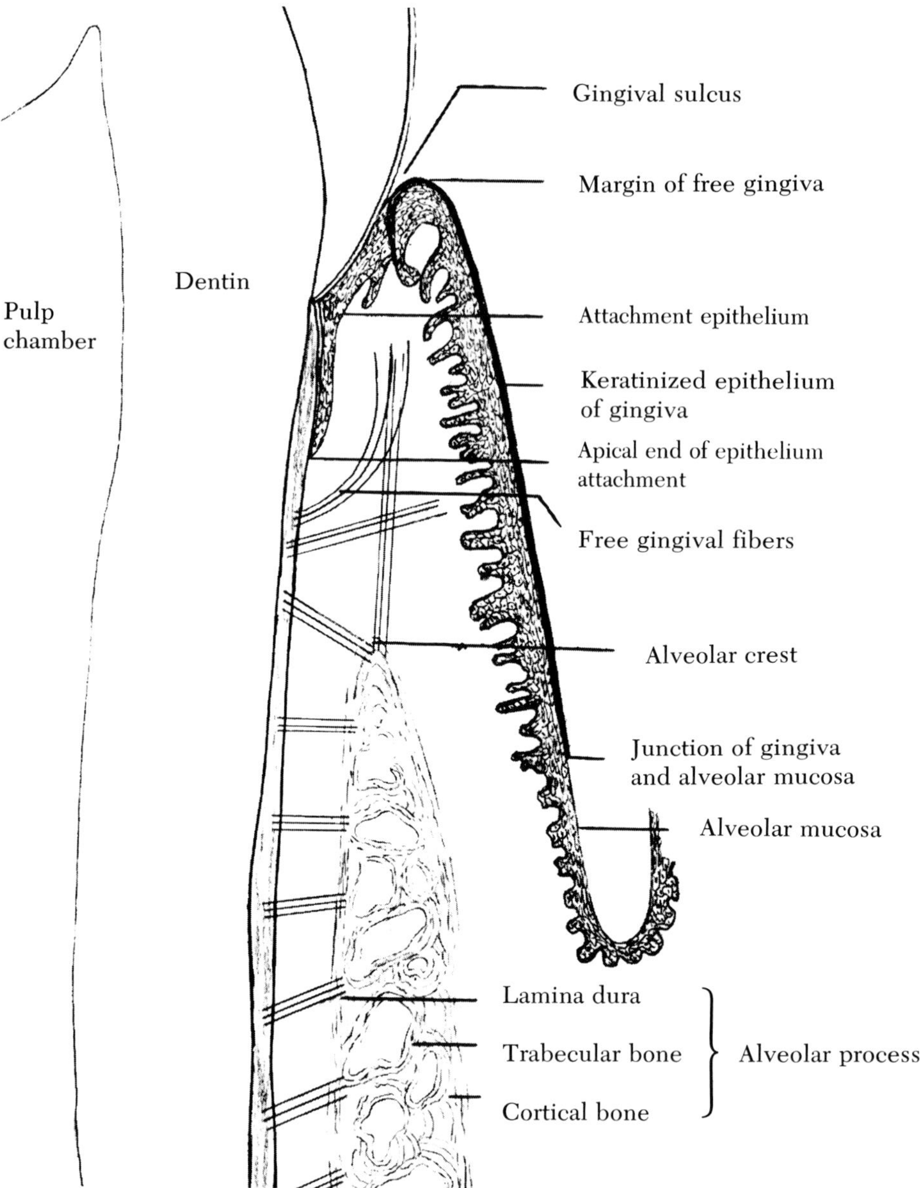

Fig. 11–6. Diagrammatic drawing of a section of the buccal cervical area of a mandibular molar tooth cut buccolingually.

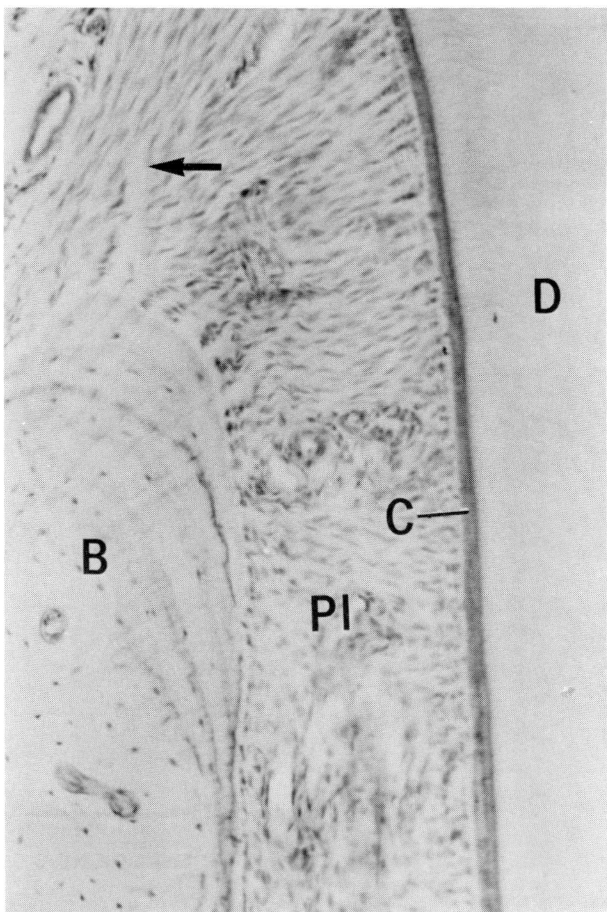

Fig. 11–7. Histologic section of the crest region of the alveolar process (bone around tooth). Connective tissue fibers of the gingiva (arrow) extend into the crest of the bone (B). These fibers are alveologingival fibers of the gingiva. (PI) Periodontal ligament. (C) Cementum. (D) Dentin. The epithelium of the gingiva, which is not seen here, is above.

sulcus is marked on the surface of the gingiva by a horizontal depression, the *free gingival groove*.

The Attachment Epithelium

The *attachment epithelium* (also called *junctional* epithelium) is the band of stratified squamous epithelium that is attached to the tooth surface around the cervical part of all teeth and that is continuous coronally with the epithelium of the gingival sulcus and on over the gingival margin with the epithelium on the outer surface of the gingiva (Figs. 11–6; 11–8; 11–9).

The epithelial cells of the attachment (junctional) epithelium that lie adjacent to the tooth surface produce a structure that resembles the basal lamina part of a basement membrane (see Chapter 1). This structure is the attaching substance between the cells of the attachment epithelium and the tooth.

In very young individuals the attachment epithelium ends apically at the cementoenamel junction (Figs. 11–10C,D). At this early stage of tooth eruption

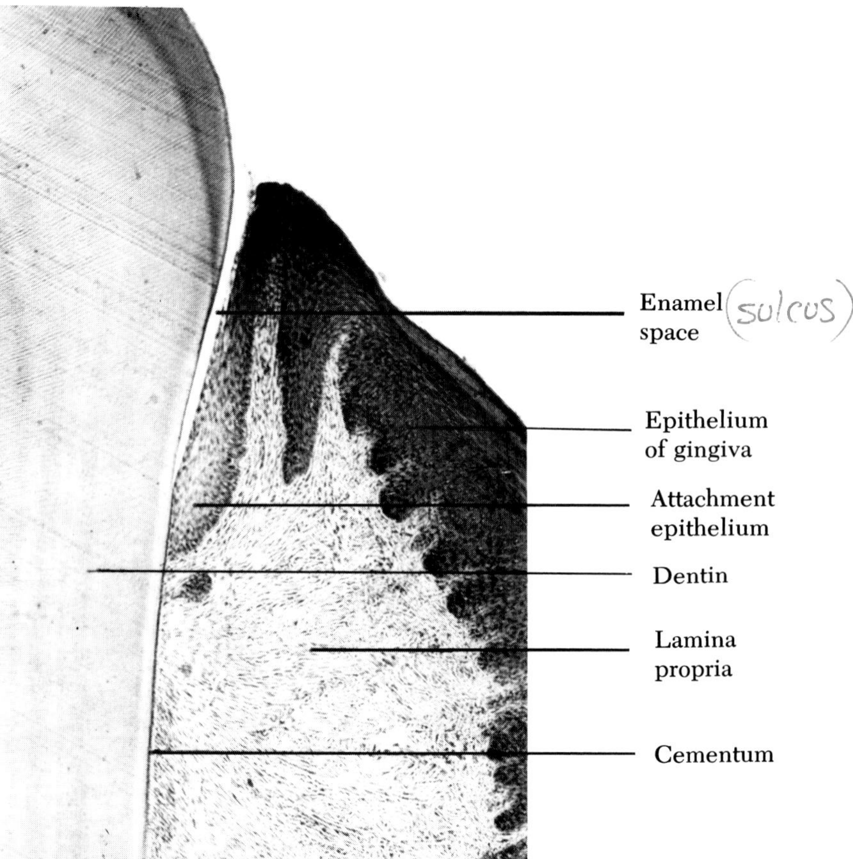

Fig. 11–8. Section of a kitten tooth and its associated gingiva. The *attachment epithelium* is adjacent to the enamel and cementum of the tooth. The enamel space is where the enamel was before the tooth was demineralized; enamel is lost during the demineralization process. (See Chapter 1.)

the clinical crown is short because the cervical part of the enamel is covered with gingiva. As tooth eruption continues the gingiva recedes cervically, exposing more of the anatomic crown; and at the same time the apical end of the attachment epithelium slowly migrates (grows by cell division) onto the cementum in the cervical part of the root. It becomes firmly attached to the cementum (Figs. 11–10E, F, G; 11–11).

With age the gingiva continues slowly to move rootward from the crown of the tooth, and the attachment epithelium continues slowly to grow apically on the cementum. This process is partly a consequence of the slow occlusal tooth movement which seems to occur, probably intermittently, throughout the life of the tooth. Chiefly, however, this apical growth of epithelium seems to take place independently of occlusal tooth movement and is referred to as the *rootward migration of the attachment epithelium.* This is a natural aging process and as such is not accompanied by inflammation. As aging continues the gingiva recedes to the point where the tooth crown is completely uncovered and exposed to the oral cavity (Fig. 11–10F). After this, continued gingival recession exposes cervical cementum and places the attachment epithelium considerably apical to the ce-

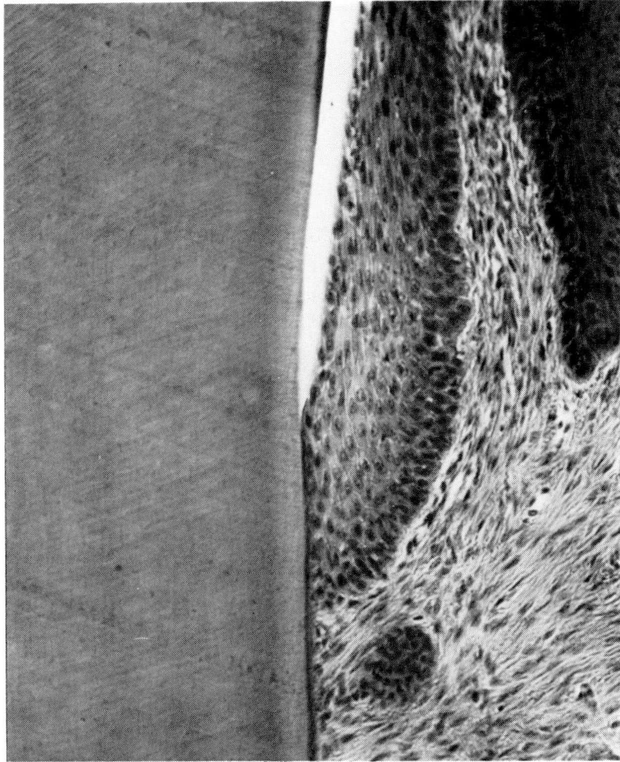

Fig. 11–9. Higher magnification of the attachment epithelium seen in Figure 11–8. The stratified squamous epithelial cells of the attachment epithelium are seen.

mentoenamel junction (Figs. 11–3; 11–10G, H, I). When the cementum is exposed, the bottom of the gingival sulcus is of course somewhere on the tooth root, but it is not necessarily at the same level on all of the teeth in a mouth nor even on all sides of the same tooth. In a healthy mouth the gingival sulcus under these conditions is ordinarily shallow.

Exposure of cementum in older individuals is to be regarded as the usual and expected condition. Such cementum exposure is not infrequently seen to a slight degree on the maxillary canines, and sometimes on other teeth, of persons less than thirty years old. After the age of thirty cementum exposure increases in frequency and extent. By forty years of age many individuals have cementum exposed on some areas of most of their teeth. By the age of sixty the amount of cementum exposure in some areas may often amount to 3 or 4 mm (Fig. 11–3). It is unusual to find an individual of middle age with no cementum exposed on any teeth.*

*Interesting references:
Carranza, F.: *Glickman's Clinical Periodontology.* 6th ed. Philadelphia, W.B. Saunders Co., 1984.
Listgarten, M.A.: Electron Microscope Study of the Gingivodental Junction of Man. Am. J. Anat., *119*:147, 1966.
Listgarten, M.A.: Changing Concepts About the Dento-epithelial Junction. J. Can. Dent. Assoc., *36*:70, 1970.
Toto P.D., and H. Sicher: Mucopolysaccharides in the Epithelial Attachment. J. Dent. Res., *44*:451, 1965.

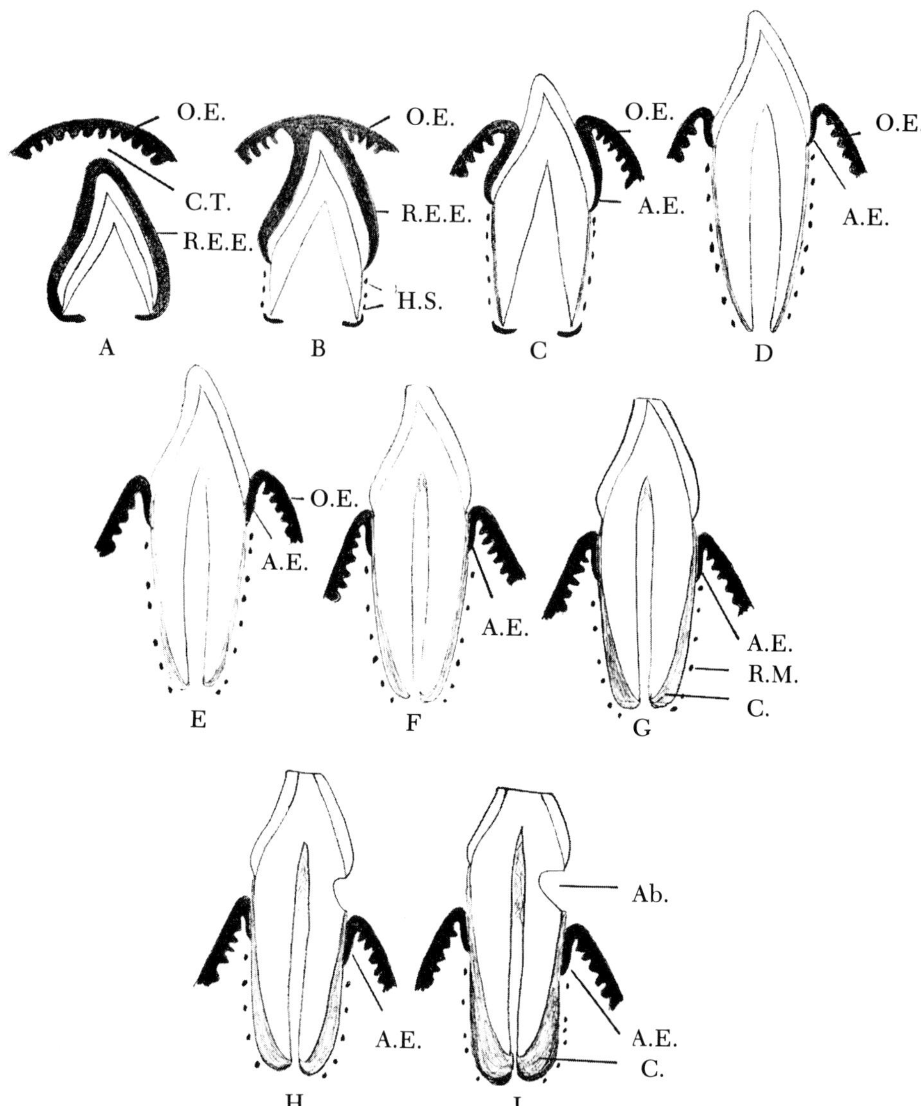

Fig. 11–10. O.E.—oral epithelium; C.T.—connective tissue; R.E.E.—reduced enamel epithelium; H.S.—Hertwig's sheath; A.E.—attachment epithelium; R.M.—rests of Malassez; C—cementum; Ab.—abrasion.

Diagrammatic illustration of the process of root formation, tooth eruption, the rootward migration of the attachment epithelium, cementum exposure, and cervical abrasion. (A) The reduced enamel epithelium covers the tooth crown and is separated from the oral epithelium by connective tissue. The root has not yet started to form. (B) Root formation has begun. The crown has moved incisally. The reduced enamel epithelium and the oral epithelium are in contact. (C) The root is longer. The incisal edge of the crown is exposed in the oral cavity. The reduced enamel epithelium (which is the remains of the enamel organ) is now continuous with the oral epithelium and is called the attachment epithelium. (D) The length of the root dentin is complete, and the crown has moved farther into the oral cavity. The attachment epithelium is still entirely on the enamel. The apical foramen is narrower. (E, F, G) The attachment epithelium grows onto the cementum at its apical border and separates from the tooth surface at its cervical border. Cementum becomes exposed. (H, I) Increased cementum exposure and improper use of an abrasive dentifrice have resulted in abrasion of cementum and dentin in the cervical area.

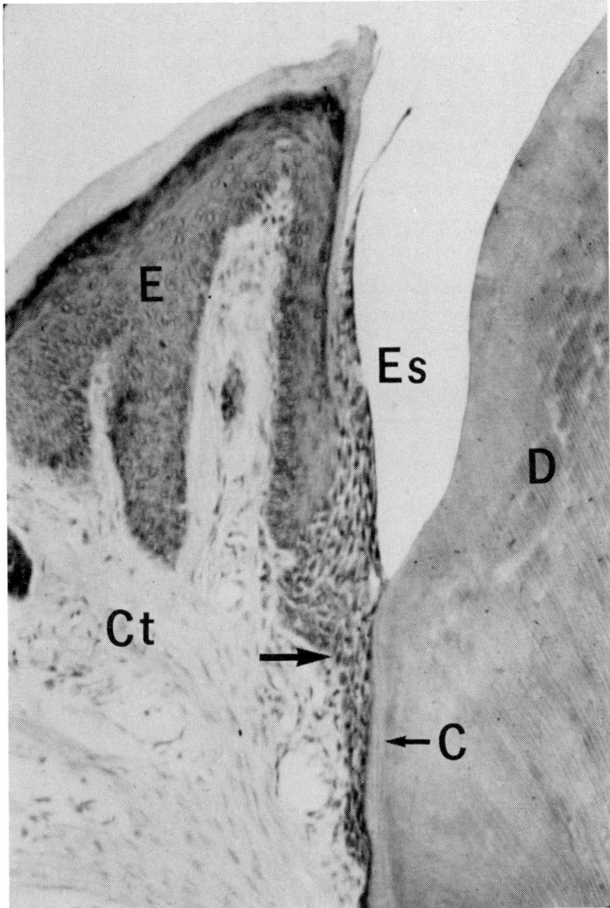

Fig. 11–11. Histologic section of the dentinogingival area. Here, the attachment (junctional) epithelium (arrow) has extended to the cementum (C). (E) Epithelium and (Ct) connective tissue of the gingiva. (Es) Enamel space, where the enamel was before it was demineralized (lost) during tissue preparation. (D) Dentin. Notice the keratin layer at the surface of the gingiva.

Clinical Considerations

The intactness of the epithelium of the gingival sulcus and attachment epithelium is important to good periodontal conditions. Since the gingival sulcus, despite the snug fit of the free gingiva to the tooth surface, is exposed to the saliva and microorganisms of the oral cavity, any damage to the epithelium of the gingival sulcus can result in damage to the underlying connective tissue. Connective tissue is not a covering tissue as is epithelium, and it does not resist injury and microorganism invasion the way epithelial tissue does. Therefore, if damage to the epithelium of the gingival sulcus is accompanied by damage to the underlying connective tissue, the ensuing effect on the tissues in this area may be inflammation, swelling, damage to the periodontal ligament fibers, resorption of the bone of the alveolar process, loosening of the tooth, and perhaps finally the necessity for tooth removal.

The presence of calculus around the cervix of a tooth is often an important factor in periodontal disease (Fig. 7–2). The calculus damages the epithelium of

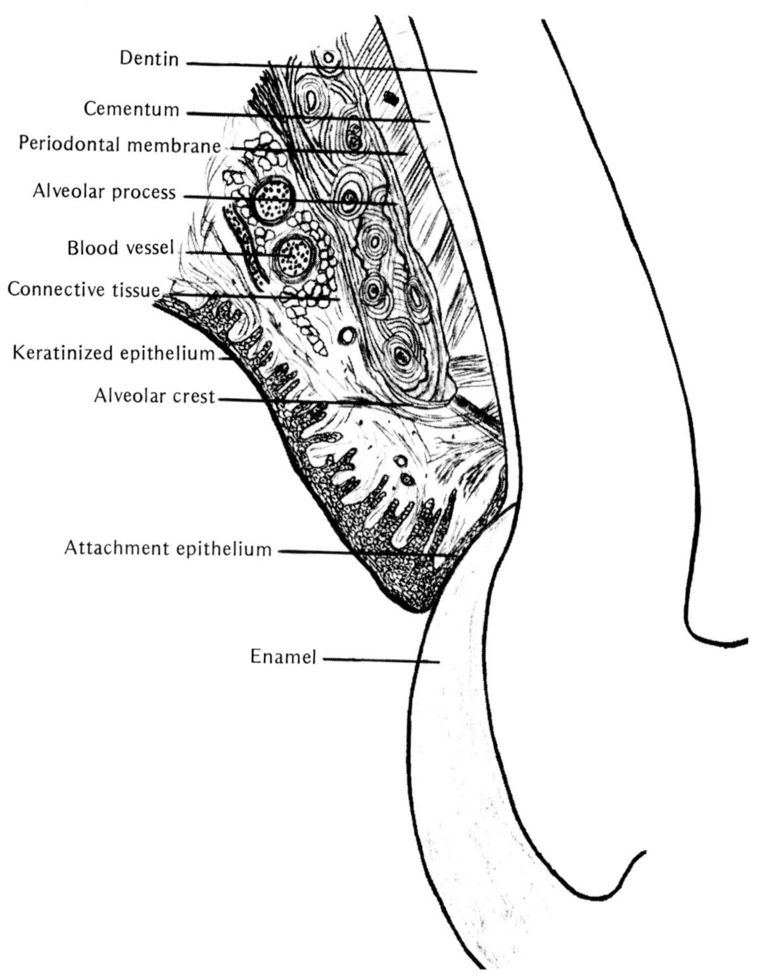

Fig. 11–12. Diagrammatic drawing of a longitudinal section cut faciolingually through a maxillary posterior tooth and the associated periodontal ligament, alveolar process, and gingiva. This is the lingual side of the tooth at the cervix. This area is free of inflammation. There is no bone resorption. The periodontal ligament fibers are well oriented.

the gingival sulcus and of the attachment epithelium. A series of consequential events follows: (1) There is inflammation of the connective tissue of the gingiva. (2) There is swelling. (3) There is damage to the periodontal ligament fibers, particularly the gingival, the transseptal, and the alveolar crest fibers.(4) There is resorption of the bone of the alveolar crest. (5) There is an increasing amount of cementum exposed in the cervical area of the tooth.

Figure 11–12 is a drawing of the cervical area on the lingual side of a maxillary molar tooth. The periodontium is in good condition: there is little or no inflammation in the gingiva; the attachment epithelium fits against the tooth; the periodontal ligament fibers are well oriented; and the alveolar crest shows no signs of resorption.

Figure 11–13 is a drawing of the cervical area on the buccal side of the same tooth. Here the presence of a mass of calculus has resulted in the formation of a gingival pocket. There has followed injury to the epithelium of the gingival

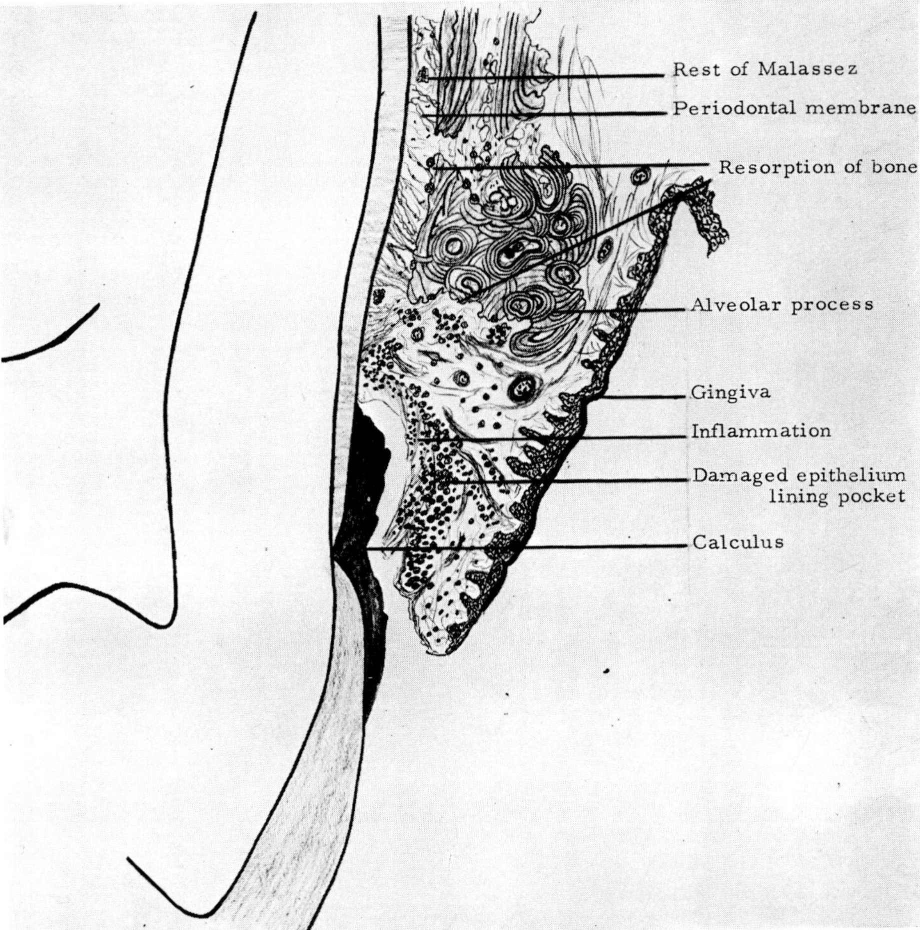

Fig. 11–13. Diagrammatic drawing of the facial side of the tooth illustrated in Figure 11–12. A large mass of calculus at the tooth cervix is responsible for the pathologic condition in this area. Here there is inflammation, destruction of the attachment epithelium, damaged peridontal ligament, and resorption of the alveolar crest and of the lamina dura.

sulcus, inflammation in the connective tissue, damage to the periodontal ligament fibers, and resorption of the alveolar crest and of the lamina dura. Continued irritation by the calculus will be accompanied by continued inflammation of the gingiva and continued bone resorption. Such pathosis sufficiently extended results in the loosening of the tooth.

Figure 11–14 is a photomicrograph of a section of the lingual side of a maxillary molar tooth and the associated periodontium. There is no calculus on the tooth surface and little inflammation in the gingiva. (Compare with Figures 11–12 and 11–13.)

Another important clinical problem is created by the presence in the mouth of exposed cervical cementum. When the extent of exposure of cervical cementum exceeds 1 mm, there frequently is found a condition known as *cervical abrasion*. Cervical abrasion is a wedge-shaped cut in the cervical cementum of a tooth. It is produced when the person uses an abrasive dentifrice and brushes his teeth with a cross-brushing stroke. The tooth enamel, due to its extreme

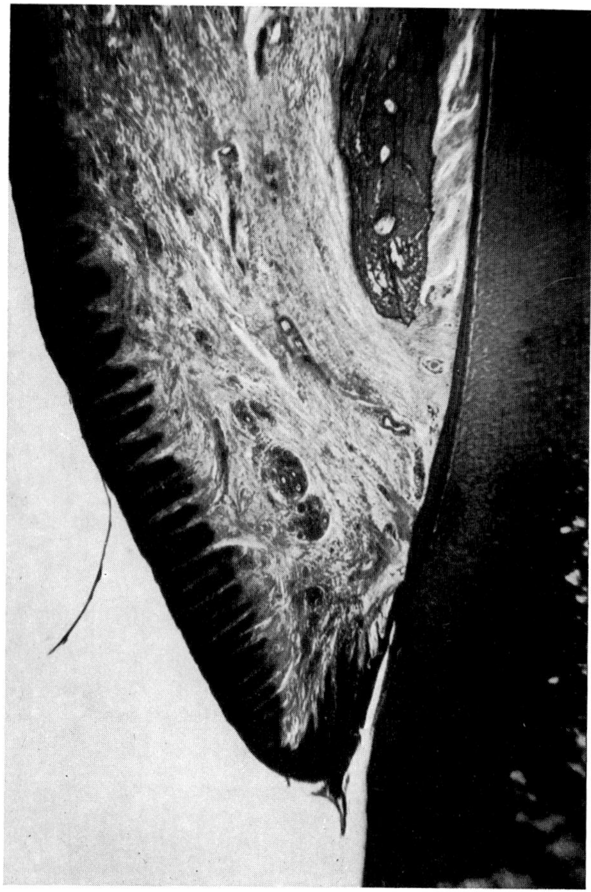

Fig. 11–14. Photomicrograph of a section cut faciolingually through a maxillary molar and the associated periodontal ligament, alveolar process, and palatal gingiva. This is the lingual side of the tooth at the cervix. The gingiva is nearly free of inflammation; there is little evidence of bone resorption; the periodontal ligament fibers are well oriented. The gingival sulcus in this specimen ends a short distance apical to the cervical margin of the cementum. (Compare with Figure 11–12). There is no enamel on this section because the preparation of the specimen for sectioning included demineralization with HNO_3 so that it could be cut with a microtome knife (Chapter 1); and demineralization completely removes the highly mineralized enamel.

hardness, is not affected by this procedure, but the cementum is abraded. Cervical abrasion is seen in its most severe form in mouths that are consistently kept clean, and on the facial sides of the teeth where most vigorous brushing has been done. A study of the process of cervical abrasion has demonstrated that the use of cross-brushing technique with a very abrasive dentifrice can result in such an amount of abrasion that a maxillary canine tooth measuring 7 mm at the cervix may be cut half through in 7.6 years; that is, in that length of time the wedge of cervical abrasion can extend half way through the 7 mm cervix.* Such cervical abrasion is illustrated on the facial side of a mandibular incisor tooth in Figure 11–10I. Figure 11–3 is a clinical photograph showing

*Interesting papers:
Kitchin, P.C., and H.B.G. Robison: How Abrasive Need a Dentifrice Be? J. Dent. Res., *27*:501, 1948.
Harte, D.B., and R.S. Manly: Effects of Toothbrush Variables on Wear of Dentin Produced by Four Abrasives. J. Dent. Res., *54*:993, 1975.

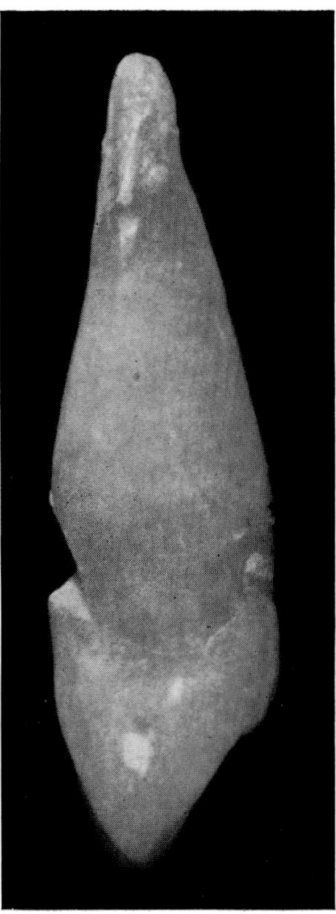

Fig. 11–15. Mesial surface of a maxillary canine tooth. There is deep abrasion of the cervical cementum on the facial surface. The enamel is not affected. Sclerotic dentin and reparative dentin (Figure 5–16) ordinarily form beneath such an area of abrasion.

cervical abrasion. Figure 11–15 is an extracted maxillary canine tooth showing deep cervical abrasion. Figure 5–16 is a picture of a ground section of a mandibular incisor tooth in which there is slight cervical abrasion on the labial side and dead tract and sclerotic dentin beneath.

Such information concerning cervical abrasion makes clear the importance of using proper tooth-brushing techniques and a dentifrice which does not contain an excessive amount of abrasive material. This is particularly important for those individuals in whom there has been considerable gingival recession leaving exposed to the oral cavity a relatively broad area of cementum.

Chapter 12

TOOTH ERUPTION AND THE SHEDDING OF THE PRIMARY TEETH

TOOTH ERUPTION

Tooth eruption is the combination of bodily movements of the tooth, both before and after the emergence of its crown into the oral cavity, which serves to bring it and maintain it in occlusion with the teeth of the opposing arch. Tooth eruption begins at the time the crown is completed and the root starts to form and continues throughout the life of the tooth.

Eruptive Movements

In its simplest form tooth eruption may be pictured as the occlusal movement of the tooth brought about, at least in part, by the lengthening of the root and the development of additional bone beneath the root. Instead of visualizing the process of root formation as one in which the root grows deeper into the jaw, it is necessary to regard the position of the apical end of the developing root as being relatively fixed. As the developing root lengthens, its growing apical end maintains its position and the crown moves occlusally. Undoubtedly this concept gives an oversimplified picture of the process.

In the development of the permanent dentition, the movements of tooth eruption vary from little more than this relatively simple process of occlusal movement in the anterior teeth, through a condition of considerable horizontal movement in the premolars, to a highly complex set of rotating and horizontal movements in the molars.

With the exception of the permanent molar teeth the enamel organ of each permanent tooth develops from the dental lamina lingual to its primary predecessor (Figs. 3–15; 3–17). By the time the primary tooth has emerged into the oral cavity the development of the permanent tooth is well advanced. In the anterior region the permanent teeth continue development lingual to their primary predecessors, but in the region of the premolars a change in relative position occurs. The premolars replace the primary molars. By the time the primary molars have come into occlusion, the crowns of the developing premolars occupy a position not lingual to, but between the roots of, the primary molars (Figs. 12–1; 12–2; 12–3). This change in relative positions occurs as a result of a vertical movement of the primary teeth and a horizontal movement of the developing permanent teeth.

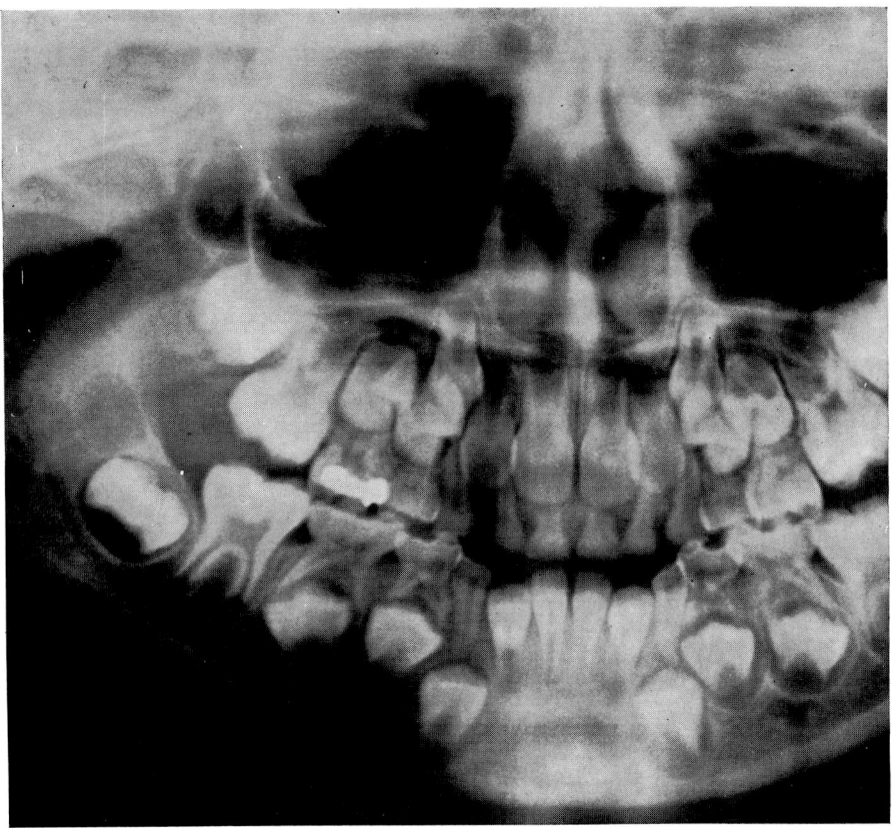

Fig. 12–1. Panoramic radiograph of a child about six years old. The permanent mandibular incisors and the permanent maxillary and mandibular first molars are present in the oral cavity. The permanent maxillary central incisors, roots still short, root canals broad, lie above the partially resorbed roots of the primary incisors. Primary teeth still present in the oral cavity are maxillary incisors, canines, and first and second molars; and in the lower jaw, canines, and first and second molars. Crowns of the permanent canines and first and second molars and their relationship to the primary teeth they will replace are best seen in the lower jaw on the left side of the picture.

Crowns of the developing maxillary and mandibular permanent second molars lie in a bone crypt (space) distal to the erupted first molars; roots have not begun to form. Distal to the crown of the permanent mandibular second molar (left side of picture) is a light circle (bone) enclosing a dark area—the location of the forming third molar.

Above the forming roots of the permanent maxillary incisors is the nasal cavity; and on either side of the nasal cavity are the orbits of the eye (large dark areas). The forming roots of the right and left permanent maxillary canines have an interesting (and important) relationship to the nasal cavity and the eye orbits. (Courtesy Dr. Gus Pappas, College of Dentistry, The Ohio State University.)

The permanent molar teeth do not have predecessors. The enamel organs of the tooth germs of the permanent molars develop from an extension of the dental lamina distal to the position of the primary molars. The first permanent molars develop in approximately the position they will hold upon emergence into the oral cavity. But the crowns of both the second and third molars form in a different position, and must undergo complicated motions of rotation and forward movement in order to emerge into correct relation to other teeth.

At the time the second and third molars begin to develop neither the maxilla nor the mandible is large enough to accommodate them. The mandibular second and third molars develop in the ramus of the mandible with their occlusal

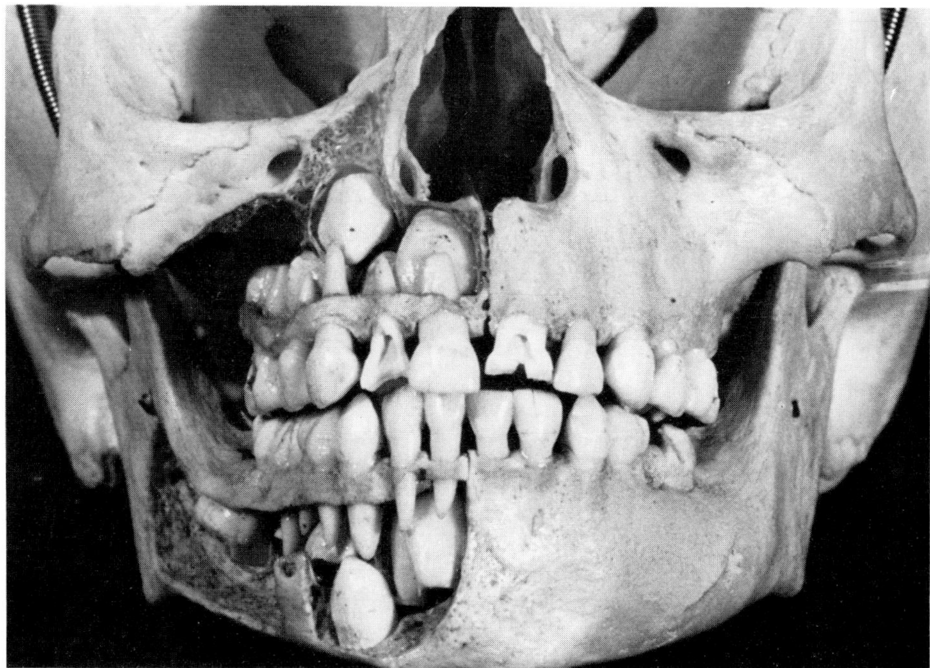

Fig. 12–2. Anterior view of dry skull of a five-year-old child. The right facial cortical plate of the maxillary and mandibular bones has been removed to show the developing permanent teeth and their relationship to the primary teeth. Crowns of the permanent anterior teeth are located lingual to the roots of the primary anterior teeth. Note the relation of the permanent maxillary central incisor to the floor of the nasal cavity; also note the permanent maxillary canine crown and its relation to the orbit of the eye. The permanent mandibular anterior teeth have a close relation to each other. Note the lingual position of the mandibular permanent lateral incisor. Compare to Figure 12–1.

surfaces directed mesially. The second molar usually emerges into the oral cavity in its correct position distal to the first molar. But inadequate jaw development and a failure of sufficient rotating movement in the early stages of eruption sometimes cause the crown of the mandibular third molar to press against the roots of the adjacent second molar. The result of such a positional relationship is an impacted third molar. In Figure 12–4 is seen a mandibular third molar crown forming in the usual position in the ramus of the mandible.

In the maxilla the second and third molars develop in the maxillary tuberosity with their occlusal surfaces directed distally and buccally. Inadequate jaw development and a failure of sufficient rotating movement in the early stages of eruption may result in the emergence of the maxillary third molar with its occlusal surface directed distally and buccally. The change in position of developing teeth in the jaws is a result of the growth of the teeth, the growth of the alveolar process, and the growth of the jaws (Fig. 12–4). Figure 12–5 is a histologic section through the region of a mandibular third molar that is in a position similar to the position of the lower third molar seen in Figure 12–4

Incidentally, in the course of the total process of tooth eruption, the tooth emerges into the oral cavity. Figure 11–10 is a diagram of some events involved in this emergence. In Figure 11–10A the tooth crown is complete, but root formation has not yet begun. The reduced enamel epithelium covering the crown

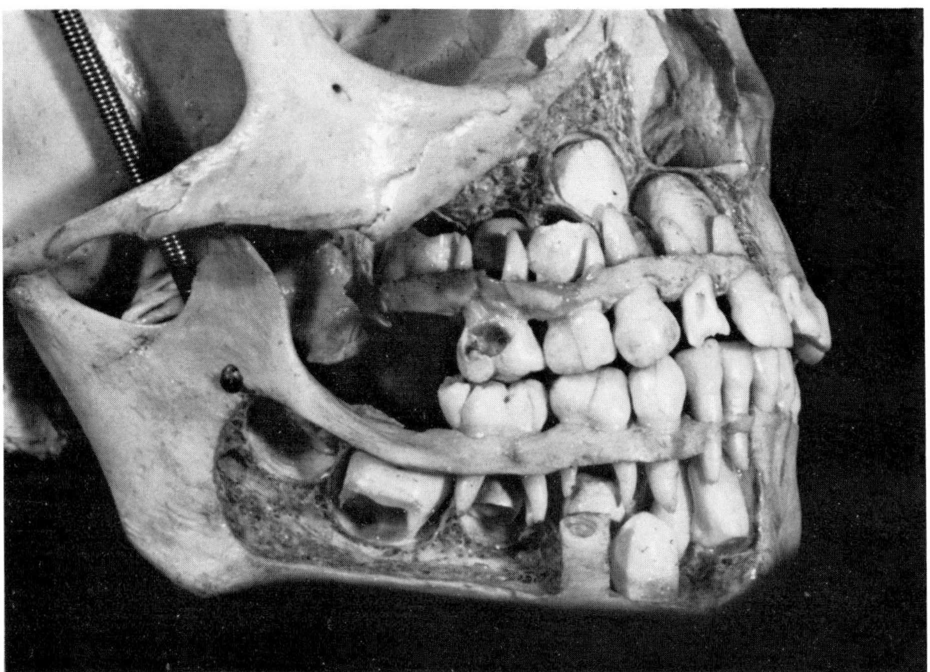

Fig. 12–3. Lateral view of the posterior region of the skull seen in Figure 12–2. Crowns of the premolars are seen between the roots of the primary molars. Note the buccal caries in the primary maxillary second molar. Crowns of the permanent first molars, surrounded by bone, are located just distal to the roots of the primary second molars. The developing crown of the mandibular permanent second molar, in its bone crypt, is seen just distal to the permanent first molar crown. Compare to Figure 12–1.

is separated from the epithelium lining the oral cavity by an area of connective tissue. In Figure 11–10B root formation is in progress and the crown has moved occlusally. With the occlusal movement of the tooth crown the reduced enamel epithelium has come in contact with the oral epithelium. At the cervical border of the reduced enamel epithelium some cells seem to have broken off and remain as an open network of epithelial cells in the periodontal ligament surrounding the tooth root. This network is *Hertwig's epithelial sheath.* In Figure 11–10C the epithelial cells which previously covered the incisal edge of the tooth have been penetrated, and the tip of the tooth has become visible in the mouth. With the emergence of the tooth into the mouth the reduced enamel epithelium becomes known as the *attachment epithelium* (Fig. 11–10D). This change is merely one of terminology. With age the cells at the apical end of the attachment epithelium proliferate onto the cementum of the root (Figs. 11–10E; 11–11).

Although the tooth comes into occlusion during the formation of the root, occlusal movement does not cease when the root is completed. Due to changes in the surrounding bone and probably also to continued cementum formation at the root end, occlusal movement may continue, at least intermittently, throughout the life of the tooth. An important need is served by this continued slow eruption. With years of use the occlusal and incisal areas of the teeth are often considerably worn off. The continued occlusal movement of the teeth with advancing years helps to compensate for loss of crown length.

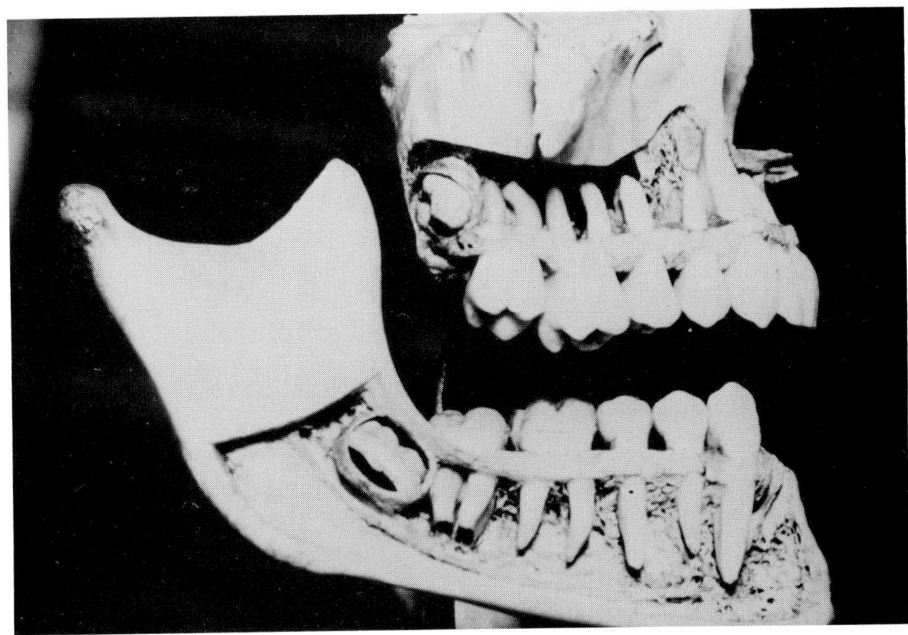

Fig. 12–4. A human maxilla and mandible with the facial parts of the alveolar process removed excepting near the cervical border. Notice the location and position of the developing mandibular and maxillary third molars. The crown of the mandibular third molar is nearly completed in the ramus of the mandible. Its occlusal surface is directed mesially and occlusally. It is surrounded by a bone crypt. The maxillary third molar is directed buccally and distally.

The Mechanism of Tooth Eruption

The mechanism of tooth eruption is difficult to explain. Early occlusal movement seems to be a result of a combination of factors: First, the tissue beneath the growing root resists apical movement of the developing root. This results in the occlusal movement of the tooth crown as the root lengthens. Second, bone formation occurs apical to the developing tooth. Other factors involved are: vascular pressures within the periodontal ligament; and traction by the cells and the fibers of the periodontal ligament.*

Cervical Exposure Without Occlusal Movement

In young individuals crowns of the teeth are smaller than the anatomic crowns (Figs. 11–10C, D). As a person ages usually there is an increase in the length of the clinical crown because some cervical cementum is exposed to the oral cavity (Fig. 11–3). More cementum exposure occurs through the years than can be accounted for by actual occlusal tooth movement. While the teeth undoubtedly do undergo occlusal movement, part of their increased exposure throughout life is a result of a progressive loss of soft tissue attachment. This occurs when the apical end of the attachment epithelium, which originally was located at the cementoenamel junction, proliferates (grows) onto the cementum (Figs. 11–10E;

---

*Interesting papers:
Marks, S.C., Jr. and Cahill, D.R.: Experimental Study in the Dog of the Non-Active Role of the Tooth in the Eruptive Process. Arch. Oral Biol., *29*:311–322, 1984.
Steedle, J.R. and Proffit, W.R.: The Pattern and Control of Eruptive Tooth Movements. Am. J. Orthod., *87*:56–66, 1985.

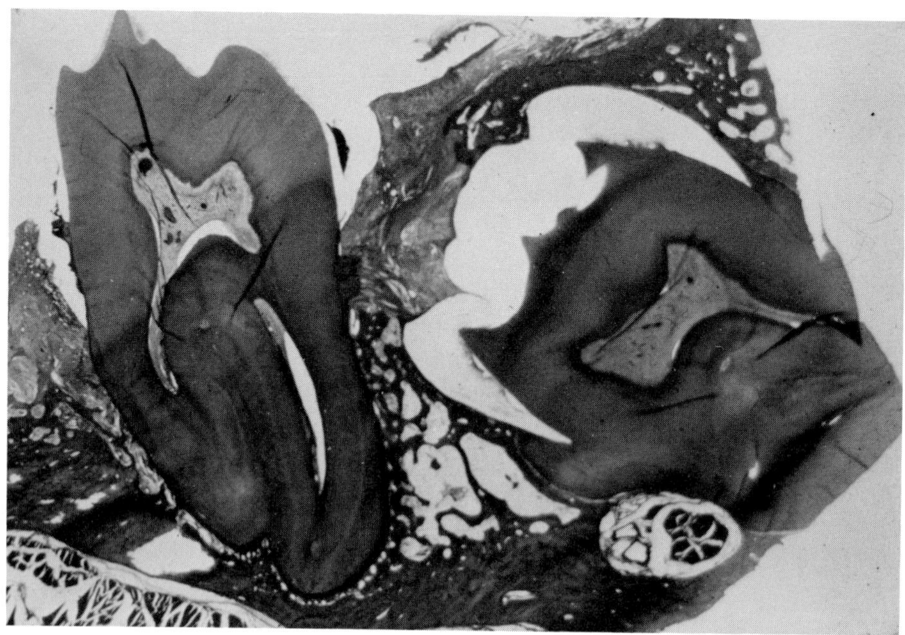

Fig. 12–5. A histologic section of a lower third molar region. The third molar, whose occlusal surface is directed mesially, is surrounded by bone of the mandible. Note the third molar's relation to the erupted second molar. The enamel of the two teeth was completely demineralized during processing. Interestingly, the enamel "space" (white area) of the third molar retains the original enamel outline because of the surrounding bone. Compare to Figure 12–14.

11–11) and the coronal end of the attachment, which is the bottom of the gingival sulcus, likewise moves apically. Eventually cementum is exposed at the cervix of the tooth (Fig. 11–10G). The apical migration of the attachment epithelium to a limited degree is a normal condition. Exposed cementum is found in the mouths of nearly all individuals who are over forty years old, and in many individuals who are younger.

This apical movement of the gingiva is called *gingival recession.*

Mesial Drift

A number of tooth movements have already been mentioned: (1) the easily recognized occlusal movement of the erupting tooth; (2) the horizontal movements which puts the developing crowns of the permanent premolars between the roots of the primary molars; and (3) the complicated combination of rotating and lateral movements which brings second and third molars into their functional position.

In addition to these tooth movements there is a type of tooth movement known as mesial drift. *Mesial drift* is the lateral bodily movement of the teeth on both sides of the mouth toward the midline of the arch. One condition leading to mesial drift may be understood if we picture the teeth in function. Since teeth are suspended in their sockets by the fibers of the periodontal ligament, they are not rigid in the jaws but undergo considerable movement during the process of mastication. This functional movement produces a rubbing of the contact areas. There is some evidence that as the proximal surfaces of adjacent teeth

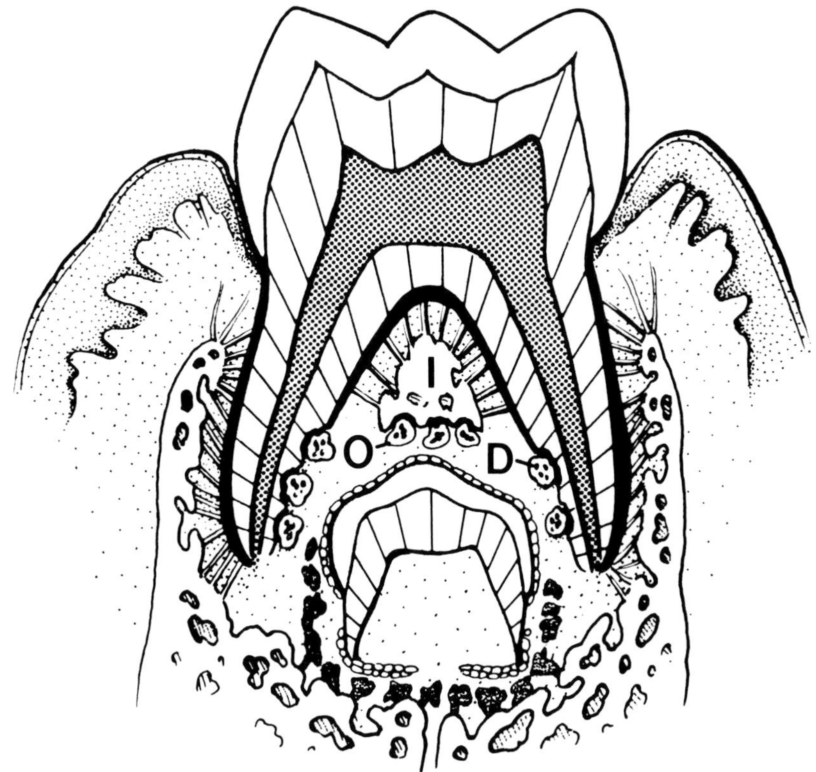

Fig. 12–6. Open diagram showing the early shedding stage of a primary tooth and the position of the precursor permanent tooth. *Dentinoclasts* (D) have resorbed through the apical interradicular cementum and have reached the dentin; also osteoclasts (O) are seen along the interradicular bone (I) of the primary tooth. Compare to Figure 12–8.

become worn as a result of functional tooth movement, the transseptal fibers of the periodontal ligament become shorter and thereby maintain tooth contact; i.e., mesial drift occurs.*

Mesial drift is possible because of the adaptability of bone tissue. Pressure on the periodontal ligament fibers results in resorption of bone, whereas pull on fibers results in bone apposition (formation). As the contact areas of the crowns wear, the teeth tend to move mesially, maintaining contact. The slight pressure thus produced on the mesial side of the socket results in slow resorption of the lamina dura. The accompanying tension of the periodontal ligament fibers on the distal side of the root induces apposition lamina dura bone in this area. As a consequence of these bone changes there is an actual shift in the position of the tooth socket.

SHEDDING OF THE PRIMARY TEETH

Primary and Permanent Dentitions

The human *primary dentition* is made up of 1 central incisor, 1 lateral incisor, 1 canine, and 2 molar teeth in each quadrant of the mouth. The first teeth to

*Interesting paper:
Picton, D.C.A., and J.P. Moss: The Part Played by the Trans-septal Fibre System in Experimental Approximal Drift of the Cheek Teeth of Monkeys (Macaca irus). Arch. Oral Biol., *18*:669, 1973.

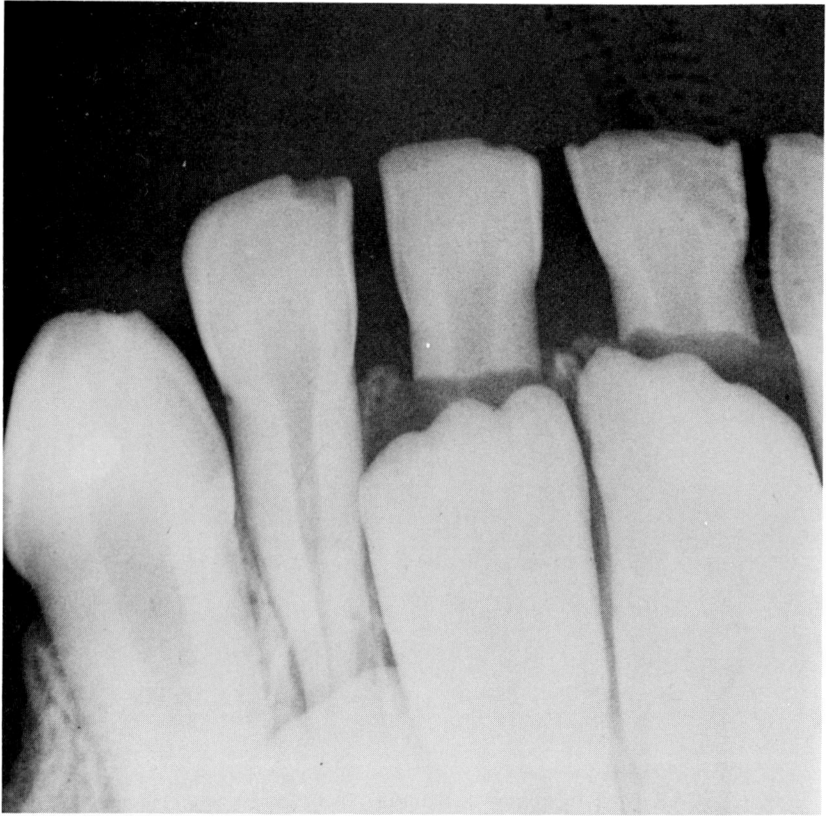

Fig. 12–7. Radiograph of the lower anterior region showing the positions of the permanent incisors apical to the resorbed roots of the shedding primary incisors.

become visible in the oral cavity are usually the primary mandibular central incisors, which emerge when the child is about six months old. The last primary teeth to appear are the maxillary second molars, which appear about the end of the second year. Each tooth of the primary dentition is eventually lost and is replaced by a tooth of the permanent dentition.

The *permanent dentition* consists of 1 central incisor, 1 lateral incisor, 1 canine, 2 premolars, and 3 molars in each quadrant of the mouth. The first permanent tooth to appear is usually a first molar, which emerges just behind the second primary molar when the child is about six years old. The last primary tooth to remain in the mouth is usually the second primary molar. This is replaced by the permanent second premolar in about the twelfth year. The permanent molars have no predecessors. Since the first permanent molars appear in the mouth during the sixth year, when the primary dentition is sometimes still intact, it is important that these teeth be recognized as teeth of the permanent dentition and not be regarded as primary teeth soon to be lost.

In Table 12–1 will be found the time of emergence into the oral cavity of the teeth of the primary and permanent dentitions, as well as the time of the beginning of hard tissue formation in each of the teeth.

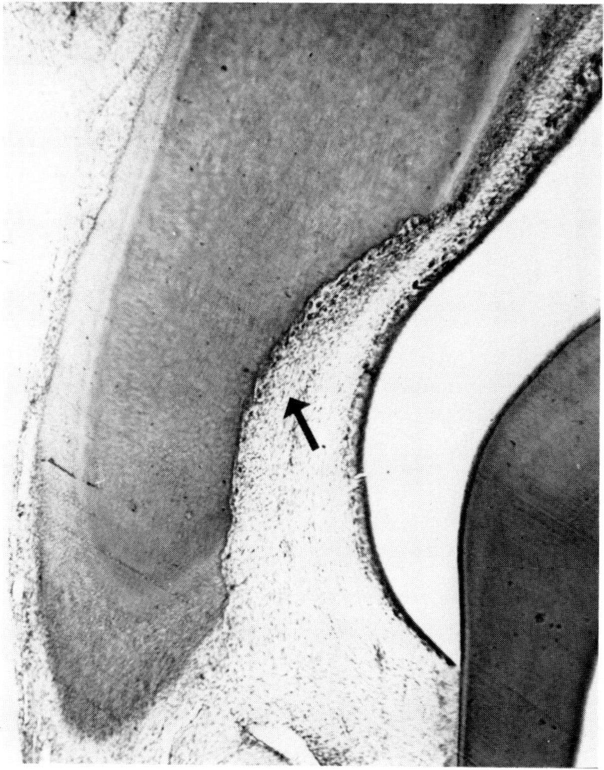

Fig. 12–8. Section of the apical end of a kitten primary tooth and its succedaneous (permanent) tooth, located between the primary tooth roots. (See Figure 12–6). A concave resorption area is clearly seen on the primary root (arrow), just adjacent to the permanent tooth crown (at right). Resorption has advanced to the root dentin; cementum of the area has been resorbed.

The Process of Shedding

The shedding of primary teeth is the result of the gradual resorption of their roots with the consequent loss of periodontal ligament attachment. The developing permanent successor, located lingual to, or beneath the root of the functioning primary tooth, probably creates sufficient pressure by its increase in size to produce resorption of the primary tooth root and of the bone surrounding the root (Figs. 12–6; 12–7; 12–8). As the root resorbs the tooth loosens. Eventually all periodontal ligament attachment is lost and the rootless crown of the primary tooth literally falls off of the jaw.

The mineralized tissues of primary tooth roots, cementum and dentin, are physiologically resorbed by large, multinucleated cells (Figs. 12–9, 12–10). These cells resemble an osteoclast (Fig. 9–13), the cell responsible for bone resorption. The cell that resorbs the mineralized tissues of a tooth is called an *odontoclast.* When the odontoclast resorbs cementum it may be called a *cementoclast,* and when it resorbs dentin it may be called a *dentinoclast.* In Figure 12–11 cementoclasts and dentinoclasts are found along the root of a primary tooth undergoing shedding.

An interesting phenomenon frequently observed in children is the alternate loosening and tightening of a primary tooth before it is finally shed. One day

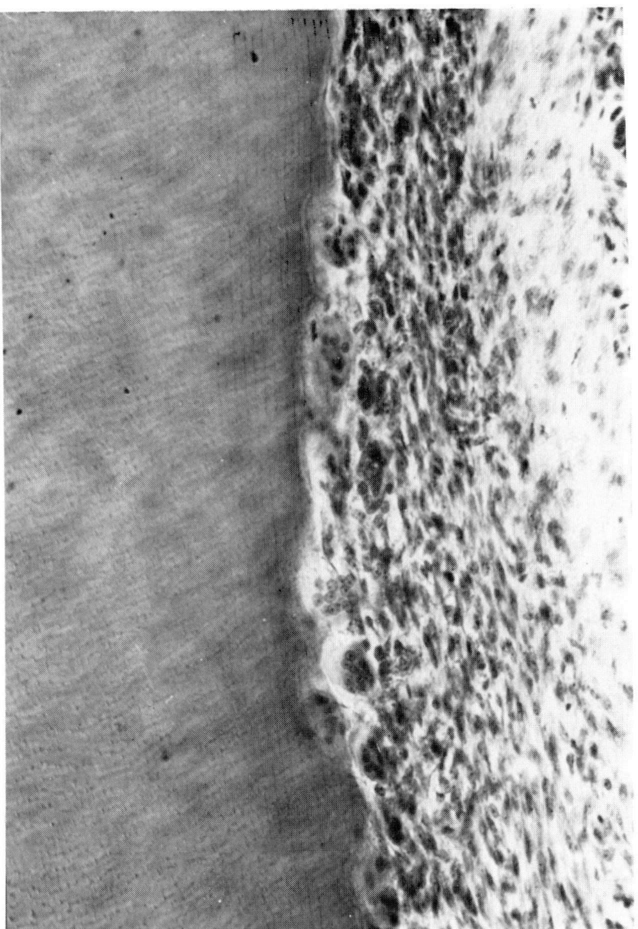

Fig. 12–9. Higher magnification of the concave resorption area of the primary tooth root seen in Figure 12–8. Dentinoclasts lie along the surface of the root dentin.

the child reports a loose tooth, and several days later the tooth seems to be firmly attached. This reattachment is due to the fact that when resorption of the primary tooth root causes the tooth to become loose, not only is pressure relieved but slight tension seems to be induced on the adjacent connective tissue. This tension stimulates the connective tissue around the resorbed root end to form new cementum on the remaining root end and new bone around the root. This results in the attachment of new periodontal ligament fibers, and the tooth tightens in the jaw. But further development of the permanent tooth soon causes more resorption of both bone and root. Loosening and reattachment may alternate several times, but as the permanent tooth continues to develop the accompanying resorption of the primary tooth root will be sufficient to bring about the shedding of the tooth.

Occasionally the relative positions of the primary tooth and its permanent successor are such that the primary tooth root is not subjected to conditions that would cause its resorption. In this case the permanent tooth may emerge into

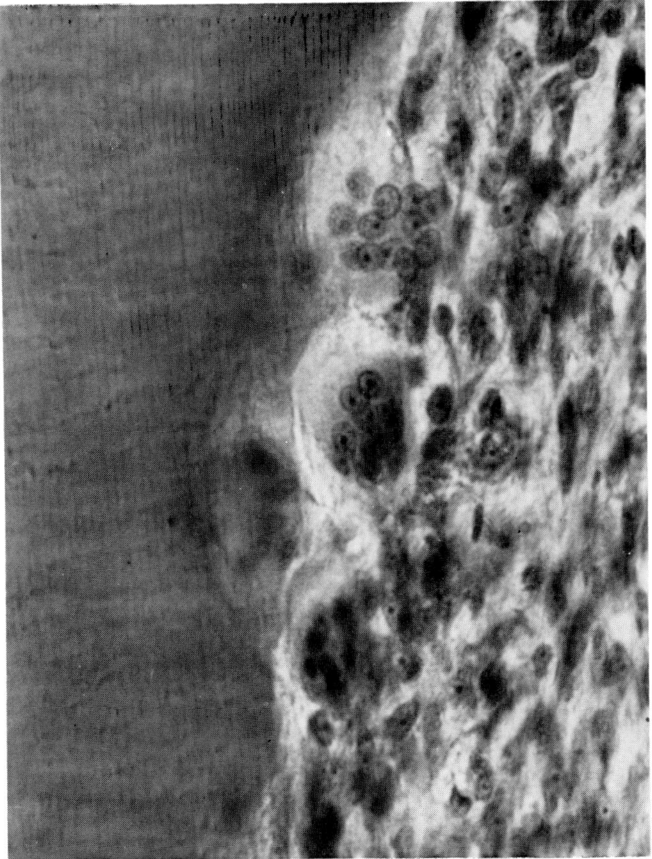

Fig. 12–10. Higher magnification of the resorption area seen in Figure 12–9. Three multinucleated *dentinoclasts* are clearly visible. Note how these cells fit into *cupped-out* sites of the dentin where resorption is actually occurring.

the oral cavity lingual to the primary tooth which it is supposed to replace. This condition is seen most often in the region of the mandibular incisors.

In cases where the permanent tooth bud has failed to develop, the roots of the primary tooth may resorb even though there is no developing permanent successor; or the primary tooth may retain its roots and continue to function in the mouth for many years.

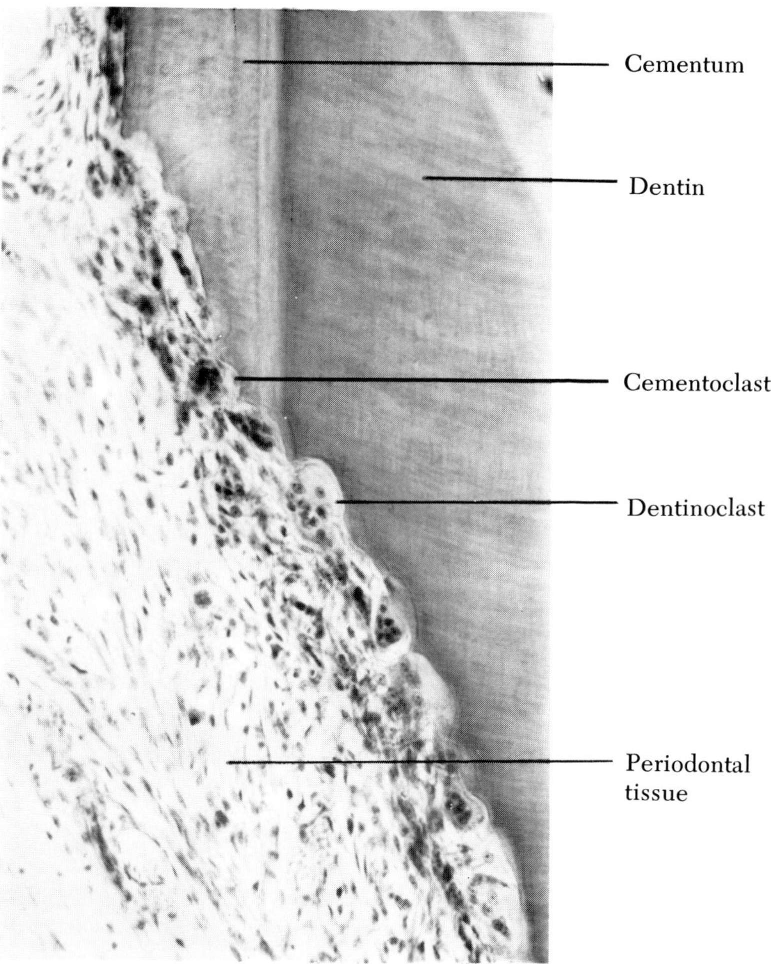

Fig. 12–11. Section through the root of a shedding primary tooth. Resorption of cementum and dentin is well advanced. *Cementoclasts* and *dentinoclasts* are found within resorption sites along the root. Where would the permanent tooth be located?

Table 12–1. The Chronology of the Human Dentition

Tooth			Formation of Enamel Matrix and of Dentin Begins	Time of Emergence Into Oral Cavity
Primary dentition	Maxillary	Central incisor	4 mos. in utero	7½ mos.
		Lateral incisor	4½ mos. in utero	9 mos.
		Canine	5 mos. in utero	18 mos.
		First molar	5 mos. in utero	14 mos.
		Second molar	6 mos. in utero	24 mos.
	Mandibular	Central incisor	4½ mos. in utero	6 mos.
		Lateral incisor	4½ mos. in utero	7 mos.
		Canine	5 mos. in utero	16 mos.
		First molar	5 mos. in utero	12 mos.
		Second molar	6 mos. in utero	20 mos.
Permanent dentition	Maxillary	Central incisor	3–4 mos.	7–8 yrs.
		Lateral incisor	10–12 mos.	8–9 yrs.
		Canine	4–5 mos.	11–12 yrs.
		First premolar	1½–1¾ yrs.	10–11 yrs.
		Second premolar	2–2¼ yrs.	10–12 yrs.
		First molar	At birth	6–7 yrs.
		Second molar	2½–3 yrs.	12–13 yrs.
		Third molar	7–9 yrs.	17–21 yrs.
	Mandibular	Central incisor	3–4 mos.	6–7 yrs.
		Lateral incisor	3–4 mos.	7–8 yrs.
		Canine	4–5 mos.	9–10 yrs.
		First premolar	1¾–2 yrs.	10–12 yrs.
		Second premolar	2¼–2½ yrs.	11–12 yrs.
		First molar	At birth	6–7 yrs.
		Second molar	2½–3 yrs.	11–13 yrs.
		Third molar	8–10 yrs.	17–21 yrs.

Adapted from Orban after Logan and Kronfeld (slightly modified by McCall and Schour)

Chapter 13

TEMPOROMANDIBULAR JOINT

Only with a thorough background of anatomy and a knowledge of occlusion can one begin to understand the functional movements of the mandible. It is not the purpose here to study the complex physiology and anatomy of the mandibular articulation and its associated muscles and ligaments. However, some concept of its design is necessary to appreciate the unique histologic composition of its parts.

ANATOMY

The temporomandibular joint is the articulation between the cranium and the mandible (Figs. 13–1; 13–2). It is a bilateral articulation, the right and left joint working as a unit, and within some limit of range its great adaptability permits virtually unrestricted movement of the mandible in speech and in the mastication of food. Proper functioning of the temporomandibular joint, with its effect on the occlusal contacts of the teeth, concerns nearly all phases of dentistry.

On either side of the head the temporomandibular joint is made up of two articulating bones, the *temporal bone* and the *mandible,* with an intervening *fibrous disc* and an enveloping *fibrous capsule.*

On the mandible the articulating area is the upper anterior slope of the *mandibular condyle;* and on the temporal bone of the cranium the articulating area is the *articular eminence* and the *anterior part of the mandibular fossa* (the *articular fossa*) (Figs. 13–2; 13–3).

The mandibular fossa is a depression on the inferior aspect of the temporal bone just posterior and medial to the posterior end of the zygomatic arch. The tip of your thumb will fit into it (Fig. 13–3). It is slightly broader mediolaterally than anteroposteriorly, and it is divided into anterior and posterior portions by the *petrotympanic fissure.* This fissure extends approximately from right to left near the posterior part of the fossa. The posterior part of the fossa (behind the fissure) is not involved in this joint. The anterior part of the mandibular fossa, the part anterior to the fissure, has an additional name, the *articular fossa.* The anterior border of the articular fossa is a smooth, round ridge, the *articular eminence,* which is oriented mediolaterally and which flattens out anteriorly. The *articular fossa* and the *articular eminence* are the parts of the temporal bone that make up the cranial articulation of the temporomandibular joint. (Locate these areas on Figure 13–3.)

The condyle of the mandible (Fig. 13–4) fits into the articular fossa of the temporal bone when the jaws are closed (Figs. 13–2; 13–3), and during certain kinds of mandibular movements it slides forward on the articular eminence; but

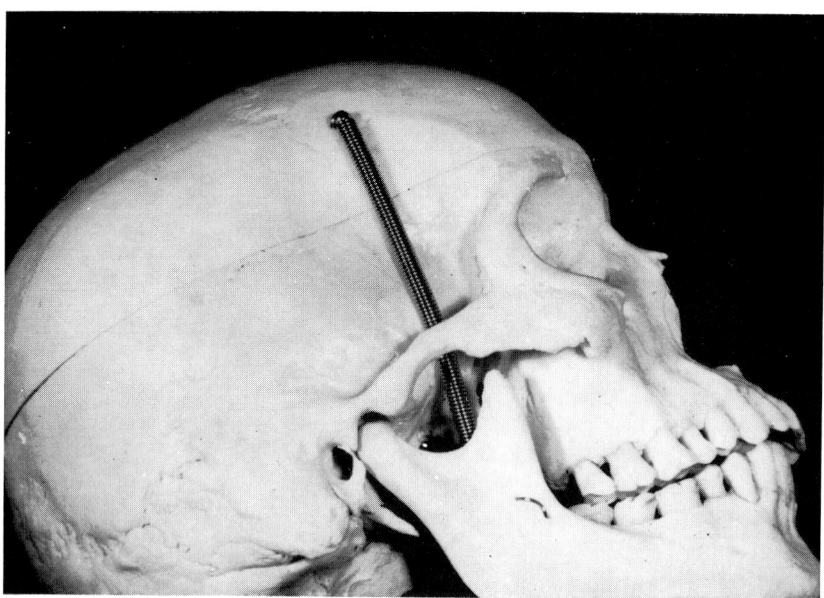

Fig. 13–1. The right side of a human skull. Recall your study of anatomy and locate the mandible, the condyloid process, the zygomatic arch, the external auditory meatus, and notice the relation of these parts to the rest of the skull.

the two bone surfaces, the condyle and the eminence, are not actually in contact: intervening is the *articular disc,* which completely divides the temporomandibular joint cavity into an upper and lower compartment (Fig. 13–5).

Figure 13–5 is a much simplified diagram of the inside of this joint from the lateral aspect. It represents the position of the joint components when the jaws are closed. Compare the diagram (Fig. 13–5) with the picture of the skull (Fig. 13–2); the styloid process is a good reference point for orientation. In the dry skull there is no disc and the condyle is in contact with the temporal bone. In life, as indicated by the diagram, there is a disc, and its interposition forms an upper space (between disc and temporal bone), and a lower space (between disc and condyle). Notice that the mandibular condyle does not fit into the deepest part of the fossa, but is somewhat forward, close to the eminence (Fig. 13–5). The disc is thin at its center, near the superior anterior surface of the condyle, and thicker at its edges. The capsule is seen here to enclose the joint anteriorly and posteriorly. Anteriorly the disc and capsule are fused. Posteriorly the disc and capsule are connected by a pad of loose connective tissue, which permits freedom of anterior movement. The capsule covers the joint in this picture. The capsule encloses the joint somewhat like a stocking attached above around the margin of the articular fossa and eminence, and below around the circumference of the mandibular condyle.

The disc is attached to the lateral and medial sides of the mandibular condyle (Fig. 13–8); it is not attached to the temporal bone. When, in functional movement, the mandible moves forward and back, the disc, attached to the condyle, moves forward and back over the anterior surface of the articular fossa and eminence (Fig. 13–5). *This gliding motion is in the upper compartment of the joint between the disc and the temporal bone.* In the lower compartment of the joint a

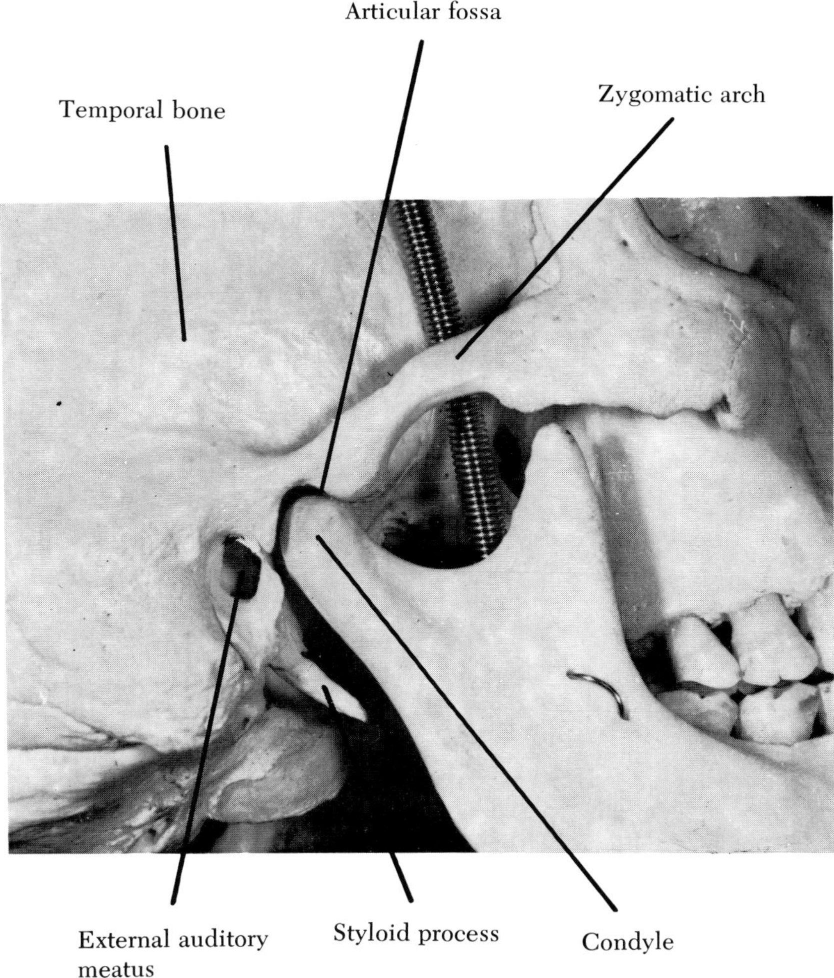

Fig. 13–2. A closer view of the temporomandibular joint of the skull pictured in Figure 13–1. If you have a human skull available for study, compare it with these illustrations.

different motion occurs: there is a backward and forward swinging motion of the mandibular condyle against the under side of the disc. The attachment of the disc to the lateral and medial sides of the condyle is loose enough to permit this swinging or hinge movement of the mandible in relation to the disc. *This hinge movement is in the lower compartment of the joint between the disc and the condyle.*

You can feel some of the movements in this joint if you place your finger tips on either side of your face just in front of the tragus of the ear. First, open and close your mouth several times just a small distance and notice the slight hinge movement in the joint. Then open your mouth wide, and close, and notice the forward movement of the condyle (with the disc attached, or course). Then place the tips of your little fingers in your ears and move the mandible from side to side.

The coordinated movements of the right and left joints are complex and will

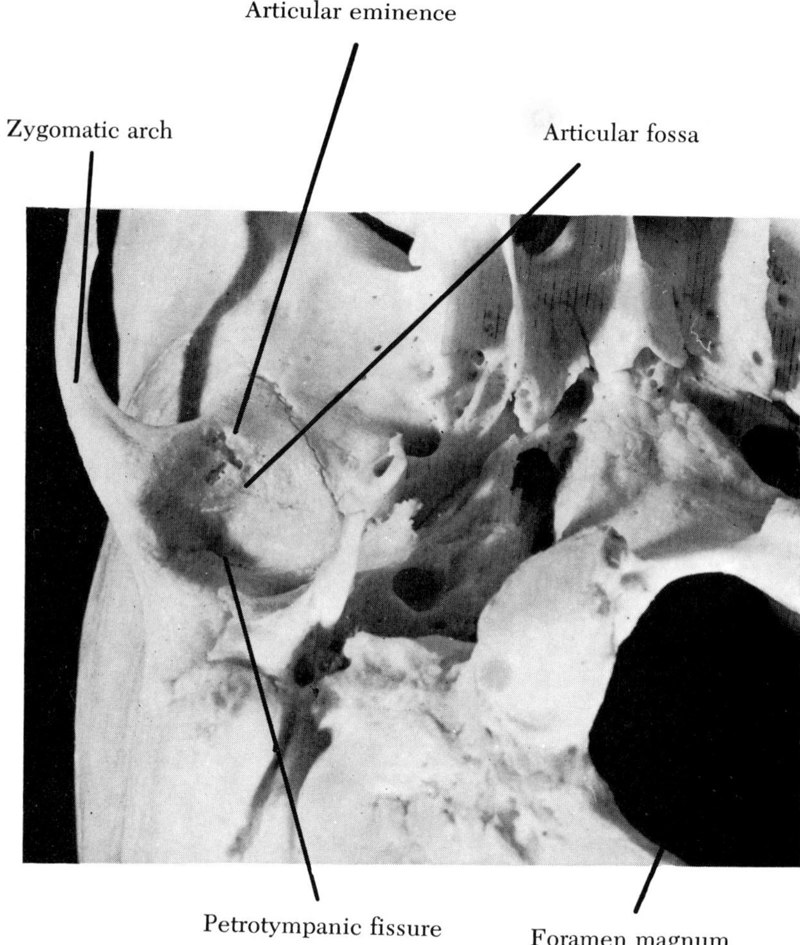

Fig. 13–3. This is a portion of the right side of the inferior surface of the skull pictured in Figures 13–1 and 13–2. Anterior is at the top. In the upper left corner of the picture is the right zygomatic arch, extending anteriorly. Medial to its posterior end is a thumb-sized depression, the *mandibular fossa.* The anterior part of this fossa is called the *articular fossa* and is the area involved in the temporomandibular articulation.

not be described here. The interested student is referred to the extensive literature on this subject.*

Histology

The *capsule* of the temporomandibular joint is composed of two layers. The outer layer is relatively firm fibrous tissue reinforced by the ligaments associated with the joint. The temporomandibular ligament on the lateral wall is particularly effective in controlling the extent of movement of the condyle.

The inner layer of the capsule, the *synovial membrane,* is thin connective tissue and contains blood vessels and nerves. *Synovial fluid* produced by this layer both lubricates the joint and furnishes nourishment to joint parts that are without a

*DuBrul, E.L.: *Sicher's Oral Anatomy,* 7th ed. St. Louis, C.V. Mosby Co., 1980.

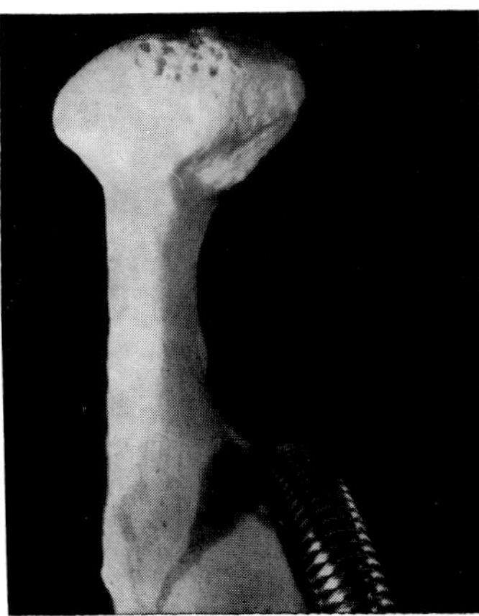

Fig. 13–4. The superior anterior surface of the mandibular condyle. Notice how this condylar head will fit into the anterior part of the mandibular fossa (the articular fossa).

blood supply: the fibrous covering of the articulating surfaces of the bones and the center of the disc.

The *disc* is composed of fibrous connective tissue (Fig. 13–6), which in older persons may have a few chondrocytes (cartilage cells). Its shape is thin in the center and thick at the anterior and posterior borders. The center has no blood supply.

On the temporal bone, the part enclosed by the capsule of the temporomandibular joint—that is, the area of the articular fossa and eminence—is covered with fibrous connective tissue (Fig. 13–6). Notice that this fibrous layer is thicker at the posterior border of the eminence than in the articular fossa. There are no blood vessels or nerves in this covering.

On the mandibular condyle the articulating surface is covered with fibrous connective tissue similar to that covering the temporal bone area (Fig. 13–6). A few chondrocytes may be found in this layer, but there are no blood vessels or nerves. Notice that the fibrous layer is very thick on the uppermost part of the curvature of the condyle.

It is the fibrous connective tissue covering of the bone surfaces of the temporomandibular joint that makes this joint different from most other such articulations. Most such movable joints have a surface of hyaline cartilage rather than of fibrous connective tissue.

In the mandibular condyle of adults compact bone is beneath the fibrous covering layer, and then, beneath this, the usual bone marrow and bone trabeculae (Fig. 13–6).

Figures 13–7 and 13–8 are photomicrographs of human fetuses about four months in utero. Figure 13–7 was cut sagittally to show the lateral aspect of the joint. Figure 13–8 was cut in a direction at right angles to the joint pictured in Figure 13–7; in this section you are seeing the joint from the front rather than from the side.

When compared to the adult temporomandibular joint, the fetal joint is found to have some different histologic features. The fetal joint has articulating surfaces that are composed of dense cellular connective tissue; the articular disc is also highly cellular (Fig. 13–9).

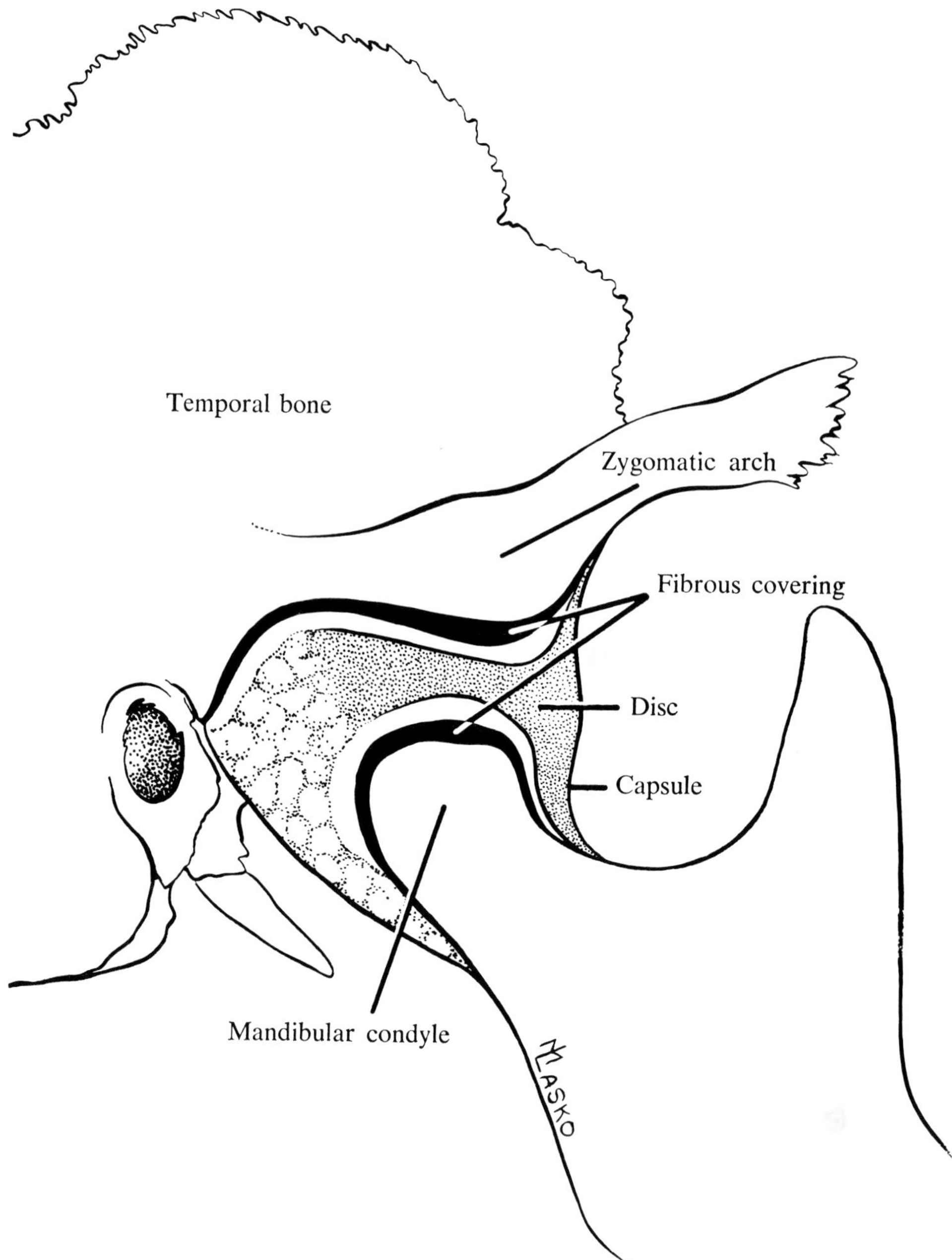

Fig. 13–5. A diagram of the temporomandibular joint. Anterior is to the right of the picture. Compare this diagram with the photograph of the section of this joint (Fig. 13–6).

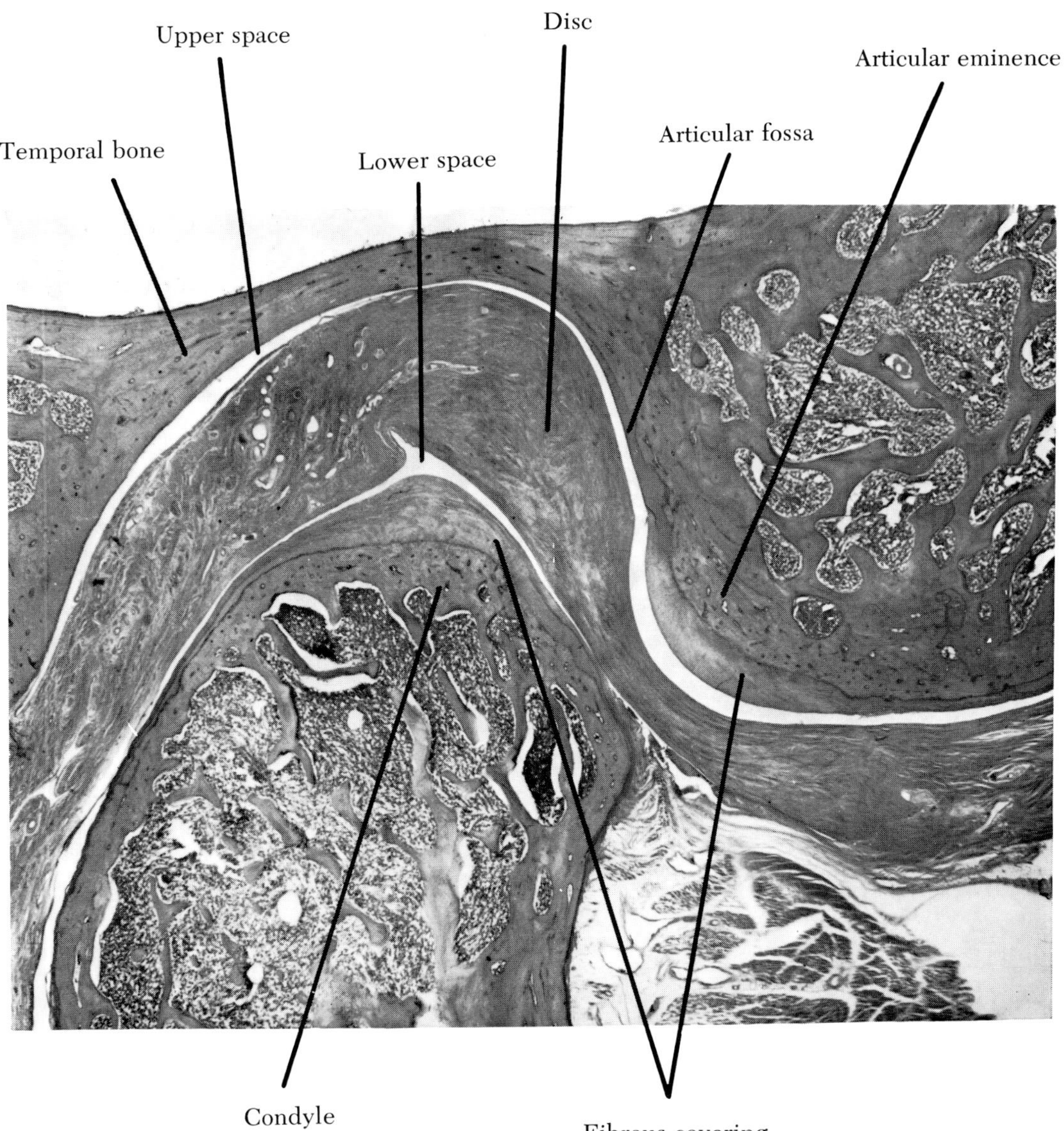

Fig. 13–6. Photomicrograph of a human temporomandibular joint. The specimen was removed in a block of tissue, fixed in formalin, demineralized, embedded in celloidin, sectioned at a thickness of about 25 microns, and stained with hematoxylin and eosin. This is the joint seen from the lateral aspect. Anterior is toward the right of the picture; the white area across the top is the space of the brain case above the articular fossa. The condyle has a surface of compact bone, inside of which is the marrow cavity with bone trabeculae and bone marrow. The same kind of bone structure is seen in the articular eminence (upper right). Notice the difference in thickness of the fibrous covering on different parts of the articular fossa and mandibular condyle.

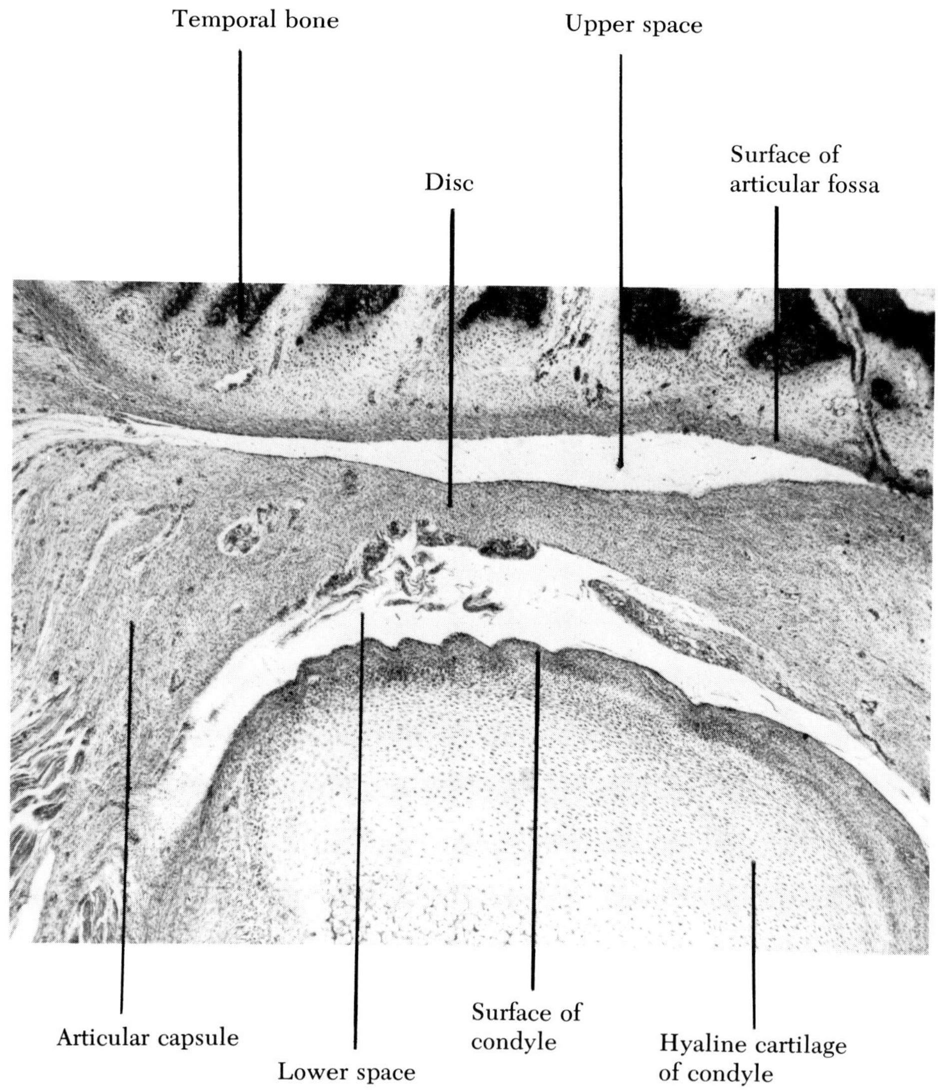

Fig. 13–7. A lateral section of the temporomandibular joint of a human fetus about four months in utero. Of interest is the soft cellular connective tissue of the articular disc. Compare this section with that of the adult temporomandibular joint seen in Figure 13–6.

Beneath the cellular covering of the fetal condyle is hyaline cartilage (Figs. 13–7; 13–8; and 13–10). This is a growth center, and in this location the cartilage increases almost entirely by appositional growth (new cartilage added to existing cartilage edges) rather than interstitial growth (cells within cartilage dividing) as in the ends of other bones (Fig. 13–10).

As development continues, the cartilage is gradually replaced by bone: compact bone forms under the fibrous connective tissue covering, and trabecular bone replaces the cartilage within the mandibular head. The condyle takes on

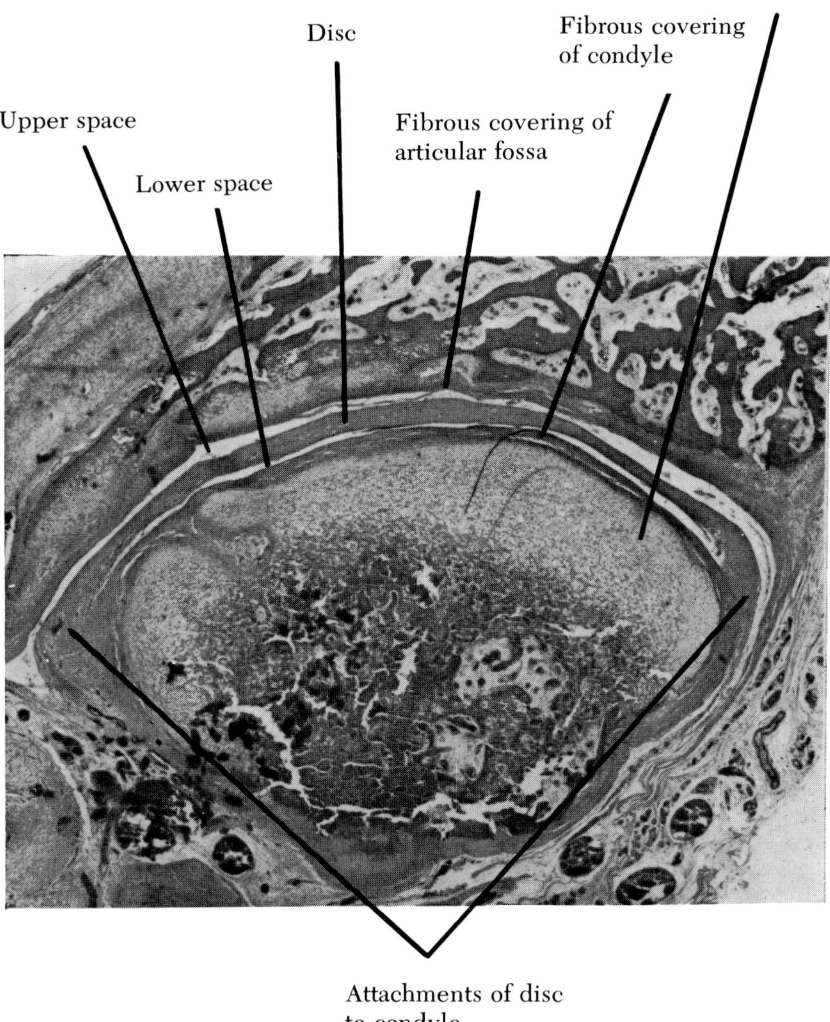

Fig. 13–8. Photomicrograph of a frontal section of the temporomandibular joint of a human fetus about four months in utero. The disc is attached to the lateral medial sides of the condyle. Due to the curvature of the bone, only the head of the condyle appears in this section. Notice the space above and below the disc, and the fibrous covering of the surfaces of both the articular fossa and the condyle. Beneath the fibrous covering of the condyle of this fetus is cartilage. This area is one of the most long-lasting growth centers of the human body.

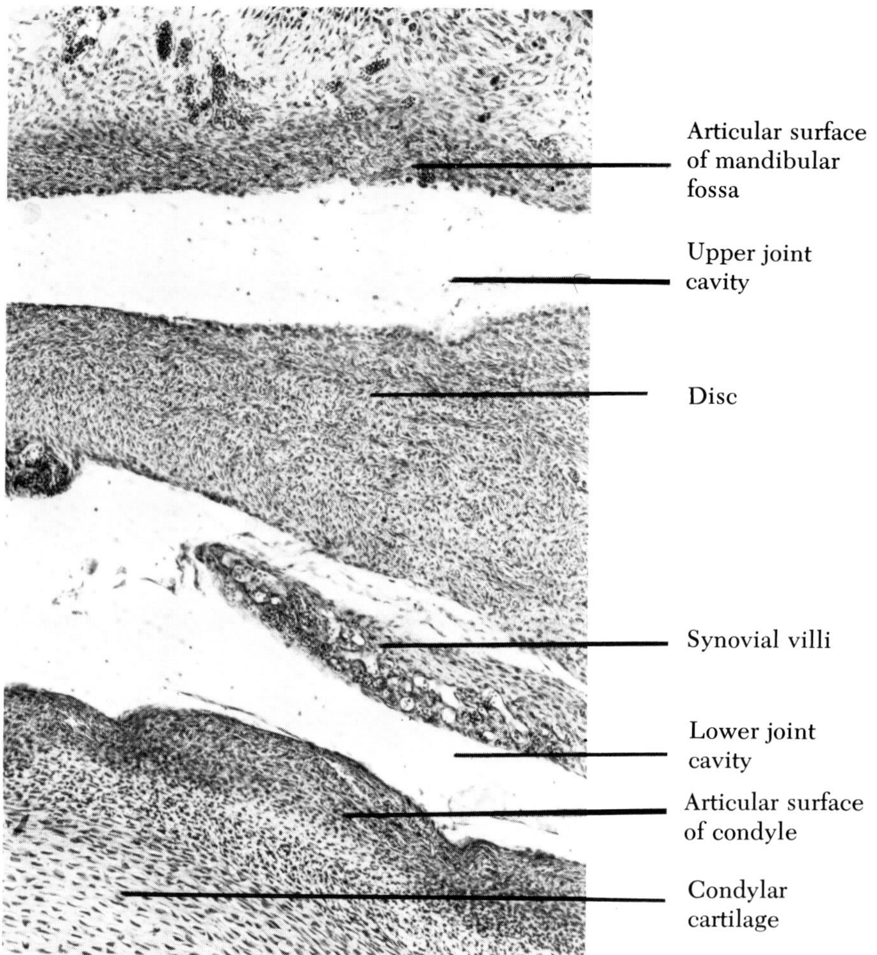

Fig. 13–9. Higher magnification of the joint components seen in Figure 13–7. Notice the dense cellular elements of the upper and lower articular surfaces and of the articular disc. Also note vascularity of the synovial villi seen in the lower space; this is a fold of the synovial membrane.

the adult histologic form, but this does not happen early in life. The condylar cartilage persists, and has growth potential, until the individual is past twenty years old. It is the longest-lasting growth center of the body.

Growth of the condylar cartilage affects the height and length of the mandible and influences the shape of the entire face. The extent of growth in the mandibular condyle may to a great extent determine the occlusion of the individual: what the orthodonist refers to as Class II and Class III occlusion.

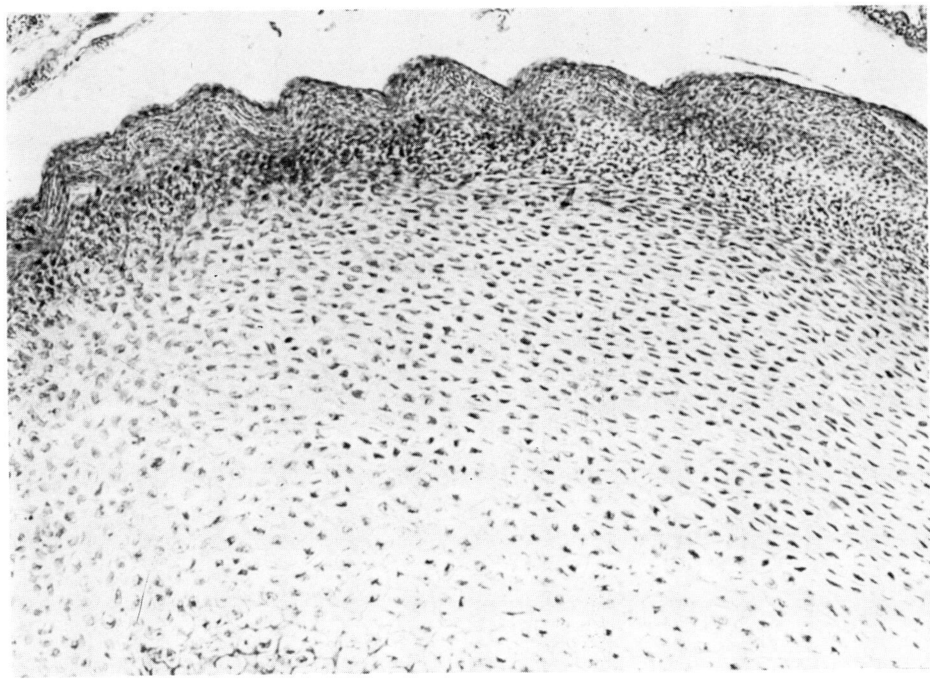

Fig. 13–10. Higher magnification of the condylar process seen in Figure 13–7. This section shows the arrangement of the cells of the articular covering and of the hyaline cartilage. Notice the cells passing from articular surface downward into the hyaline cartilage; this is appositional growth. The clear area at the top of photo is the lower joint space.

Index

Page numbers in *italics* indicate figures.